THE ORIGINS AND CONSEQUENCES OF OBESITY

Ciba Foundation Symposium 201

THE ORIGINS AND CONSEQUENCES OF OBESITY

1996

JOHN WILEY & SONS

Chichester · New York · Brisbane · Toronto · Singapore

Published in 1996 by John Wiley & Sons Ltd,
Baffins Lane, Chichester,
West Sussex PO19 1UD, England

National 01243 779777
International (+44) 1243 779777
e-mail (for orders and customer service enquiries): cs-books@wiley.co.uk
Visit our Home Page on http://www.wiley.co.uk
or http://www.wiley.com

Other Wiley Editorial Offices

John Wiley & Sons, Inc., 605 Third Avenue,
New York, NY 10158-0012, USA

Jacaranda Wiley Ltd, 33 Park Road, Milton,
Queensland 4064, Australia

John Wiley & Sons (Canada) Ltd, 22 Worcester Road,
Rexdale, Ontario M9W 1L1, Canada

John Wiley & Sons (Asia) Pte Ltd, 2 Clementi Loop #02-01,
Jin Xing Distripark, Singapore 0512

Ciba Foundation Symposium 201
x+278 pages, 37 figures, 26 tables

Library of Congress Cataloging-in-Publication Data

The origins and consequences of obesity / [edited by] Derek J.
Chadwick, Gail Cardew.
 p. cm. — (Ciba Foundation symposium ; 201)
 "Symposium on the Origins and Consequences of Obesity, held at the
Wyndham Kingston Hotel, Kingston, Jamaica, 28–30 November 1995" —
Contents p.
 ISBN 0 471 96506 5
 1. Obesity—Epidemiology—Congresses. 2. Obesity—Etiology—
Congresses. I. Chadwick, Derek. II. Cardew, Gail. III. Ciba
Foundation. IV. Symposium on the Origins and Consequences of
Obesity (1995 : Kingston, Jamaica) V. Series.
RA645.023075 1996
616.3'98—dc20   96-24161
                                                        CIP

British Library Cataloguing in Publication Data

A catalogue record for this book is available from the British Library

ISBN 0 471 96506 5

Typeset in 10/12pt Garamond by Dobbie Typesetting Limited, Tavistock, Devon.
Printed and bound in Great Britain by Biddles Ltd, Guildford.
This book is printed on acid-free paper responsibly manufactured from sustainable forestation, for which at
least two trees are planted for each one used for paper production.

Contents

Participants

D. B. Allison   Obesity Research Center, St Luke's Roosevelt Hospital Center, 14th Floor, 1090 Amsterdam Avenue, New York, NY 10025, USA

A. Astrup   The Research Department of Human Nutrition & Centre of Food Research, The Royal Veterinary and Agricultural University, Rolighedsvej 30, DK-1958 Frederiksberg C, Copenhagen, Denmark

F. Bennett   Tropical Metabolism Research Unit, University of the West Indies, Mona, Kingston 7, Jamaica, West Indies

P. Björntorp   Department of Heart and Lung Diseases, University of Göteborg, Sahlgren's Hospital, S-413 45 Göteborg, Sweden

J. E. Blundell   BioPsychology Group, Department of Psychology, University of Leeds, Leeds LS2 9JT, UK

C. Bouchard   Physical Activity Sciences Laboratory, Laval University, Sainte-Foy, Québec G1K 7P4, Canada

G. A. Bray   Pennington Biomedical Research Center, Louisiana State University, 6400 Perkins Road, Baton Rouge, LA 70808-4124, USA

L. A. Campfield   Department of Metabolic Diseases, Hoffmann-La Roche Inc, Nutley, NJ 07110, USA

A. Ferro-Luzzi   National Institute of Nutrition, Via Ardeatina 546-00178 Rome, Italy

T. Forrester   Tropical Metabolism Research Unit, University of the West Indies, Mona, Kingston 7, Jamaica, West Indies

H. S. Fraser   Department of Medicine, Faculty of Medical Sciences, University of the West Indies, Queen Elizabeth Hospital, Bridgetown, Barbados, West Indies

J. S. Garrow   The Dial House, 93 Uxbridge Road, Rickmansworth, Herts WD3 2DQ, UK

B. L. Heitmann   Research Associate Professor, Danish Epidemiology Science Center at the Institute of Preventive Medicine, Copenhagen Hospital Corporation, Kommunehospitalet, DK-1399 Copenhagen K, Denmark

S. B. Heymsfield   Obesity Research Center, St Luke's-Roosevelt Hospital Center, 14th Floor, 1090 Amsterdam Avenue, New York, NY 10025, USA

G. A. Hitman   Medical Unit, Royal London Hospital, Royal Hospitals NHS Trust, Whitechapel, London E1 1BB, UK

A. A. Jackson   Department of Human Nutrition, University of Southampton, Biomedical Sciences Building, Bassett Crescent East, Southampton SO16 7PX, UK

W. P. T. James   The Rowett Research Institute, Greenburn Road, Bucksburn, Aberdeen AB2 9SB, UK

N. McFarlane-Anderson   Tropical Metabolism Research Unit, University of the West Indies, Mona, Kingston 7, Jamaica, West Indies

P. M. McKeigue   Department of Epidemiology and Population Sciences, London School of Hygiene and Tropical Medicine, Keppel Street, London WC1E 7HT, UK

A. M. Prentice   MRC Dunn Clinical Nutrition Centre, Hills Road, Cambridge CB2 2DH, UK

E. Ravussin   Clinical Diabetes and Nutrition Section, NIDDKD Room 541-A, National Institutes for Health, 4212 North 16th Street, Phoenix AZ 85016, USA

A. M. Rissanen   Department of Psychiatry, University of Helsinki, Tukholmankatu 8C, FIN 00290 Helsinki, Finland

S. B. Roberts   Energy Metabolism Laboratory, USDA Human Nutrition Research Center into Aging, Tufts University, 711 Washington Street, Boston, MA 02111, USA

A. G. Shaper   Department of Primary Care and Population Sciences, Royal Free Hospital School of Medicine, Rowland Hill Street, London NW3 2PF, UK

P. S. Shetty   Human Nutrition Unit, Department of Public Health and Policy, London School of Hygiene and Tropical Medicine, Keppel Street, London WC1E 7HT, UK

A. J. Stunkard   Department of Psychiatry, University of Pennsylvania, 3600 Market Street, PA 19104, USA

B. A. Swinburn   Department of Community Health, School of Medicine, University of Auckland, Private Bag 92 019, Auckland, New Zealand

S. Walker   Tropical Metabolism Research Unit, University of the West Indies, Mona, Kingston 7, Jamaica, West Indies

R. Wilks   Tropical Metabolism Research Unit, University of the West Indies, Mona, Kingston 7, Jamaica, West Indies

D. A. York   Pennington Biomedical Research Center, Louisiana State University, 6400 Perkins Road, Baton Rouge, LA 70808-4124, USA

Preface

Those who know the work of the Ciba Foundation well will acknowledge that although based in London, the Foundation is a truly international organization. Participants from all corners of the globe take part in our meetings and experience the hospitality of 41 Portland Place and our books are sold worldwide. To underscore this commitment to fostering scientific co-operation internationally we try, at least once a year, to hold one of our symposia outside the UK.

So it was that the Autumn of 1995 found us in Kingston, Jamaica for our first ever foray to the Caribbean, for a symposium on The origins and consequences of obesity, a topic originally suggested to us by Professor Gerry Shaper.

It gives me very great pleasure to record here the invaluable help and support given to the Foundation by Dr Terrence Forrester and his colleagues at The Tropical Metabolism Research Unit, University of the West Indies, Mona, Kingston. Dr Forrester responded to our invitation to collaborate in the holding of a symposium and open meeting on this topic with energy and enthusiasm and gave his time generously in the selection of an appropriate location and in identifying interested local participants; no Ciba Foundation symposium can have had a more inspirational setting than that afforded by the backdrop of the Blue Mountains on the one hand and the Caribbean sea on the other!

I very much hope that this record of the wide-ranging papers presented at the symposium and the discussions they stimulated, guided by the skilful chairmanship of Professor Philip James, will inspire further research in this important area of public health where science, medicine and social policy meet.

Derek J. Chadwick
Director, The Ciba Foundation

The epidemiology of obesity

W. P. T. James

The Rowett Research Institute, Greenburn Road, Bucksburn, Aberdeen AB2 9SB, UK

Abstract. An agreed definition of obesity as a body mass index (BMI) of 30 kg/m² or more seems to be accepted everywhere except in North America. Recent data confirm the importance of setting an upper individual BMI limit of 25 kg/m² and a population optimum of 20–23 kg/m². Some adjustment of BMI should be made in individuals and populations with disproportionate shapes, e.g. short or long legs, and morbidity and mortality risks are especially important in those with a waist measurement of about 102 cm or more, the risk increasing from 88 cm. Waist measurements should probably now be substituted for the waist/hip circumference ratio. Diabetes is universally closely linked to increases in BMI, and cardiovascular disease is amplified by obesity, particularly in western societies where other dietary factors contribute substantially. Industrialization with reduced physical activity and higher fat diets lead to obesity first in middle-aged women, then in men, with younger adults and children eventually being affected. Physiological studies display the interaction of physical activity and energy dense, high fat diets and explain the secular, age- and social class-related trends throughout the world. Intergenerational amplification of obesity may be underway, so the public health implications of obesity are immense.

1996 The origins and consequences of obesity. Wiley, Chichester (Ciba Foundation Symposium 201) p 1–16

The epidemiology of obesity is concerned not only with the population distribution of an index of adiposity but also with an effort to use population data to assess the impact of the problem and indeed to provide clues to its basis. This is what will be attempted with a global overview of obesity.

The definition of obesity in adults

The use of the body mass index (BMI) as the height-independent measure of weight allows morbidity and mortality analyses to be condensed effectively. The robust nature of the measurements and the widespread routine inclusion of weights and heights in clinical and population health surveys mean that a more selective measure of adiposity, such as skinfold thickness measurements, has been set aside as providing additional rather than primary information. In practice, the squaring of the height is an arbitrary use of a power value ideally to be assessed in each population (Benn 1971). Women often require a height power value of 1.6 to produce a height-independent

1

measure of weight-for-height, and normal values based on Metropolitan Life Insurance figures were originally specified in terms of frame size (James 1974). Our further analyses, which set aside frame size, revealed that the optimum BMI was not height independent at the extremes of height (Royal College of Physicians 1983). Short people are more prone to illness and premature death than tall people, but the real issue is whether differences in body composition have the same significance across the height spectrum and whether the estimate of BMI is still appropriate at the extremes of height.

Some racial groups have unusual body proportions that affect their BMI values and in turn imply (wrongly) differences in body fat content. Within a BMI category there is, of course, a substantial variation in body fat content, but in general the proportion of the variance in body fat (as a percentage of weight rather than in absolute terms) reflected in the BMI amounts to 50–70%. The very tall and lean Australian Aborigines or Dinkas in Africa with their long legs tend to have a spuriously low BMI (by about two units), whereas the stocky American Indians living in Mexico and Central America with their short legs and thick trunks will qualify as obese on the basis of a high BMI. Analyses by Norgan & Jones (1995) could allow an adjustment in BMI if the sitting heights of adults are also measured. The ratio of sitting height to standing height, known as the CORMIC index, varies within the UK population from 0.48 to 0.56, with an effect on BMI of five units within that range. Each 0.01 difference in ratio from 0.52, taken as a typical European or Indo-Mediterranean value, can be used to adjust the BMI by 0.9 units. Norgan now accepts the value of individual group adjustment: recalculating Aboriginal data to allow for their unusual body proportions increased the percentage with a $BMI > 25 \, kg/m^2$ from 8% to 15%.

Reference values

In the Royal College of Physicians (1983) report on obesity I used the specifications of weight-for-height presented in the Metropolitan Life Insurance tables (adjusted for a clothing and shoe allowance) to calculate BMI. With frame size neglected, reference points were $18.7–23.8 \, kg/m^2$ for women and $20.1–25.0 \, kg/m^2$ for men. Garrow (1982) then, sensibly, rounded the values for both sexes to $20–25 \, kg/m^2$ because the slope of the relationship between morbidity or mortality and BMI was minimal in this BMI range. There is also an advantage in having a simple index for both sexes which can be established in everyday practice so that overweight or Grade I obesity with a BMI of $25–29 \, kg/m^2$ and obesity grades (Grade II, BMI $30–39 \, kg/m^2$; and Grade III, $\geqslant 40 \, kg/m^2$ for extreme obesity) become standard measures readily accepted by the public and health professions.

In the USA there is a persisting muddle because a BMI percentile distribution is used to determine cut-off points for obesity; as the population fattens so the BMI range or crude tables of weight-for-height are raised, thereby minimizing the problem of obesity in an almost ludicrous Orwellian manner. The need for specific reference values of universal applicability was established by auxologists dealing with global analyses on children in the 1960s and was perhaps at that time acceptable in the USA because the reference population was American! It is time the USA accepted the World Health Organization's (WHO 1990) recognition of Garrow's definition.

There is also confusion on smoking in relation to BMI and mortality. If cohorts of middle-aged adults are assessed, then there seems to be an advantage in being moderately overweight with BMIs in the range of 26–$28\,kg/m^2$. This reflects not only the fact that early deaths are to be expected in those who are inadvertently losing weight but also that smokers, with their high death rates, tend to be slim. Simple recalculations of the American Cancer Society data reveal two parallel curves for smoking and non-smoking adults with a nadir in mortality in the range of 20–$25\,kg/m^2$ for both groups, the smokers, of course, having a much higher mortality rate (Royal College of Physicians 1983). New USA data in women (Manson et al 1990) confirm the old analyses in men (Royal College of Physicians 1983), showing that a BMI of 20–$21\,kg/m^2$ is the ideal range, provided that one is a non-smoker and one considers the long-term impact of different weights in young adults. Young overweight or obese adults carry risks that may be greater than those observed by modest weight gain into middle age (Royal College of Physicians 1983). Yet in western societies there is evidence that weight gain leads to disadvantageous increases in at least two principal risk factors: blood cholesterol and blood pressure. There seems little reason, therefore, to revise the European and WHO convention of specifying a normal BMI as within 20–$25\,kg/m^2$; this range may be defined more strictly in the future, but it may not be raised.

Waist measurements and waist/hip circumference ratios as a measure of risk

Vague (1956) originally pointed out that abdominally distributed fat was a much greater risk factor than similar amounts of fat distributed on the hips. This is now widely accepted with the suggestion that there is an interaction between the waist/hip circumference ratio (WHR) and the BMI in terms of risk (Björntorp 1993), so that a high WHR (> 1.0 in men and > 0.85 in women) is hazardous even in modestly overweight adults. A re-examination of the old data and new analyses suggest that by simply using the waist measurement one achieves nearly as good (Lapidus et al 1984) or, in larger data sets, even a greater discrimination of risk than by including the hip measurement to produce a ratio (Chan et al 1994). This finding implies that a simple waist measurement—taken at the mid-point between the lower border of the rib cage and the iliac crest—may not only be a useful simple guide for individuals to assess their risk, but also a valuable additional tool for combining with a BMI measurement in epidemiological analyses. It seems likely that measures of abdominal obesity and perhaps specifically of intra-abdominal fat (Sjostrom 1993) are likely to be more effective discriminators of risk than measurements of truncal subcutaneous skinfold thickness, which correlate with but are not direct measures of intra-abdominal fat.

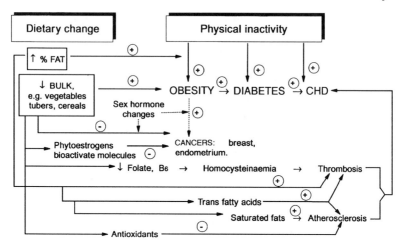

FIG. 1. The interlinking of physical inactivity and dietary effects on obesity and the progression of disease with industrialization. CHD, coronary heart disease.

Morbidity and mortality in relation to obesity

Almost all analyses have depended either on insurance data collected and re-analysed in relation to mortality or on cohort studies conducted for the prime purposes of understanding the basis of cardiovascular disease or cancer in affluent western societies. This may bias our evaluation of the role of obesity because, in the developing world, factors that lead to obesity do not necessarily also induce cardiovascular disease or cancers. Indeed, it has become conventional to consider a sequence of obesity, diabetes, coronary heart disease (CHD) and cancer as a portfolio of public health problems that emerge over decades as developing countries become westernized and industrialized (Fig. 1). It seems clear, however, that rates of non-insulin-dependent diabetes mellitus are closely related in time to the prevailing level of obesity in all societies. CHD emerges as saturated and *trans*-fatty acid intakes rise and have their impact on atherosclerosis and thrombosis over two to three decades. The DNA instability that predisposes to carcinogenesis also seems to be linked to diet, both in terms of processes that activate or dispose of xenobiotic or free radical-induced changes in DNA and in terms of DNA repair mechanisms. Cumulative DNA change proceeds from birth onwards but it would seem that the cancers relating particularly to obesity, e.g. breast and uterine cancers, are those which are heavily influenced by reproductive hormones. These are recognized to be deranged both in obesity and by the intake of fibre-rich vegetables with their phytooestrogen content, e.g. in soya beans. Thus, some cancers as well as CHD may be promoted by the development of obesity, but both conditions are probably dominated by dietary factors, only some of which are linked to obesity.

If these arguments are accepted then epidemiological cohort data on the importance of obesity are relevant worldwide in relation to diabetes but may not apply to CHD and cancers and other conditions, e.g. gallstones or menstrual abnormalities. Modest weight gains seem to impact universally on diabetes rates, particularly if there is intra-abdominal fat accumulation, e.g. in Samoans (Galanis et al 1995). Indians and other groups are particularly susceptible to intra-abdominal fat increases for reasons that are explored elsewhere, e.g. James (1995a) and McKeigue (1996, this volume). The risk of diabetes increases with modest weight gains from a BMI of less than $25 \, kg/m^2$ and rates escalate markedly above a BMI of $30 \, kg/m^2$, so there is now epidemiological validity in using the simple BMI classification universally.

Children's obesity

A recent WHO re-evaluation of children's weight-for-height (WHO 1995) emphasizes the arbitrary nature of the original reference data, which were based on the growth data of children from societal groups in the USA with limited disease rates and where food sufficiency could reasonably be assumed. These data properly replaced the British Tanner graphs which, although based on meticulous longitudinal measurements, included only a small number of children measured after the Second World War. From these analyses have stemmed simplifying schemes for assessing individual children in percentile or Z scores, where the Z score for weight or height refers to the location in standard deviation units of a child on the carefully defined percentile charts.

These charts and the system of specifying a child's weight, height and weight-for-height have been systematized on a global basis (Waterlow et al 1977) because of a primary concern to document the impact of environmental conditions, such as infections and diet, on a child's growth. International analyses have been made of the problem of stunting and the prevalence of wasting (where the weight-for-height Z score is low) (Waterlow 1992).

These cumbersome charts, which require the age as well as the child's measurements to be related to the reference values, are somewhat analogous to the original Metropolitan Life Insurance tables, so clearly it would be convenient if there were some simplifying system, e.g. based on BMI, which could also be applied. Rolland-Cachera et al (1991) established appropriate BMI standards for young children and adolescents as well as adults, and Cole et al (1995) have produced BMI reference curves for the UK from birth to 20 years. Nevertheless, these developments mark a welcome attempt to cope with specifying children's weights at different ages in a coherent and systematic way. The difficulty in including data on adolescence is likely to remain a problem given the substantial international differences in the age of onset of the pubertal spurt and the differential interindividual rates of fat accumulation.

In addition to these difficulties, there is still confusion about the appropriate cut-off points for designating a child as obese. Thus, 85th and 90th percentiles have been used, as have a Z score of 2.0 and a weight-for-height of 120% above the median for age, as the limit of normal. A variety of more direct measures of adiposity, such as triceps skinfold thickness, have also been tried (Chinn & Rona 1994). The principal international analyses so far conducted by Gurney & Gorstein (1988) on childhood obesity use a cut-off point of two Z scores, i.e. more than two standard deviations above the reference mean as the cut-off point. This seems reasonable in that two standard deviations should correspond approximately to the 97th percentile and therefore conform with the classic choice of cut-off point for many nutritional indices. Such a limit is probably also appropriate given our re-analyses of the BMIs of physically fit and healthy young British adults in the army (James et al 1988); few, if any, of these recruits had a BMI above 25.0 kg/m^2 so, as far as overweight is concerned, a two standard deviation limit derived from a suitable reference population seems to be appropriate.

Prevalence studies: global analyses and time trends

A recently established WHO international task force is setting about the daunting task of attempting to generate systematic data on the prevalence of obesity in both children and adults and to assess the rate at which obesity is increasing. The data of Gurney & Gorstein (1988) on children of 0–5 years of age demonstrate, for example, very high rates of obesity in Jamaican and Chilean children, and in the same publication they summarized data on men and women from the Americas, Europe and Australia. A more recent and comprehensive review by Hodge & Zimmet (1994) highlights the extraordinary range of obesity rates in different parts of the world. In these analyses only a portion of the surveys have chosen the new WHO international classification of BMI with 30 kg/m^2 as the cut-off point for obesity, but Table 1 extracts a range of these values to illustrate the diversity of rates. A further problem in comparing rates is that weight gain in most societies occurs in adult life, so the precise age groups chosen affect the proportion of obese cited and few analyses have standardized the rates for age. Nevertheless, several features become clear. First, in Micronesia obesity rates are astonishingly high with Naurans having rates of 60–70% with BMIs > 30 kg/m^2. Polynesians are nearly as badly affected with clear rural–urban differences. Melanesians have intermediate prevalences, and Asian Indians, Creoles and Chinese have the lowest.

Gurney & Gorstein (1988) set out a preliminary analysis of the proportion of children who exceed the mean plus two standard deviation limit of the National Center for Health Statistics (NCHS) standards of weight-for-height and again showed a very wide range in the prevalence of obesity with surprisingly high rates in several developing countries.

A link between the population's mean BMI and the prevalence of obesity was clearly established by Rose (1991), and this has important implications for the analysis of the basis for the change in the prevalence of obesity. When the average BMI of a population is in the range of 20–22 kg/m^2 there are few, if any, individuals with a BMI > 30 kg/m^2. However, for BMIs of > 23 kg/m^2, there is a 4.66% increase in the prevalence of obesity for every single unit increase in the population's average BMI.

TABLE 1   Recent age-standardized prevalences of obesity (BMI > 30 kg/m^2) in adults aged 25–69[a]

Population	Year of study	Men	Women
Micronesians			
Nauru	1987	64.8	70.3
Kiribati (urban)	1981	29.8	34.5
Kiribati (rural)	1981	11.8	13.1
Polynesians			
Western Samoa (urban)	1991	58.4	76.8
Western Samoa (rural)	1991	41.5	59.2
Melanesians			
Papua New Guinea (urban)	1991	36.3	54.3
Papua New Guinea (rural)	1991	23.9	18.6
Papua New Guinea (highlands)	1991	4.7	5.3
Asian Indians			
Mauritius	1992	5.1	16.2
Bombay	1992	6.5	9.6
Creoles			
Mauritius	1992	8.0	20.7
Rodrigues	1992	9.8	31.1
Chinese			
Mauritius	1992	2.1	6.0
China (urban)	1992	2.2	5.2
China (rural)	1992	1.4	3.1
Caucasians			
Finland	1988	8.3	17.4
Australia	1989	11.1	12.7
UK	1993	13.0	16.0
USA	1976–1980	12.0	12.0

[a]Except for Bombay (31–52 years), both urban and rural China ($\geqslant$40 years) and UK (16–64 years). Extracted in part from Hodge & Zimmet (1994) with additional data for Caucasians. Some of the data, particularly for Caucasians, Indians and Chinese, are not age standardized.

An average BMI of 25 kg/m^2 brings with it a prevalence of obesity of approximately 10% for all adults aged 20–59 years. Women, in general, tend to have a broader distribution of BMIs with higher obesity rates. When the average BMI rises to 27.5 kg/m^2, obesity rates escalate to about 22%, and with an average rather than a median BMI of 30 kg/m^2, then 30–40% of the population is obese. Figure 2 displays

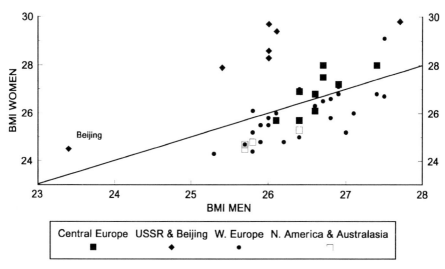

FIG. 2.   A comparison of the average body mass index (BMI) of men and women in the World Health Organization MONICA (MONItoring of trends and determinants in CArdiovascular diseases) Study Centres, aged 35–64 in 1979–1987. Data taken from WHO (1988).

the average BMIs of a large number of populations aged 35–64 taking part in the global WHO MONICA (MONItoring of trends and determinants in CArdiovascular diseases) studies. Note that: in most populations women tend to have a higher average BMI than men; Beijing has a low BMI and only 1–2% obesity; in general, western European societies have far lower BMIs than central or eastern Europe; and Russians and the people of Kaunas in Lithuania have such high values that perhaps 30–50% of the women are obese. These rates, however, are still well below those for the Pacific Islanders (Table 1).

Epidemiological and physiological analyses of the basis for the development of obesity

Physiological principles governing energy balance in humans require that both energy intake and physical activity are considered. Recent data (Stubbs et al 1995) on the control of energy intake in relation to physical activity are illuminating because they reveal that a high fat diet, which is dense in energy, is readily eaten with little evidence of immediate short-term down-regulation of intake as excess energy is consumed. Young adults tend to eat the same amount of food whatever its energy content, so high fat diets promote over-consumption, positive energy balance and weight gain. These effects are minimized if physical activity is encouraged, so very inactive subjects are only in approximate energy balance when eating a 20% fat diet whereas, when moderately active, the individuals are almost in balance on a 40% fat diet (Stubbs et al 1995). Thus, there seems to be a dual effect of a high energy density diet, particularly if high in fat, and the level of physical inactivity on promoting fat storage.

This concept can then be used to interpret many epidemiological analyses. In China not only are obesity rates negligible but there is also little evidence of the problem of adult chronic energy deficiency with BMIs $< 18.5 \, \mathrm{kg/m^2}$ (Shetty & James 1994). The Chinese are still relatively active and their dietary fat content is about 15% of energy with little or no sugar being consumed. The first increases in BMI are seen in middle-aged women as societies 'develop', and an increasing relationship with physical inactivity and high fat diets is becoming apparent (Francois & James 1994). Thus, urban dwellers are more inactive than those living in rural areas (Table 1) and secular trends in physical activity are linked particularly to increasing obesity rates (Prentice & Jebb 1995). Surveys in the UK also reveal that there is an association between low activity and obesity rates, and between the decline in activity with age and weight gain. It is possible to show that adults with a positive energy balance of only 50–100 kcal/day will slowly gain weight for 3–5 years before re-establishing a new plateau weight at a higher level. Thus, we estimate that in the UK physical activity has dropped by up to 800 kcal/day on average over a 20-year period with behavioural changes, such as eating smaller meals and the avoidance of breakfast, reflecting the intrinsic physiological drive to eat less. However, on our high fat diets we have only managed to reduce our intakes by 750 kcal/day, the net balance of 50 kcal daily explaining the average adult weight gain of 2–3 kg. Those who are particularly inactive, expose themselves to an energy-dense, high fat diet and are genetically susceptible, will be those who, within society, display the greatest weight gain (James 1995b).

International and national analyses show a good relationship between the fat content of the diet and obesity rates, but with the two major interacting factors of diet and activity a single effect is inevitably not always apparent. Nevertheless, the physiological data are coherent and imply the need to re-evaluate all our policies that relate to physical activity and diet. Indeed, we have set out a large number of proposals to promote physical activity in society as a whole and to reduce the fat content of the diet (James 1995b).

Conclusions

Given the global emergence of obesity as a major public health problem, we will need to become much more effective in ensuring that the basis for the population changes in adiposity is documented and evaluated. Emerging concern that an intergenerational effect may be becoming apparent as overweight, glucose-intolerant women in pregnancy produce ever larger babies with an increased risk of obesity in adult life adds to the pressure to rethink our approach to this escalating problem. Our analyses suggest that the optimum population average BMI needs to be 20–22 kg/m² to avoid both undernutrition and obesity, so the challenge will be to provide policies for transport and other physical activity, and dietary changes to allow adults to maintain an optimum weight throughout adult life.

Acknowledgement

I thank the Scottish Office Agriculture, Environment and Fisheries Department for their support.

References

Benn RT 1971 Some mathematical properties of weight-for-height indices used as measures of adiposity. Br J Prev Soc Med 25:42–50

Björntorp P 1993 Visceral obesity: a 'civilization' syndrome. Obesity Res 1:206–222

Chan JM, Rimm EB, Colditz GA, Stampfer MJ, Willett WC 1994 Obesity, fat distribution and weight gain as risk factors for clinical diabetes in men. Diabetes Care 17:961–969

Chinn S, Rona RJ 1994 Trends in weight-for-height and triceps skinfold thickness for English and Scottish children, 1972–1982 and 1982–1990. Paed Perin Epid 8:90–106

Cole TJ, Freeman JV, Preece MA 1995 Body mass index reference curves for the UK, 1990. Arch Dis Child 73:25–29

Francois PJ, James WPT 1994 An assessment of nutritional factors affecting the BMI of a population. Eur J Clin Nutr (suppl 3) 48:110S–114S

Galanis DJ, McGarvey ST, Sobal J, Bansserman L, Levinson PD 1995 Relations of body fat and fat distribution to the serum lipid, apolipoprotein and insulin concentrations of Samoan men and women. Int J Obes 19:731–738

Garrow JS 1982 Treat obesity seriously: a clinical manual. Churchill Livingstone, Edinburgh

Gurney M, Gorstein J 1988 The global prevalence of obesity: an initial overview of available data. World Health Stat Q 41:251–254

Hodge AM, Zimmet PZ 1994 The epidemiology of obesity. In: Caterson ID (ed) Obesity. Baillière Tindall, London, p 577–599

James WPT 1974 Research on obesity. A report of the DHSS/MRC group. HMSO, London

James WPT 1995a Coronary heart disease in Indians. Possible role of nutritional factors. Bull Nutr Found India 16:1–4

James WPT 1995b A public health approach to the problem of obesity. Int J Obes (suppl 3) 19:37S–45S

James WPT, Ferro-Luzzi A, Waterlow JC 1988 Definition of chronic energy deficiency in adults. Report of a Working Party of the International Dietary Energy Consultative Group. Eur J Clin Nutr 42:969–981

Lapidus L, Bengtsson C, Larsson B, Pennert K, Rybo E, Sjöstrom L 1984 Distribution of adipose tissue and risk of cardiovascular disease and death: a 12 year follow-up of participants in the population study of women in Gothenberg, Sweden. Br Med J 289:1257–1261

Manson JE, Colditz GA, Stampfer MJ et al 1990 A prospective study of obesity and risk of coronary heart disease in women. N Engl J Med 322:882–889

McKeigue PM 1996 Metabolic consequences of obesity and body fat pattern: lessons from migrant studies. In: The origins and consequences of obesity. Wiley, Chichester (Ciba Found Symp 201) p 54–67

Norgan NG, Jones PRM 1995 The effect of standardizing the body mass index for relative sitting height. Int J Obes 19:206–208

Prentice AM, Jebb SA 1995 Obesity in Britain: gluttony or sloth? Br Med J 311:437–439

Rolland-Cachera MF, Cole TJ, Sempe M, Tichet J, Rossignol C, Charraud A 1991 Body mass index variations: centiles from birth to 87 years. Eur J Clin Nutr 45:13–21

Rose G 1991 Population distributions of risk and disease. Nutr Metab Cardiovasc Dis 1:37–40

Royal College of Physicians 1983 Obesity: a report of the Royal College of Physicians. J R Coll Physicians Lond 17:1–58

Shetty PS, James WPT 1994 Body mass index. A measure of chronic energy deficiency in adults. Unipub, Lanham, MD (FAO Food and Nutrition Paper Series 56)

Sjostrom L 1993 Impacts of body weight, body composition and adipose tissue distribution on morbidity and mortality. In: Stunkard AJ, Warren TA (eds) Obesity: theory and therapy, 2nd edn. Raven, New York, p 13–41

Stubbs RJ, Ritz P, Coward WA, Prentice AM 1995 Covert manipulation of the ratio of dietary fat to carbohydrate and energy density: effect on food intake and energy balance in free-living men eating *ad libitum*. Am J Clin Nutr 62:330–337

Vague J 1956 The degree of masculine differentiation of obesities: a factor determining predisposition to diabetes, atherosclerosis, gout and uric-calculous disease. Am J Clin Nutr 4:20–34

Waterlow JC 1992 Protein-energy malnutrition, 2nd edn. Arnold, London

Waterlow JC, Buzina R, Keller W, Lane JM, Nichaman MZ, Tanner JM 1977 The presentation and use of height and weight data for comparing nutritional status of groups of children under the age of 10 years. Bull WHO 55:489–498

WHO 1988 Geographical variation in the major risk factors of coronary heart disease in men and women aged 35–64 years. The World Health Organization MONICA project. World Health Stat Q 41:115–140

WHO 1990 Diet, nutrition and the prevention of chronic disease. World Health Organization, Geneva (Technical Report Series 797)

WHO 1995 Physical status: the use and interpretation of anthropometry. Report by a WHO expert committee. World Health Organization, Geneva (Technical Report Series 854) p 368–369

DISCUSSION

Shetty: I assume that we all agree that when we talk about body mass index (BMI), we're really using it as a proxy for the amount of adipose tissue. However, identical or similar BMIs of different population groups (that have different sitting heights) may represent different percentages of body fat. Philip James, could you clarify whether the adjustment of BMIs for sitting heights corrects for this variation in body fat of different population or ethnic groups?

James: I do not have these data. The adjustment is simply a technique for standardizing BMI using a modelling approach with sitting height. It's difficult to get data on body composition as well.

Garrow: I would like to make a point relating to the problems of defining obesity in terms of a desirable BMI. We should discuss the results of the Nurses' Health Study (Manson et al 1995), which involved a follow-up of 115 000 nurses who were between 35–50 years of age in 1976. If nurses who either died within the first four years of follow-up or smoked cigarettes are removed from the statistical analysis, then rather than getting a J-shaped curve, a curve is obtained which starts to climb from 20 kg/m^2

and the multivariate risk of death is significantly increased by 27 kg/m². In my opinion, 25–30 kg/m² is not a good range to move into.

McKeigue: We seem to have overestimated or imagined spurious hazards associated with BMI at the lower end of the normal range because of our failure to control for the confounding effect of people who are underweight either because they're sick or because they smoke heavily. Even the Nurses' Health Study does not adjust fully for people who are underweight because they're either sick or heavy smokers. If one looks at Seventh-day Adventists, who do not smoke for religious reasons, there is a positive linear relationship between BMI and mortality down to a BMI of 20 kg/m² (Linsted et al 1991). J-shaped and U-shaped relationships are observed in older populations that generally have a higher prevalence of morbidity and smoking (McKeigue & Davey 1995). These relationships are not just observed for BMI but also for blood pressure and cholesterol, and they have led epidemiologists to raise a number of concerns about hazards associated with low blood pressure, low cholesterol or low BMI.

Swinburn: One of the concerns in terms of population targets for BMI is that the Nurses' Health Study showed a linear relationship between BMI and the development of diabetes through the normal range so that a BMI of 20–22 kg/m² carried the lowest risk. There was a doubling of risk just over the normal range, which is quite alarming.

Bray: In the Multiple Risk Factor Intervention Trial, the lowest mortality is associated with the lowest levels of cholesterol, i.e. below 162 mg/dl. A similar relationship is seen for blood pressure of 120/80 mmHg, where values below 80 mmHg diastolic blood pressure have the lowest risk, and for a BMI of less than 20 kg/m². The National Cholesterol Education Programme has not tried to lower people's cholesterol to a target level of 163, 182 or 195 mmHg, but to round numbers, such as 200 and 240 mmHg. We have to make some similar judgements about where the benefit/risk effects can be most useful. It would be nice if everyone's BMI was 20 kg/m², but I suggest that this is not realistic. We need to consider the practicalities versus the theoretical issues. In the Nurses' Health Study, the risks increase significantly at about 27 kg/m², so I suggest that we should draw a line at 25 or 27 kg/m². We also have to consider not just total BMI, but the distribution of fat and weight gain.

Heitmann: I would like to make several similar comments to those already made. For instance, Williamson et al (1995) studied intentional weight loss and mortality in never-smoking overweight Caucasian women aged 40–64 years and found that intentional weight loss was associated with decreased total mortality and cancer mortality in women with pre-existing illness, such as obesity-related cancer, heart disease and stroke. However, intentional weight loss among non-smoking women without pre-existing disease was associated with increased total mortality and cancer mortality. In this context, it must be mentioned that the group studied by Williamson et al (1995) included about 50 000 women, which represented a subset selected from a much larger study (Hammond et al 1969). This study originally included half a million women and 400 000 men so, as such, this subgroup of women may have been highly selected. For instance, why were only women aged 40–64 years included, and not younger or older women, or why were associations not given for the men?

Also, in relation to the need to consider effects of body composition rather than BMI, I would like to focus your attention on some intriguing data on the associations between body fat and cardiovascular mortality, versus BMI and cardiovascular mortality, which were presented by Ellsinger et al (1991) at the European Congress of Obesity, France 1991. They showed that when body fat was analysed in relation to mortality there was a two to three times stronger relative risk of either developing myocardial infarction or stroke compared to the risk associated with BMI. Furthermore, they showed that the association between body fat and myocardial infarction was, in fact, linear, whereas the association between BMI and myocardial infarction was U-shaped. In my opinion, it is fairly logical that it is the amount of body fat, and not the degree of overweight, that determines risk. We need data indicating that the risk is associated with body fat mass rather than body weight.

Finally, I would like to make a comment related to a recent committee report from the American Institute of Nutrition (AIN) (Blackburn et al 1994) which concluded that, based on the world literature, the lowest total mortality risk seemed to be for a BMI of 18–25 kg/m². However, the AIN also recognized that even lower BMIs may be associated with fitness and health. In fact, their recommendation for intervention at the low end of BMI was directed towards individuals with weight below a BMI of 16 kg/m².

Allison: I would like to comment on the issue of the U-shaped curve, in the light of both the Nurses' Health Study and the Seventh-day Adventist Study. Many questions have been raised about how the latter study was analysed. For example, Sorkin et al (1994) suggested that age effects were analysed inappropriately. Also, it's important to bear in mind that in the Nurses' Health Study the linear effect was only observed in Caucasian women between the ages of 30 and 55 in 1976 who had a stable weight and who had never smoked. This represents only a small per cent of the total number analysed. One must be cautious in making generalizations from that reduced population to the broader population. The assumption is, in making these generalizations, that smoking and pre-existing disease are confounding variables and not modifiers of effect (Andres 1980, 1985). However, it is plausible that smoking and pre-existing disease are modifiers of effect as much as they are confounders. Also, there are other data sets addressing this issue that do not show a linear relationship (e.g. Rissanen et al [1989]), and other studies have tried to control for pre-existing disease issue by excluding subjects who died early (Troiano et al 1996).

Rissanen: Despite the well-documented U-shaped or J-shaped relationship between BMI and longevity, there seems to be a positive linear relationship between BMI and many measures of morbidity and functional incapacity, such as premature work disability. In the Finnish population, premature work disability and mortality have linear and J-shaped relationships, respectively, with BMI (Rissanen et al 1990).

Björntorp: The waist circumference measurement is a good measure of visceral fat mass, particularly in men. Visceral fat mass has a particular significance because there is a strong relationship between this and conventional risk factors, such as for diabetes and cardiovascular disease. We calculated waist circumference as a risk factor in the Gothenburg population and it was not as strong a risk factor as the waist/hip circumference ratio (WHR) (Larsson et al 1984, Lapidus et al 1984). One point in favour of measuring the WHR is that the hip circumference is a measurement of the amount of muscle, and muscle plays a role in the regulation of insulin sensitivity.

James: Although the Gothenburg Study found a slightly better index with the WHR than measurements of waist circumference, other studies have not found this and, pragmatically, one probably gains more by having a simple measurement.

Heymsfield: What is obesity? How can we define it? My most basic understanding about obesity is that it's a functional disturbance, and that in turn leads to increased morbidity and mortality. However, we seem to have equated it with a static measure, which is either body weight, BMI or even body fat. One of the questions that came to my mind is that considering a 20-year-old and an 80-year-old that have different amounts of body fat but the same BMI, is the 80-year-old person obese? There is also the question of sitting versus standing height, as was mentioned by Prakash Shetty at the beginning of this discussion, i.e. two individuals of the same height may have different leg lengths and this might influence the use of BMI as a measure of fitness and obesity.

Campfield: But the reason we're trying to define the optimal BMI is to obtain a BMI where people are free of the associated risk factors. A more direct approach may be to quantify the presence and magnitude of the risk factors of individual obese patients and just take note of the BMIs. There are many people with different BMI values who do not have the well-known complications or risk factors associated with obesity. Therefore, ultimately, the mortality associated with obesity may not be well represented by BMI. Metabolic risk factors have to be considered in addition to BMI.

Ravussin: Waist circumference correlates relatively well with the percentage of body fat in Pima Indians ($r = 0.72$, $P < 0.0001$; R. E. Pratley, personal communication 1995) and I suspect also in other populations. Regarding Steve Heymsfield's comment on age and BMI, I believe that BMI may not always change with age but that waist circumference definitely increases with age. Therefore, this indicates the need to characterize obesity not only by BMI, but by multiple phenotypes including waist circumference and possibly per cent body fat.

Bouchard: Waist circumference has been an anthropometric variable of interest in our laboratory for many years. We have reported that waist circumference was the best surrogate measurement for visceral fat. Of course, the relationship between visceral fat and risk factors is well documented. In our hands, the risk factors are worst when the surface area of visceral fat, measured by computed tomography at the level of L4/L5, exceeds 130 cm^2 (Pouliot et al 1994). We can use this cut-off value to derive the best waist circumference value to predict this particular amount of visceral fat. Lemieux et al (1993) have done this for various age groups for both sexes. They have found that for women a larger waist circumference is required for the same amount of visceral fat as men because women, on average, have less visceral fat for a given waist girth.

Ferro-Luzzi: I wish to call your attention to the problem of classifying younger adults as obese on the basis of BMI. This issue has not yet received the attention that it requires. The age 18–24 years represents a transition to adulthood after which the body reaches the final stages of maturation. Using adult BMI cut-off points to screen obesity in this as yet immature age group has intrinsic limitations and might lead to misclassification of a large proportion of normal youths as undernourished. This issue has been discussed by the World Health Organization Expert Committee on Physical Status (WHO 1995).

Garrow: And I would like to discuss the situation in children. Philip James pointed out that the relationship of BMI to fatness is highly complicated. However, you didn't mention triceps skinfold. If we're aiming at a simple clinical measure that people can use, then tricep skinfold is a good measure of fatness in children, although this is not true for adults.

James: I was told by my epidemiological friends in London that it was not a practical option to measure triceps skinfold measurements routinely in children.

Bray: In our study of children in Baton Rouge, we used skinfold measurements in children and their correlation with dual energy X-ray absorptiometry measurements was extremely good. I have changed my mind about skinfold measurements in children: they are really quite good correlates of total fat.

James: So you're an advocate of triceps skinfold measurements in children?

Bray: For children yes, but preferably multiple skinfold measurements.

Campfield: How do you define 'children'?

Bray: We actually define children as being pre-pubertal, but we do follow them through puberty.

Hitman: Finally, I have reservations about using the same weighting of risk factors for coronary heart disease in all ethnic groups. Are the risk factors the same in developing countries as so-called westernized countries? Ramachandran's studies of rural and urban India suggest that, for instance, impaired glucose tolerance in men is present in 8.7% of the rural population and 8.8% of the urban population (Ramachandran et al 1992). However, despite very similar WHRs they have markedly different BMIs and the prevalence of diabetes is four times more common in the urban environment. This suggests that there is no relationship between BMI and impaired glucose tolerance in a rural setting but that impaired glucose tolerance may relate stronger to WHR. Therefore, in this context it is the distribution of body fat rather than the BMI itself which is predicting the risk factor for ischaemic heart disease, and furthermore it is only of relevance in the urban setting.

References

Andres R 1980 Effect of obesity on total mortality. Int J Obes 4:381–386

Andres R 1985 Mortality and obesity: the rationale for age-specific height–weight tables. In: R Andres, EL Bierman, WR Hazzard (eds) Principles of geriatric medicine. McGraw-Hill, Maidenhead, p 311–318

Blackburn GL, Dwyer J, Flanders WD et al 1994 Report of the American Institute of Nutrition (AIN) Steering Committee on Healthy Weight. J Nutr 124:2240–2243

Ellsinger B-M, Welin L, Svärdsudd K, Eriksson H, Tibblin G 1991 Is body fat mass, calculated from total body potassium determination, a stronger predictor of myocardial infarction and stroke than anthropometric indices? Int J Obes 15:18

Hammond EC, Garfinkel L 1969 Coronary heart disease, stroke and aortic aneurysm. Arch Environ Health 19:167–182

Lapidus L, Bengtsson C, Larsson B, Pennert K, Rybo E, Sjöström L 1984 Distribution of adipose tissue and risk of cardiovascular disease and death: a 12 year follow-up of participants in the population study of women in Gothenburg, Sweden. Br Med J 288:1257–1261

Larsson B, Svärdsudd K, Welin L, Wilhelmsen L, Björntorp P, Tibblin G 1984 Abdominal adipose tissue distribution, obesity and risk of cardiovascular disease and death: 13 year follow-up of participants in the study of men born in 1913. Br Med J 288:1401–1404

Lemieux S, Prud'homme D, Bouchard C, Tremblay A, Després JP 1993 Sex differences in the relation of visceral adipose tissue accumulation to total body fatness. Am J Clin Nutr 58:463–467

Linsted K, Tonstad S, Kusma JW 1991 Body mass index and patterns of mortality among Seventh-day Adventist men. Int J Obes 15:397–406

Manson JE, Willett WC, Stamfer MJ et al 1995 Body weight and mortality among women. N Engl J Med 333:677–685

McKeigue PM, Davey G 1995 Associations between insulin levels and cardiovascular disease are confounded by co-morbidity. Diabetes Care 18:1294–1298

Pouliot MC, Després JP, Lemieux S et al 1994 Waist circumference and abdominal sagittal diameter: best simple anthropometric indexes of abdominal visceral adipose tissue accumulation and related cardiovascular risk in men and women. Am J Cardiol 73:460–468

Ramachandran A, Snehalatha C, Dharmaraj D, Viswanathan M 1992 Prevalence of glucose intolerance in Asian Indians. Urban–rural difference and significance of upper body adiposity. Diabetes Care 15:1348–1355

Rissanen A, Heliövaara M, Knekt P, Aromaa A, Reunanen A, Maatela J 1989 Weight and mortality in Finnish men. J Clin Epidemiol 42:781–789

Rissanen A, Heliövaara M, Knekt P, Reunanen A, Aromaa A 1990 Risk of disability and mortality in a Finnish population. Br Med J 30:835–837

Sorkin JD, Muller D, Andres R 1994 Body mass index and mortality in Seventh-day Adventist men. A critique and re-analysis. Int J Obes 18:752–754

Troiano RP, Frongillo EA, Sobal J, Levitsky DA 1996 The relationship between body weight and mortality: quantitative analysis of combined information from existing studies. Int J Obes 20:63–75

Williamson DF, Pamuk E, Thun M, Flanders D, Byers T, Heath C 1995 Prospective study of intentional weight loss and mortality in never-smoking overweight US white women aged 40–64 years. Am J Epidemiol 141:1128–1141

WHO 1995 Physical status: the use and interpretation of anthropometry. Report of a WHO expert committee. World Health Organization, Geneva (Technical Report Series 854) p 368–369

Obesity in the Caribbean

Terrence Forrester, Rainford Wilks, Franklyn Bennett, Norma McFarlane-Anderson, Daniel McGee*, Richard Cooper* and Henry Fraser†

*Tropical Metabolism Research Unit, University of the West Indies, Mona, Kingston 7, Jamaica, West Indies, *Department of Preventive Medicine and Epidemiology, Loyola University, Stritch School of Medicine, South First Avenue, Maywood, IL 60153, USA, and †Department of Medicine, Faculty of Medical Sciences, University of the West Indies, Queen Elizabeth Hospital, Bridgetown, Barbados, West Indies*

Absract. People of African origin who live in the Caribbean share a common genetic heritage but live in socioeconomic environments that diverge widely. A cross-cultural study of males and females from Jamaica, St. Lucia and Barbados investigated the prevalence of hypertension and its environmental determinants. Standardized measurement techniques allowed comparable measurements of weight, height, waist and hip circumferences, and blood pressure. The population values for body mass index (BMI), per cent overweight (males BMI $\geqslant 27.8$ kg/m^2; females BMI $\geqslant 27.3$ kg/m^2) and per cent obese (males BMI $\geqslant 31.1$ kg/m^2; females BMI $\geqslant 32.3$ kg/m^2) are presented. Prevalence of hypertension is based on the age-adjusted total population. The gradient in per capita gross national product in Jamaica, St. Lucia and Barbados parallels the gradient in the proportions of populations in those countries who are obese. BMI explained 26% of the variance in blood pressure in females and 13% in males. Obesity is a significant problem in the Caribbean, as it is in many other developing countries, and it is associated with a high prevalence of hypertension, particularly in women.

1996 The origins and consequences of obesity. Wiley, Chichester (Ciba Foundation Symposium 201) p 17–31

Weight gain occurs when energy balance is consistently positive. Fat is deposited under these circumstances, and when the proportions of lean body mass and fat mass are altered sufficiently such that metabolism is affected, and risk of poor health from a variety of diseases is increased, we define that body compositional state as obesity.

Within populations, body mass index (BMI) is an acceptable indicator for the degree of fatness. Populations from different societies show wide variations in BMI. The mean body mass of a population represents the average level of fatness which exists when energy balance is achieved, and so represents the steady-state condition in which dietary energy intake equals energy expenditure. The major contributor to the variation in energy expenditure is activity.

In general, the BMI in poorer societies is lower than that in more affluent ones. This reflects, among other factors, the differences in caloric intake and energy expenditure, both of which are associated with the level of economic development. In developing countries, however, different strategies for achieving food security at the household level give rise to variation in caloric intake. Although obesity is not a problem for some of these countries, it is in others, and within countries there is unevenness in the distribution of obesity (James 1989). In the Caribbean there is a wide variation in the strength of economies that affect household income and probably also household food consumption. For example, in 1990 the per capita gross national product (GNP) was US $5965 in Barbados, US $1500 in St. Lucia and US $1103 in Jamaica. Therefore, the problem of obesity in the Caribbean is likely to be distributed unevenly, following economic lines.

The results of a recently concluded epidemiological survey support this hypothesis. These studies estimated the prevalence of hypertension against the background of the risk factors for developing hypertension. They were part of a larger undertaking to determine the prevalence of hypertension and its risk factors across cultures in West Africa, the Caribbean and the USA. The cross-cultural study design among peoples with substantial genetic similarity facilitated a distinction between environmental and genetic contributions to the variance of blood pressure, and the risk of hypertension (International Collaborative Study of Hypertension in Blacks).

In Jamaica, St. Lucia and Barbados samples of adults aged 25–74 years were drawn from defined communities using probabilities proportional to size methodology (Lemeshow & Robinson 1985). Measurements of weight, height, waist and hip circumferences, and blood pressure were made at all three sites. In Jamaica, in addition, an oral glucose tolerance test was performed on all participants. In a subgroup of participants, body composition was further studied with measurements of impedance and total body water using deuterium dilution. We report here our findings relating body weight and composition in men and women across Caribbean sites to major physiological outcomes, blood pressure and blood glucose.

Prevalence of obesity in Jamaica, St. Lucia and Barbados

We observed a gradient for males in the direction, Jamaica, Barbados and St. Lucia for weight, BMI, waist circumference and waist/hip circumference ratio (WHR) (Table 1). A similar gradient was present among females. In addition, mean BMI was greater among females compared with males at all sites. Waist circumference was almost as large in these shorter women as it was in men, but WHRs were lower among females.

Table 1 also shows the percentage of males and females who were overweight. We defined overweight using the National Institutes of Health consensus values: $BMI \geqslant 27.8 \text{ kg/m}^2$ for males; and $BMI \geqslant 27.3 \text{ kg/m}^2$ for females. Females had twice the rate of overweight as males in all three territories. Almost 70% of Barbadian females were overweight compared with 38% of Jamaican females and 15% of Jamaican males.

We defined obese males as having a $BMI \geqslant 31.1 \text{ kg/m}^2$, and obese females as having a $BMI \geqslant 32.3 \text{ kg/m}^2$. The frequency of obesity among Jamaican females was fourfold higher than Jamaican males; whereas the frequency of obesity among Barbadian

TABLE 1 Summary of the prevalence of obesity in males and females of Jamaica, St. Lucia and Barbados

Country	Number of participants	Weight (kg)	Height (cm)	BMI (kg/m²)	Waist (cm)	Hip (cm)	WHR	MUAC (cm)	Overweight (%)	Obese (%)
Jamaica										
Males	337	69.4	172.4	23.4	79.6	95.1	0.84	29.4	15.4	3.9
Females	481	70.4	160.4	27.3	82.0	103.0	0.77	30.8	37.5	15.6
St. Lucia										
Males	489	73.0	173.5	24.2	82.4	95.2	0.86	28.9	20.8	7.6
Females	590	72.4	162.9	27.2	85.1	103.7	0.82	29.3	42.7	16.1
Barbados										
Males	329	76.4	172.0	25.8	85.8	97.8	0.88	31.5	30.8	11.0
Females	481	75.2	160.2	29.3	86.9	106.6	0.81	32.2	69.2	34.6

BMI, body mass index; MUAC, mid-upper arm circumference; WHR, waist/hip circumference ratio.

females was threefold higher than their male counterparts. More than a third of all
Barbadian females were obese (Table 1). Figures 1 and 2 show the percentage of
males and females who were found to be overweight or obese in the different age
categories. Overweight and obesity increased steadily with age.

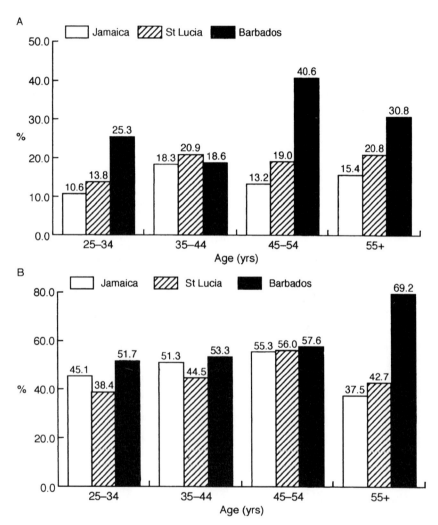

FIG. 1.   Percentage of males (A) and females (B) from Jamaica, St. Lucia and Barbados who
were classified as overweight, i.e. those with a body mass index of at least 27.8 kg/m² and 27.5 kg/
m² for males and females, respectively.

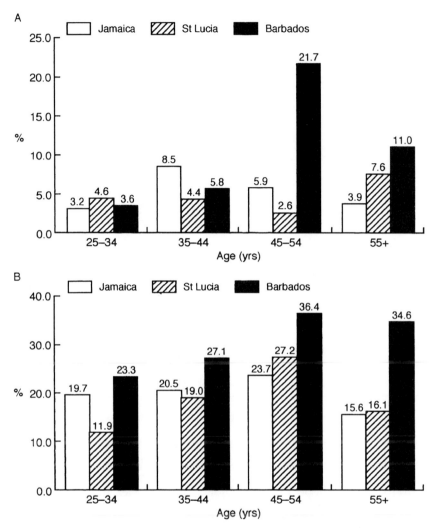

FIG. 2.   Percentage of males (A) and females (B) from Jamaica, St. Lucia and Barbados who were classified as obese, i.e. those with a body mass index of at least 31.1 kg/m² and 32.3 kg/m² for males and females, respectively.

Examination of body composition

We measured bioelectrical impedance in a subgroup of 64 Jamaican women and 56 Jamaican men, and compared the results for total body water derived from the impedance measurements with those derived from deuterium dilution using another

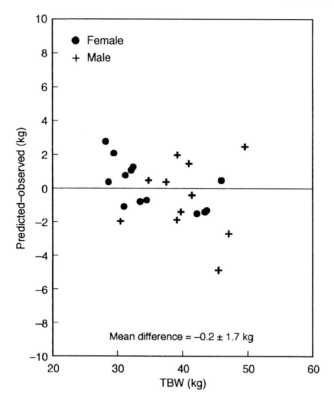

FIG. 3.   Mean differences between total body water (TBW) estimated using deuterium dilution and bioelectrical impedance.

subgroup of 13 Jamaican females and 11 Jamaican males. Figure 3 shows the plot of the mean differences between these measurements, which was not different from zero. Impedance estimates of per cent body fat in men and women are plotted in Fig. 4. Women at any BMI had a greater per cent body fat. The relationship between BMI and per cent body fat was linear in men but curvilinear in women, tending to flatten out at the higher values of BMI. It is interesting that 40% of women were misclassified as non-overweight on the basis of BMI although they had over 30% body fat. This suggests that although BMI was a good index of total fat in this population, it was not for per cent body fat, and this is consistent with the literature (Spiegelman et al 1992).

The cost of obesity in the Caribbean

What is the cost attending this level of obesity in the Caribbean? Our data show associations between prevalence of hypertension and diabetes and the measures of fatness and fat distribution.

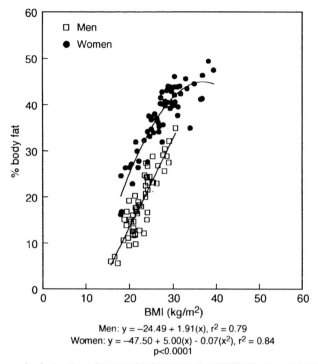

Men: y = −24.49 + 1.91(x), r² = 0.79
Women: y = −47.50 + 5.00(x) - 0.07(x²), r² = 0.84
p<0.0001

FIG. 4. Per cent body fat plotted against body mass index (BMI) for men and women. Curves fitted using regression analysis.

TABLE 2 Summary of the prevalence of hypertension in males and females of Jamaica, St. Lucia and Barbados

Country	Number of participants	Systolic blood pressure	Diastolic blood pressure	% Hypertensives (≥140/90)	% Hypertensives (≥160/95)
Jamaica					
Males	337	123.1 (21.6)	70.3 (14.9)	18.4	13.0
Females	481	122.3 (21.9)	70.4 (14.5)	27.2	19.3
St. Lucia					
Males	489	126.8 (18.9)	75.9 (13.9)	24.1	13.9
Females	590	122.7 (22.5)	73.4 (14.6)	27.4	20.8
Barbados					
Males	329	125.5 (17.0)	77.0 (10.9)	25.9	18.0
Females	481	122.0 (19.9)	73.5 (11.5)	28.2	22.9

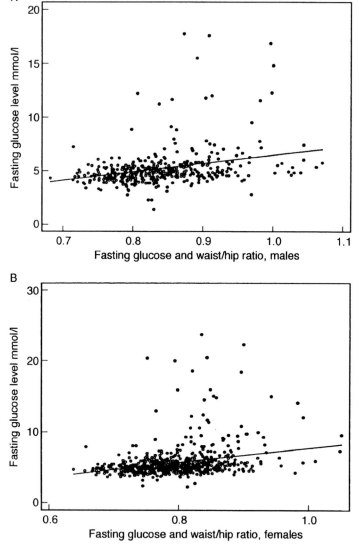

FIG. 5.   Fasting blood glucose level versus waist/hip circumference ratio in males (A) and females (B).

Trained personnel measured blood pressure using standard mercury sphygmomano-meters. Systolic and diastolic pressures were taken as Korotkoff sounds 1 and 5, respectively. Mean blood pressures among men were lowest in Jamaica and highest in Barbados (Table 2). Age-adjusted prevalence of hypertension was lowest in Jamaica, intermediate in St. Lucia and highest in Barbados. Prevalence of hypertension was greater among females in all territories. These figures for prevalence are lower than for Afro-Americans (Burt et al 1995). Linear regression analysis showed that BMI accounted for 26% of the variance of blood pressure in females and 13% in males.

We defined diabetes by the World Health Organization criteria after a 75 g oral glucose challenge. In a sample of 1058 subjects, which included the sample used for blood pressure relationships, 12.5% of males and 14.9% of females with no previous history of diabetes were shown to have impaired glucose tolerance. The per cent of previously undiagnosed diabetes was 3.6% for males and 6.7% for females. The overall prevalence for previously undiagnosed diabetes was 5.4%, and this compares with 3.2% in North American Caucasians and 4.8% in North American Blacks from the National Health and Nutrition Examination Surveys (NHANES) II study. WHR was more strongly associated with fasting glucose than BMI (if both are included in the regression model, BMI is no longer significant). Similar relationships were seen with 2 h postprandial glucose. Female sex, WHR, age and systolic pressure were significantly related to diabetes diagnosed on oral glucose tolerance tests. These data reveal that the per cent of males with impaired glucose tolerance and diabetes is 12.5% and 3.6%, respectively; whereas for females the figures are 14.9% and 6.7%, respectively. However, while the coefficients indicated statistical significance, very little of the variance was explained ($R^2 = 0.15$). Figure 5 shows the relationships between fasting glucose and WHR in men and women. There was extreme variation about the regression line. These observations suggest that although body fat and fat distribution might contribute to glucose intolerance and diabetes, other more potent underlying factors are operating. These data are, of course, cross-sectional, and they do not address the issue of the prognostic importance of body composition for glucose intolerance and emergence of diabetes.

In the Caribbean, therefore, obesity is a significant problem. It is more common in countries with a higher per capita GNP, and it affects women disproportionately. It is associated with a parallel increase in the prevalence of hypertension and diabetes. However, the proportions of the variance of blood pressure and blood sugar explainable by body mass or fatness are small. This suggests that body compositional changes in populations and physiological outcomes, blood pressure and blood glucose might be related through other undescribed metabolic influences.

Acknowledgements

We wish to thank Maria Jackson, Audrey Smith, Marsha Ivey and Paul Mattocks for invaluable assistance in the field. The study was funded by the National Institutes of Health grant HLB 45508 and the Wellcome Trust.

References

Burt VL, Whelton P, Roccella E J et al 1995 Prevalence of hypertension in the US adult population: results from the 3rd National Health and Nutrition Examination Survey, 1988–1991.
Hypertension 25:305–313

James WPT 1989 A European view of nutrition and emerging problems in the Third World. Am J Clin Nutr 49:985–992

Lemeshow S, Robinson D 1985 Surveys to measure programme coverage and impact: a review of the methodology used by the expanded programme on immunization. World Health Stat Q 38:65–75

Spiegelman D, Israel RG, Bouchard C, Willett W 1992 Absolute fat, percent body fat, and body fat distribution: which is the real determinant of blood pressure and serum glucose? Am J Clin Nutr 55:1033–1044

DISCUSSION

Garrow: I am distressed by the increasing tendency to use bioelectrical impedance as a measure of body fat because different machines give different answers, and comparisons cannot therefore be readily made between studies. I'm voting against using bioelectrical impedance as a primary method for measuring body fat.

Ferro-Luzzi: I agree. In my opinion bioelectrical impedance should be used only to predict water content and not to measure body fat.

Heymsfield: Although water content is probably the best component measured by bioelectrical impedance, different instruments and prediction equations will still produce variable results. However, one can control this by calibrating the instrument and carefully selecting cross-validated water-prediction equations.

James: The earlier bioelectrical impedance systems were more variable, but now there are more sophisticated multifrequency analysers, so that with correct calibration of individual techniques one can produce far more robust results.

Ferro-Luzzi: They may be more robust when predicting water content, but this may not necessarily be the case for predicting body fat.

James: The water content measurements are robust and reproducible, although one probably needs to specify the length of the legs, for example. Transforming the measurements of water to obtain a value for fat is a separate issue. Terrence Forrester, which machines were used for your studies?

Forrester: We used a machine obtained from RJL Systems Inc (MI, USA) to measure impedance.

Swinburn: Bioelectrical impedance has some value if there are large differences in resistance measurements for a given body mass index (BMI), even though this approach is not as accurate as other methods and needs population-specific equations.

Heitmann: In my opinion, the use of population-specific equations for calculating body composition from bioelectrical impedance will be more robust than using just height and weight (Heitmann 1990). In this regard, we may need population-specific equations for different ethnic groups, but I believe that equations developed in a British population or an American population of Caucasians can be applied to other Caucasian groups. Theoretically, the use of multifrequency bioelectrical impedance implies that the population specificity is less of an issue, and ethnic comparisons using multifrequency bioelectrical impedance for calculating body composition should be possible. Therefore, we might come closer to comparing body composition measurements in populations if the theoretical rationale behind multifrequency bioelectrical impedance holds water, making it a more universal technique than single frequency bioelectrical impedance. However, this is not yet fully known.

James: Are you suggesting that repeated validations should be made in the appropriate context?

Heitmann: It is not a question of validations, it is a question of whether single frequency bioelectrical impedance is a sufficient technique for measuring body composition in different populations. This is due to a possible difference in extracellular to intracellular water distribution in different ethnic populations (Heitmann 1994). In theory, this may be overcome with multifrequency bioelectrical impedance, but there are not enough data to document this yet.

Campfield: This tool may be more useful for intervention purposes within a population, rather than for epidemiological studies between populations.

Heymsfield: We have found that there is a small difference in the prediction of total body water in African-American Blacks in New York compared with Caucasians (Heymsfield 1993). In large samples of 2000–3000, for example, ethnicity is a statistically significant covariant in total body water prediction in addition to stature and impedance. This is largely due to differences between Blacks and Caucasians in arm and leg lengths. The majority of bioelectrical impedance originates from the extremities.

James: The trunk is about 10% and the extremities make up the rest, so the length of trunk-to-limb ratio is an important factor.

Shetty: I would like to change the subject and raise the issue of having simple, round numbers for BMI cut-off values for grades of obesity to avoid misinterpretations by the public. My concern is how does one agree on cut-off values that are acceptable and hence are used commonly worldwide. I would like to ask Terrence Forrester what is the basis for using the cut-off values in his study?

Forrester: We used criteria for overweight and obesity based on the National Health and Nutrition Examination Surveys (NHANES) II data: at least 27.8 kg/m^2 for males and 27.2 kg/m^2 for females for overweight, and at least 31.1 kg/m^2 for males and 32.3 kg/m^2 for females for obesity.

Bray: The National Center for Health Statistics (NCHS) used these BMI values. To most Americans, these numbers are uninterpretable, and I would not like to see them used any more broadly than they now are. The numbers are strictly arbitrary and based on the 85th BMI percentile of 20–29 year-old Americans in the 1976–1980 NCHS survey. If the 85th percentile was used for each survey, there would be a steady increase in BMI with every population survey, since weights continue to rise. However, the NCHS decided to fix it to the 1976–1986 population survey. I hope that we will be able to escape from some of these values and adopt simpler ones. For example, the values 25 and 30 kg/m^2, would be useful numbers to use for both genders in all populations, with 25 kg/m^2 being the upper limit for normal weight and 30 kg/m^2 the value separating overweight and obesity.

I would like to ask Terrence Forrester a question about his data on glucose levels versus BMI. Glucose levels are tightly controlled unless you're diabetic. Did you measure the levels of insulin in this population, which may turn out to be a more interesting measurement?

Forrester: No, we have not done this yet.

Garrow: BMI may not be a good predictor of diabetes. For example, in the Pima Indians there isn't a good correlation between BMI and diabetes, although there is a good correlation between BMI measured before the onset of diabetes because there is weight loss once diabetes is established (Knowler et al 1981).

Ravussin: Terrence Forrester presented data showing that only about 15% of the variation in glucose was explained by BMI, age and sex. However, because of the weight loss occurring with the development of non-insulin dependent diabetes mellitus (NIDDM), one should exclude diabetic subjects from the analysis. If one does that, it is likely that BMI, age and sex might explain more than 15% of the variance in fasting plasma glucose. Insulin resistance is the best predictor of the development of NIDDM in Pima Indians (Lillioja et al 1993). Therefore, insulin resistance is likely to be more strongly related to BMI than plasma glucose.

Astrup: I would like to ask whether the Tropical Metabolism Research Unit (TMRU) has any data on the ethnic differences in susceptibility to ischaemic heart disease and stroke?

Wilks: We have had the opportunity at the TMRU to collaborate with the World Health Organization to look at cardiovascular diseases and hormonal contraception in women, particularly in the age group 15–49 years. We found that the incidence of stroke was 12.4 per 100 000 women (95% confidence interval 8.7–16.1), but we don't have any information on the incidence in the general population.

Fraser: At present, the best data on this in the Caribbean is that of the St. James coronary risk factor study by Beckles et al (1986). This was a large, seven-year study of 2400 men and women in a suburban section of the Port of Spain in Trinidad and Tobago. They studied Afro-Caribbeans, defined as Black by their grandparental origin, Indian populations and a smaller group of mixed populations. They showed that there were clear relationships between weight, blood pressure and stroke in the Black population, and that there was a strong relationship between coronary heart disease (CHD) and mortality in the Indian population. Finally, they showed that there was a marked difference between the two populations in the levels of high density lipoprotein–cholesterol (HDL–C).

James: Which population had the higher level of HDL–C?

Fraser: The Black population, i.e. the population that was not susceptible to CHD.

Bray: Terrence Forrester has presented data on populations that have an increased prevalence of obesity, and Philip James has presented data on the increase in mortality rates with obesity. From this, one would expect to observe a higher mortality rate in Barbados than in St. Lucia or Jamaica. Is that true?

Fraser: Barbadians have the longest life expectancy out of these three countries. There is some preliminary evidence to suggest that for both the Trinidadians and Barbadians the increase in life expectancy has plateaued.

Shaper: Diabetes is common in obese or overweight East Africans, but because people in this community have a low fat diet, they have a relatively low level of blood cholesterol and there is virtually no CHD. This suggests that diet is an important factor that influences which obesity-related complications develop. In a sense, the issue that we're all skirting around is that the pathway by which one becomes fat is critical. For instance, in southern Italians there is a high prevalence of obesity but a low prevalence of CHD.

Jackson: Please can you elaborate on these different pathways?

Shaper: One often talks about becoming fat in a western society, but what exactly do we mean by that? One may become fat as a result of consuming a high saturated fat diet, which raises blood cholesterol level and increases the risk of developing coronary complications. In contrast, if one becomes fat by consuming a predominantly high carbohydrate diet, one may have relatively low levels of blood cholesterol and have a low risk of CHD.

Garrow: Is there any evidence that the gradient in obesity-related problems between Jamaica and Barbados is related to the levels of exercise?

Forrester: We do not have any data on this as yet, but the study is continuing and we intend to measure the activity of our subjects.

York: Are the diets of these three countries similar? Are the indigenous foods and the way that they are prepared similar? Or are the changes that you are observing related to the introduction of the American-style fast foods which become more available as the population increases its wealth?

Shetty: And a related question to this is: how is income related to the differences in the prevalence of adult obesity?

Wilks: There are large differences between Jamaica and Barbados in terms of per capita income, i.e. about US$1103 in Jamaica and US$6000 in Barbados. Therefore, we can make assumptions about the westernization of the countries and relate this to dietary influences, but as yet we have not done a detailed dietary analysis of these countries.

Jackson: I have two points. Firstly, the data in the presentation were cross-sectional and therefore could not give any sense of trends in the prevalence of obesity with time. I am not convinced that there have been changes in the relative rates, as Barbados has always appeared to have higher rates compared with other islands such as Jamaica (Sinha 1995). Therefore, there is an underlying difference between the two societies, unrelated to the more recent relative affluence in Barbados or the penetration of 'fast foods' from the USA. Changes in food habits might have accentuated an underlying difference.

Secondly, Rainford Wilks could not comment on dietary differences between the two societies because they have not yet analysed their dietary data. However, it is known from the St. James study in Trinidad that there are different patterns of mortality and morbidity between those of Indian descent and those of African descent, which have been attributed to differences in dietary patterns. Although complete information is not available, certain obvious differences have been identified in the past; for example, the limited domestic production of fresh fruits in Barbados. Nevertheless, I agree that in a more detailed analysis of diets there may be important factors which play an important role and are not evident from a simple overview.

Fraser: A slightly different perspective is the sociocultural aspects of emerging societies: they have a perception that fat is not just associated with affluence but also with health and with beauty. In the Caribbean, and particularly in the lower socioecomonic strata, men prefer fatter women. We have clear data from the 1980s showing that the majority of overweight women think they're normal and very few want to lose weight. Those in the obese strata who want to lose weight, want to lose only a mean of nine pounds. This is the opposite of most western societies: a western woman may look in the mirror and see herself as too fat, and a West Indian woman may see herself as too thin.

Blundell: As a corollary to that one would predict a low incidence of eating disorders in the West Indies.

Fraser: Yes, these are rare. Our psychiatrist said he had only experienced four cases of anorexia nervosa, and all of these were in Caucasian women, two of whom were expatriates.

James: What is the incidence of bulimia in the Caribbean?

Fraser: This is also very rare.

Campfield: Is the social perception changing with time?

Fraser: It is changing, but it is fastest in the higher socioeconomic groups.

Campfield: Is there a difference between urban and rural populations in the Caribbean or is it just along socioeconomic status?

Fraser: We can't answer that specifically but it is chiefly socioeconomic.

Campfield: Given these changes, the prediction would then be that eating disorders should now become apparent in the higher social classes.

Allison: We've done some research in the USA comparing men's views of desirable female body shapes (Allison et al 1993, 1995). We expected to find that African-American and Hispanic men preferred overweight women, but we found that this was not the case. We also found that when we studied women's views of themselves, African-American women were tolerant of being overweight: being overweight did not seem to affect their self-esteem or their perceptions of beauty.

References

Allison DB, Hoy K, Fournier A, Heymsfield SB 1993 Can ethnic differences in men's preferences for women's body shapes contribute to ethnic differences in female obesity? Obesity Res 1:425–432

Allison DB, Kanders BS, Osage GD et al 1995 Weight-related attitudes and beliefs of obese African-American women. J Nutr Edu 27:18–23

Beckles GLA, Miller G J, Kirkwood BR et al 1986 High total of cardiovascular disease morbidity in adults of Indian descent in Trinidad. Lancet I:1298–1300

Heitmann BL 1990 Evaluation of body fat estimated from body mass index, skinfolds or electrical impedance. A comparative study. Eur J Clin Nutr 44:831–837

Heitmann BL 1994 Impedance: a valid method in assessment of body composition? Eur J Clin Nutr 48:228–240

Heymsfield SB, Wang ZM 1993 Human body composition: the five level model of body composition and its relation to bioimpedance analysis. Rivista Italiana Di Nutrizione Parenterale Ed Enterale 11:71–77

Knowler WC, Pettit D J, Savage P J, Bennett PH 1981 Diabetes incidence in Pima Indians: contributions of obesity and parental diabetes. Am J Epidemiol 113:144–156

Lillioja S, Mott DM, Spraul M et al 1993 Insulin resistance and insulin secretory dysfunction as precursors of non-insulin-dependent diabetes mellitus. N Engl J Med 329:1988–1992

Sinha DP 1995 Food, nutrition and health in the Caribbean: a time for re-examination. Caribbean Food and Nutrition Institute, Kingston, Jamaica

General discussion I

Björntorp: I would like to discuss whether environmental temperature can play a role in the development of obesity. In Europe there is an increased prevalence of obesity from north to south. It's possible that energy expenditure is lower in the south because of the higher environmental temperature, so that the need to eat is less and it becomes easier to overeat.

Astrup: A decrease in the environmental temperature by about 8 °C would increase one's 24 h energy expenditure by 2%, which may not be sufficient to exert any important effect on energy balance.

Ferro-Luzzi: Consolazio (1963) has studied the energy requirement of soldiers exercising in cold conditions. He concluded that the insulating material of their clothes provided a microclimate, which he used to explain the 2–5% increase in energy expenditure. The increase in obesity from north to south in Europe is a recent trend, which has occurred concurrently with the shift from a rural to a city-based lifestyle. This suggests that changes in lifestyle might be responsible, rather than the temperature gradient across Europe.

Prentice: The issue of temperature may be important in a behavioural context rather than in a metabolic context, which is probably not significant. Heat may be important in European cultures in terms of inducing lethargy rather than having an effect on thermoregulation. This may also be important in African and tropical environments, but people in these countries have an obligatory requirement for work in spite of the high temperatures. There may be some permissive socioeconomic situations in which people do not have to be active, because one can argue that in many populations the natural state is to expend as little energy as possible. We need to understand more about these new socioeconomic conditions that are now allowing people to seek out that state of minimal physical activity.

Fraser: The Barbadians don't necessarily have to work. In fact, there is a large difference in the activity levels between Barbadians and Jamaicans. In Barbados there are a large number of cars, and people no longer walk. Also, if you don't have to work and you get too hot then you sit down, it's a fundamental social response.

James: Are you suggesting that we ought to be focusing on leisure time activity, where behavioural responses and attitudes to temperature might be more important?

Fraser: Absolutely.

Forrester: You may well need data on this in Barbados; however, we still need data on work-related activities in Jamaica.

Bouchard: In my opinion, temperature is not a major issue for several reasons. The anthropological literature over many years has demonstrated that there is a reasonably

32

consistent gradient from north to south of an increase in body mass index (BMI). The consequent average increase in body surface area associated with this increase in mass becomes one way to dissipate heat. In Canada the contemporary prevalence of overweight and obesity (BMI $\geqslant$ 27 kg/m^2) ranges from 28% in Quebec and British Columbia to 41% in Newfoundland, and this difference can certainly not be accounted for by differences in climate.

Garrow: Buskirk et al (1957) did a study on army recruits being trained at different units, some of which were cold and some of which were hot, and they found negligible changes in energy expenditure. In Jamaica there is an opportunity for doing an interesting study because of the changes in temperature with altitude.

Hitman: One would have to be careful doing such a study because it would be difficult to control for social class and income per household.

Ravussin: Whilst working in our laboratory, Steve Lillioja showed that Pima Indians born during the summer (when it is very hot in Arizona) had higher BMI than those born during the winter (personal communication 1993). In addition, Jim Young (personal communication 1995) found that cold exposure at a young age has a significant impact on the activity of the sympathetic nervous system at a later stage of life in animals.

Roberts: Recent studies have shown seasonal variations in body fat in the USA that are the opposite to what one may predict, i.e. that people are fatter in the winter than in the summer (Dawson & Harris 1992). There are also changes in the distribution of fat in post-menopausal women: when they go through a winter cycle they gain weight in the abdominal region and in the summer they lose it at peripheral sites.

York: The weight gain in winter may not be related to temperature but to changes in day length.

Shaper: There are differences in seasonal dietary intake that appear to account for the differences in seasonal weight.

Stunkard: There may also be seasonal changes in behaviour that may affect a person's ability to lose weight. For example, it is easier to start a weight reduction programme on New Year's Day, after the over-indulgences at Christmas, or in the Spring, when one is looking forward to wearing light clothes. Many people are susceptible to these strong behavioural controls.

Campfield: The Euronut–Seneca multicentre study in Europe was originally funded by the European Economic Community to look at nutrition in the elderly. They published a report in 1991 (de Groot et al 1991), and they are now doing the follow-up study at fewer sites. This study is not a strict north–south analysis of BMI, but there are some surprises. Study sites in Switzerland, for example, which is not one of the most southerly countries studied, had the third highest BMI of the sites studied. Therefore, there are differences between sites, but there is no apparent latitudinal gradient. The follow-up data should be available soon.

James: What is the age group of these people?

Campfield: They are older people (70–75 years) who live in the more rural areas.

Shetty: I recently saw some data (M. E. J. Valencia, personal communication 1995) on the prevalence of obesity and non-insulin dependent diabetes among the Pima Indians in Mexico, (Maycoba Pimas in Sonora, Mexico) who are thought to have come from the same genetic stock as the Pima Indians in Arizona. The prevalence of obesity in these Indians seems to be much less, although they have similar gender differences. The Maycoba Pima Indians have traditional agricultural lifestyles with a high degree of physical activity which may account for the lower incidence of obesity.

Ferro-Luzzi: We seem to be taking it for granted that physical activity is important for either the prevention or treatment of obesity. Although this may be true, information is still lacking on the intensity and amount of physical activity required to avoid becoming obese. To speak about physical activity and obesity in general terms is, in my opinion, unproductive and frustrating.

Roberts: We hear more about the importance of physical activity than the importance of diet, and I wonder whether that's because in epidemiological studies it's much easier to quantify changes in physical activity. One can quantify how many hours people watch television, whereas quantifying what people eat is more difficult because you have to rely on what they tell you. I would be interested to compare the incidences of obesity between physically active and inactive communities that eat either high or low fat diets.

Shaper: The only data I know in relation to that is from the Masai-speaking Nomads (Samburu) in northern Kenya, who apparently have a high fat intake in terms of meat and milk, but they eat it on an intermittent basis. They are lean, physically active and their average body weight does not increase with age after the age of 20 years. However, overall they may not consume a very high fat diet (Shaper & Spencer 1961).

Roberts: Unpublished studies by Penelope Nestel showed that the perception that they ate a lot of milk and meat was erroneous. They were actually selling those products and buying corn, so their diet was much higher in carbohydrates.

Shaper: Even if this is so, our data from the 1960s suggest that they still have a low level of blood cholesterol (Shaper et al 1963).

Swinburn: Prior et al (1981) studied migrant Polynesians in the 1960s who were living on coral atolls, on which it was difficult to grow root vegetables. Their diet consisted of fats from coconuts and proteins from fish, and it was about a 50% fat diet. When these populations moved to New Zealand, their fat intake decreased but their weight increased.

James: What was their level of physical activity?

Swinburn: It was undoubtedly higher on their home islands before migration.

Jackson: I am not sure that it is useful to equate the pattern of energy intake and weight without some measure of expenditure or activity.

Rissanen: In the 1960s and early 1970s the average fat intake of Finns was close to 40% of the total energy intake, but now it is 34%. At the same time, the percentage of the population who are obese has increased, but less so than in many other countries. The most important factor here is the decline in physical activity, which is overriding any advantage that a lower fat intake may have in terms of weight development.

Shaper: But their levels of blood cholesterol and their coronary heart disease rates are lower.

Heitmann: It is important to recognize that there may be an interaction between fat intake and physical activity in promoting weight gain. It may very well be that you can eat a high fat diet if you are physically active without gaining weight, whereas the same high fat diet may cause weight gain if you are physically inactive. In my opinion, there is a need to be more specific with the recommendations for the public. Although the problem is the identification of specific groups—and more research needs to be put into this area—we may need to direct our recommendations to those subgroups who are at particular risk, rather than go for the whole population.

Astrup: Denmark has the highest levels of fat intake, but it does not have the highest prevalence of obesity. The high levels of physical activity in Denmark are therefore probably important here too. From experimental studies, we know that the level of physical activity is a modifier of the interaction between dietary composition and body weight.

We have also looked at the 24 h energy expenditure and spontaneous physical activity in a cohort of adult siblings, and we obtained the same results as reported by Erik Ravussin in the Pima Indians (Zurlo et al 1992); that is, that the strongest risk factor for weight gain is a low level of spontaneous physical activity.

Campfield: What is the percentage of total energy as fat in the Caribbean diet, and does it vary from Jamaica to Barbados?

Forrester: There are some preliminary results which suggest that this is 35–38% in Jamaicans.

Fraser: We don't have any data on this in Barbados.

Heymsfield: If there is a reduction in physical activity, why does this not produce a physiological down-regulation of food intake, assuming that there is some interaction between the two?

Garrow: To do sums about the increasing prevalence of obesity and the decreasing food intake, you have to postulate a decrease in physical activity which is worth about 800 calories/day. For example, the studies by Garry et al (1955) on coal miners, showed that their average energy expenditure was five calories per minute, so to account for that extra 800 calories, they would have had to do an extra two and a half hours of coal mining per day (Garry et al 1955). I do not believe this is possible. It is due, as Susan Roberts suggests, to errors in the estimated food intake.

References

Buskirk ER, Iampietro PF, Welch BE 1957 Variations in resting metabolism with changes in food, exercise and climate. Metabolism 6:144–153

Consolazio F 1963 The energy requirements of men living under extreme environmental conditions. In: Bourne GH (ed) World review of nutrition and dietetics, vol 4. Pitman Medical, London, p 54–57

Dawson-Hughes B, Harris S 1992 Regional changes in body composition by season and overall in healthy postmenopausal women. Am J Clin Nutr 56:307–313

de Groot LCPGM, Sette S, Zajkas G, Carbajal A, Cruz JAA 1991 Nutritional status: anthropopmetry. Eur J Clin Nutr 45:31–42

Garry RC, Passmore R, Warnock GM, Durnin JVGA 1955 Studies on expenditure of energy and consumption of food by miners and clerks, Fife, Scotland, 1952. MRC Special Report 289. HMSO, London

Prior IA, Davidson F, Salmond CE, Czochanska Z 1981 Cholesterol, coconuts and diet on Polynesian atolls: a natural experiment. The Pukapuka and Tokelau Island studies. Am J Clin Nutr 34:1052–1561

Shaper AG, Spencer P 1961 Physical activity and dietary patterns in the Samburu of Northern Kenya. Trop Geogr Med 13:273–280

Shaper AG, Jones KW, Jones M, Kyobe J 1963 Serum lipids in three nomadic tribes of Northern Kenya. Am J Clin Nutr 13:135–146

Zurlo F, Ferraro R, Fontvieille AM, Rising R, Bogardus C, Ravussin E 1992 Spontaneous physical activity and obesity: cross-sectional and longitudinal studies in Pima Indians. Am J Physiol 263:296E–300E

Obesity in peoples of the African diaspora

Rainford Wilks, Norma McFarlane-Anderson, Franklyn Bennett, Henry Fraser†, Daniel McGee*, Richard Cooper* and Terrence Forrester

*Tropical Metabolism Research Unit, University of the West Indies, Mona, Kingston 7, Jamaica, West Indies, *Department of Preventive Medicine and Epidemiology, Loyola University, Stritch School of Medicine, South First Avenue, Maywood, IL 60153, USA, and †Department of Medicine, Faculty of Medical Sciences, University of the West Indies, Queen Elizabeth Hospital, Bridgetown, Barbados, West Indies*

Abstract. People of African descent in the Caribbean and the USA originated from the Bight of Benin in West Africa. Although these populations share a common genetic heritage, they now live under different socioeconomical conditions. Assuming genetic similarity, a cross-cultural examination of these peoples in West Africa, the Caribbean and the USA may attenuate the effect of genetic factors and allow the assessment of environmental contributions to a biological outcome. We carried out an epidemiological survey to determine the prevalence of hypertension and the contribution of risk factors to the variation in blood pressure. We measured the height, weight, waist and hip circumferences, and blood pressure of adults in Nigeria, Cameroon, Jamaica, St. Lucia, Barbados and the USA. In urban populations there was a trend towards increasing weight, height, body mass index, and proportions of those overweight and obese going from West Africa to the USA, with the Caribbean being intermediate. The prevalence of hypertension lay on a similar gradient. Given a common genetic susceptibility, urbanization and western acculturation are therefore associated with increasing hypertension and obesity.

1996 The origins and consequences of obesity. Wiley, Chichester (Ciba Foundation Symposium 201) p 37–53

In poor societies diseases of malnutrition continue to be important causes of morbidity and mortality. Notwithstanding this, there has been a definite epidemiological transition in disease pattern in countries such as Jamaica since the 1970s. Since then, the chronic diseases — in particular cardiovascular disease and cancer — have emerged as the leading causes of death. This transition mirrors a similar situation seen in the USA in the 1920s. A change in diet towards more energy-dense food and an increase in the prevalence in obesity have been correlated with this change in disease pattern (WHO 1990).

Obesity may be defined as an increased mass of adipose tissue resulting from a systematic imbalance between calorie intake and energy expenditure (Weigle 1994).

Considerable evidence has been accumulated on the adverse effect of obesity on health. This evidence has come from a variety of sources including actuarial studies by life insurance companies, cohort studies, such as the Framingham study, and secular trends in societies. (Garrow 1988).

Measurement of the excess fat that constitutes obesity is a subject of some controversy. Among the measures available, the body mass index (BMI), or quetelet index, in kg/m^2 and the waist/hip circumference ratio (WHR) are two indices used at the individual level. At the level of the population, the percentage of people overweight, or obese, or the mean BMI are measures that can be used for comparison.

Obesity has therefore taken on the role of a marker for chronic diseases, of which cardiovascular diseases and cancer are the major contributors to morbidity and mortality. Obesity has been shown to be positively correlated with average annual income and is therefore likely to be influenced by the sociocultural gradient (P. J. Francois, unpublished FAO document 1989). Between 1970 and 1980 there has been a relative increase of 21% in mortality due to chronic diseases in the Caribbean area. Central America and South America have experienced 56% and 105% increases, respectively, over the same period of time. (Litvak et al 1987).

In West Africa, the source of the Africa diaspora, the effect of westernization is less pronounced, but distinct urban elite groups have emerged that show features of increased obesity and the associated chronic diseases.

The secular trend in the prevalence of obesity has been seen in the Caribbean, and Barbados is the best documented example. In the Barbadian population from 1968 to 1981, obesity has increased from 7.0% to 16.2% in males and 31.0% to 37.9% in females. An even more dramatic increase is observed in women over 40 years old. The prevalence of obesity in this group increased from 32% to 50% in 13 years. In 1981 the prevalence of obesity among adolescent females was 20% (Hagley 1990, Hoyos 1993). At the clinical level, the prevalence of obesity among Barbadian women attending general practices was 47%, and 63% in female hospital medical outpatients.

Table 1 illustrates the impact of chronic diseases on the Jamaican population. In 1990 diseases of the circulatory system accounted for 33.3% and 39.2% of male and female deaths, respectively. Rheumatic heart disease accounted for less than 1% of these deaths, whereas neoplasms accounted for 16% and 14.4% of deaths overall in males and females, respectively (Demographic Statistics 1990).

Morbidity and mortality associated with obesity include:

(1) cardiovascular disorders (hypertension, stroke and ischaemic heart disease);
(2) gastrointestinal disorders (colon cancer, diverticulosis coli, gall stones and hae-morrhoids);
(3) metabolic disorders (diabetes mellitus and dyslipidaemia); and
(4) musculoskeletal disorders (degenerative joint disease).

These correlations and associations do not constitute cause. All the diseases mentioned are multifactorial in their aetiology, as is obesity. Among the aetiological factors is

TABLE 1 **Cause of death profile in Jamaica in 1990 (Demographic Statistics Jamaica 1990)**

Cause of death	Total number	Percentage of total number
Circulatory system		
males	2204	33.3
females	2570	39.2
Neoplasms		
males	1058	16.0
females	942	14.4
Endocrine, metabolic nutritional and immunity		
males	606	9.2
females	882	13.5
Communicable disease		
male	468	7.1
female	389	5.9
Injury and poisoning		
males	152	2.3
females	45	0.7
Ill-defined conditions		
males	1034	15.6
females	1043	15.9

genetic predisposition. A study across a sociocultural gradient but within the same genetic stock should provide some answers to the question of obesity and its relationship to the chronic diseases at the population level.

The International Collaborative Study of Hypertension in Blacks

The International Collaborative Study of Hypertension in Blacks (ICSHIB) is an international collaborative study of populations that have formed through the course of the African diaspora (Harris 1993). These peoples share a common history but live under widely different socioeconomic circumstances. The genetic contribution to any variance in outcome measures are likely to be attenuated, thus allowing the focus to be on environmental factors. In this paper we examine the pattern of obesity in a cross-cultural comparison within the same genetic stock and relate this to one of the obesity-associated diseases, i.e. hypertension. The study aimed to measure the prevalence of hypertension and various risk factors for the disease. We postulate that hypertension increases across the African diaspora from West Africa to the USA.

Methods

We studied populations from Nigeria, the Cameroons, Jamaica, St. Lucia, Barbados and Maywood, Chicago. In Nigeria and the Cameroons we examined both rural and urban populations; whereas in the Caribbean and the USA, we studied peri-urban and urban populations, respectively. The urban Cameroon population consisted of Civil Servants from the capital Yaounde, an affluent segment of the population, and it represents a perturbation in the sociocultural gradient from Africa to the USA. Source populations varied in size from 10 000 to 40 000 adults aged 25–74 years old.

We selected samples using single-stage cluster sampling by probability proportionate to size. This was facilitated by a predetermined sampling interval aimed at obtaining a sample of 1600 individuals in eight age–sex categories i.e. males/females aged 25–34, 35–44, 45–54 and 55+ years. Clusters varied between countries. For example, in St. Lucia and Maywood, they were city blocks while in Jamaica and Barbados they were census districts provided by the respective National Statistical Institutes.

Trained staff canvassed each cluster door-to-door. We used the number of eligible participants who were contacted in person as the denominator to determine the rate of participation. Participation rates were: USA, 61%; Jamaica, 60%; Barbados, 63%; and 90–99% in St Lucia, Nigeria and the Cameroons. We visited households repeatedly in an effort to improve the participation rates.

Training and certification

The comparability of measurements across the sites was crucial to the study. At least one person was brought to the coordinating centre in the USA where training and certification took place in questionnaire administration, anthropometric and blood pressure measurements.

Blood pressure was measured by mercury sphygmomanometer and particular care was taken to avoid digit preference. The first and fifth Korotkoff sounds were interpreted as the systolic and diastolic blood pressures, respectively. Appropriate cuff size was used in every situation.

Anthropometric measurements included height, weight, waist and hip circumferences, and mid–upper arm circumference.

Details of the protocol are reported elsewhere (Ataman et al 1996). Recertification was carried out at intervals of three months or after every 400 subjects were recruited, whichever was the earliest.

Results

Table 2 shows the distribution of participants by site, gender and age group. Males are fewer in numbers in almost all categories. Participation was lowest in the 45–54 age group. Weight varied consistently in both sexes across the postulated sociocultural gradient in the order: Nigeria, rural Cameroon, Jamaica, St. Lucia, urban Cameroon,

TABLE 2 Distribution of male (A) and female (B) participants by age and site

A

| Site | Total number of subjects | Number in each age group | | | |
		25–34	35–44	45–54	55+
West Africa	2528	806	554	511	657
Nigeria	1171	374	202	182	413
Cameroon (urban)	612	233	178	140	61
Cameroon (rural)	745	199	174	189	183
Caribbean	1161	330	274	254	303
Jamaica	340	96	72	68	104
St. Lucia	491	151	116	116	108
Barbados	330	83	86	70	91
USA (Maywood)	708	207	198	139	164

B

| Site | Total number of subjects | Number in each age group | | | |
		25–34	35–44	45–54	55+
West Africa	2809	895	669	580	665
Nigeria	1338	456	285	215	382
Cameroon (urban)	749	247	226	183	93
Cameroon (rural)	722	192	158	182	190
Caribbean	1561	426	364	339	432
Jamaica	480	123	118	114	125
St. Lucia	598	186	139	126	147
Barbados	483	117	107	99	160
USA (Maywood)	810	203	207	193	207

Barbados and Maywood, USA (Table 3). Pairwise comparisons were all significant at the 1% level except for urban Cameroon versus St. Lucia (males), and Jamaica versus St. Lucia and urban Cameroon (females).

A similar trend was seen in BMI and there was no significant difference between Jamaica, St. Lucia and urban Cameroon (Table 3). This was in accordance with a similar trend in their gross national products.

TABLE 3   Distribution of anthropometric variables in males (A) and females (B) by site

A

Site	Total number of subjects	Weight (kg)	BMI (kg/m²)	Waist circumference (cm)	Hip circumference (cm)	WHR
Nigeria	1171	61.5 (11.0)	21.7 (3.6)	77.3 (8.4)	88.3 (8.2)	0.88 (0.06)
Cameroon (rural)	745	68.1 (10.4)	23.5 (3.1)	80.4 (7.1)	90.7 (6.7)	0.89 (0.05)
Jamaica	340	69.4 (12.7)	23.4 (4.0)	79.9 (11.3)	95.1 (7.8)	0.84 (0.07)
St. Lucia	491	73.0 (11.4)	24.3 (3.7)	82.7 (9.5)	95.3 (7.4)	0.87 (0.06)
Cameroon (urban)	612	74.5 (12.5)	25.1 (3.6)	83.3 (9.1)	96.8 (8.1)	0.86 (0.06)
Barbados	330	76.4 (13.2)	25.9 (4.3)	86.2 (11.3)	97.8 (7.7)	0.88 (0.07)
USA (Maywood)	708	84.5 (18.0)	27.1 (5.5)	92.4 (14.0)	103.4 (10.7)	0.89 (0.07)

B

Site	Total number of subjects	Weight (kg)	BMI (kg/m²)	Waist circumference (cm)	Hip circumference (cm)	WHR
Nigeria	1338	56.6 (12.3)	22.6 (4.7)	73.9 (9.6)	93.5 (10.8)	0.79 (0.06)
Cameroon (rural)	722	60.6 (11.9)	23.5 (4.3)	80.9 (9.2)	92.6 (9.3)	0.87 (0.06)
Jamaica	480	70.4 (17.6)	27.8 (6.5)	82.2 (13.0)	103.0 (12.8)	0.80 (0.07)
St Lucia	598	72.3 (17.0)	27.3 (6.2)	85.5 (13.4)	103.7 (13.1)	0.82 (0.07)
Cameroon (urban)	749	71.0 (13.6)	27.0 (4.7)	82.5 (9.8)	102.5 (11.0)	0.81 (0.07)
Barbados	483	75.2 (16.3)	29.4 (6.4)	87.1 (12.6)	106.7 (12.8)	0.82 (0.07)
USA (Maywood)	810	82.4 (20.9)	30.8 (7.7)	91.4 (15.4)	111.8 (15.0)	0.82 (0.08)

BMI, body mass index; WHR, waist/hip circumference ratio. Values given are: mean (S.D.).

There was a consistent increase in waist and hip circumferences across the diaspora. As a result WHRs were similar across sites. (Table 3). This indicates that body proportions were similar in all the study sites.

Figure 1 shows the 85th percentile of BMI, a measure of the population burden of overweight persons, in males and females for each country. This is lowest in Nigeria at

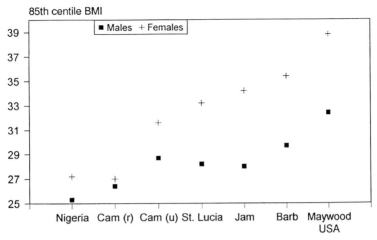

FIG. 1.   The 85th percentile of body mass index (BMI, kg/m²) in countries across the African diaspora. Barb, Barbados; Cam, Cameroon; Jam, Jamaica; r, rural; u, urban.

25.3 kg/m² and 27.2 kg/m² (for males and females, respectively), increases steadily across the diaspora and is highest in Chicago at 32.4 kg/m² and 38.8 kg/m² (for males and females, respectively).

Figure 2 shows the family of curves for the percentage of the population which is obese by age group and gender. This was calculated using a BMI of 31.2 kg/m² for males and 32.3 kg/m² for females (the National Health and Nutrition Examination Surveys [NHANES] II data). Two points are noteworthy: the increasing burden of obesity from Africa to the USA; and the consistent fall-off in the prevalence of obesity after the age of 55 years.

The mean blood pressures by gender across the diaspora is shown in Table 4. The mean values are similar and reflect the fact that many hypertensives are treated effectively and that the proportion of controlled hypertensives is greatest in the USA.

Figure 3 shows the prevalence of hypertension by the World Health Organization and the fifth Joint National Committee on Detection, Evaluation and Treatment of High Blood Pressure criteria (Gifford et al 1993). There is a steady increase in blood pressure across the diaspora (sociocultural gradient), which coincides with the increase in BMI. Figure 4 shows the relationship between the prevalence of hypertension by the latter criteria and the mean BMI for each gender. In both genders there is a strong positive relationship between the percentage of hypertension and mean BMI. The urban Cameroon sample falls below the expected values in both genders but this is more marked in females.

Discussion

The epidemiological transition in disease incidence has been attributed to several risk factors (Stamler et al 1975). Of these, obesity is one of the major risk factors for chronic

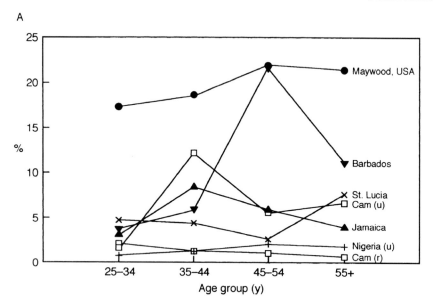

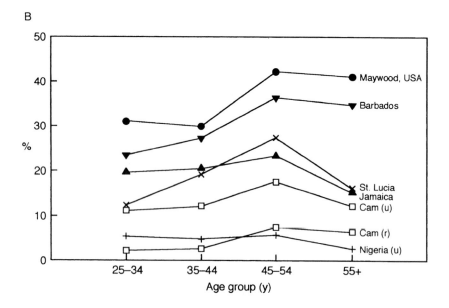

FIG. 2.   The percentage of obese males (A) and females (B) by age group (years) in countries of the African diaspora. r, rural; u, urban.

TABLE 4 Mean blood pressure in males (A) and females (B) of the African diaspora

A

Site	Systolic (mmHg)	Diastolic (mmHg)
Nigeria	121.5 (19.7)	73.3 (13.0)
Cameroon (rural)	119.9 (17.9)	74.3 (10.4)
Jamaica	123.1 (21.6)	70.3 (14.9)
St. Lucia	126.8 (18.9)	75.9 (13.7)
Cameroon (urban)	123.7 (13.5)	78.0 (13.0)
Barbados	125.5 (17.0)	77.0 (10.9)
USA (Maywood)	125.3 (19.5)	73.9 (13.4)

B

Site	Systolic (mmHg)	Diastolic (mmHg)
Nigeria	119.1 (21.8)	73.3 (13.0)
Cameroon (rural)	119.4 (24.8)	72.6 (11.9)
Jamaica	122.3 (21.9)	70.4 (14.5)
St. Lucia	122.7 (22.5)	73.4 (14.6)
Cameroon (urban)	118.4 (18.8)	73.4 (13.8)
Barbados	122.0 (19.9)	73.5 (11.5)
USA (Maywood)	122.4 (19.6)	72.7 (11.8)

Values given are: mean (S.D.).

diseases (such as hypertension and diabetes). Both hypertension and obesity are multifactorial syndromes that are influenced by genetic predisposition and environmental interaction. In this study, the standardized training and certification of study personnel allow effective data comparisons across sites. Response rates were more than acceptable (over 90%) in St. Lucia, the Cameroons and Nigeria. In Jamaica, Barbados and Chicago the 60% response rate is likely to introduce some bias with an over-representation of those who were conscious about their health and who also had one of the outcome illnesses. This was offset by the reluctance (because they perceived no benefit from the study) of some individuals who were on treatment to participate. Our results show that obesity increases linearly across the African diaspora along the postulated socioeconomic gradient. This increase across sites is consistent with increasing westernization, which may be explained by a change in diet (access to more energy-dense food) and less physical activity. The perturbation in trends from West Africa to the USA, where urban Cameroon has a higher mean BMI than Jamaica

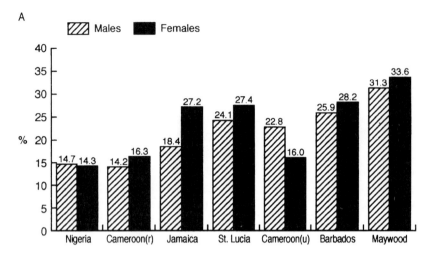

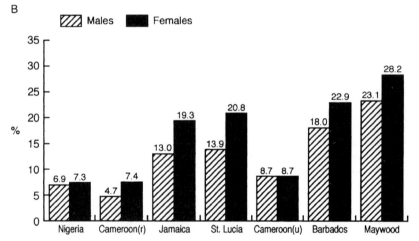

FIG. 3.   Age-adjusted prevalence (represented by percentage on y-axis) of: (A) Hypertension-1 (systolic blood pressure $\geqslant 140$, diastolic blood pressure $\geqslant 90$ or taking antihypertensives); and (B) Hypertension-2 (systolic blood pressure $\geqslant 160$, diastolic blood pressure $\geqslant 95$ or taking antihypertensives) by gender. r, rural; u, urban.

and St Lucia, may be explained by the peculiarity of the sample. This was drawn solely from civil servants, whereas those from Jamaica and St Lucia were drawn from a wider spectrum of social classes.

Obesity is strongly associated with hypertension (Foster et al 1993), although the proportion of the variance in blood pressure that is explained by obesity is consistently less than 20% (Willet 1990). This estimate may be influenced by the population in which the study takes place and the impact of other risk factors.

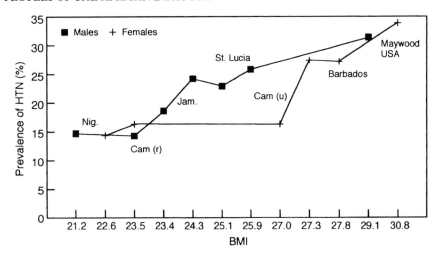

FIG. 4. The prevalence of hypertension (HTN) by mean body mass index (BMI). Cam, Cameroon; Jam, Jamaica; Nig, Nigeria; r, rural; u, urban.

Our findings confirm this association because we show that hypertension increases across the diaspora in a manner which mirrors the trend in obesity. We are unable to estimate the proportion of the blood pressure variance that is due to obesity because the impact of treatment on high blood pressure results in similar mean blood pressures across the sites. As a result, blood pressure cannot be analysed as a continuous variable.

The prevalence of hypertension among the civil servants in the Cameroons is lower than might be expected according to the postulated trend. This may be explained by the observation by Shaper (1996, this volume) that the development of hypertension lags behind the development of obesity.

The populations studied have a common genetic background (Cooper & Rotimi 1994). Therefore, the gradient in prevalence of hypertension points to the role of environmental exposure. These include changes in diet and physical activity, which are also linked to the development of obesity. These data do not exclude the possibility of a genetic predisposition to both disorders but clearly indicate the impact of social factors.

Among the other obesity-related diseases, such as diabetes and dyslipidaemia, the demonstration of a similar gradient would support the central role of obesity as a risk factor.

Acknowledgements

We wish to thank Maria Jackson, Audrey Smith, Marsha Ivey and Paul Mattocks for invaluable assistance in the field. The study was funded by grants from the National Institutes of Health grant HLB 45508 and the Wellcome Trust.

References

Ataman SL, Cooper RS, Rotimi C et al 1996 Standardisation of blood pressure measurements in an international comparative study. J Clin Epidemiol, in press

Cooper R, Rotimi C 1994 Hypertension in populations of west African origin: is there a genetic predisposition? J Hypertens 12:215–227

Foster C, Rotimi C, Fraser H et al 1993 Hypertension diabetes and obesity in Barbados: findings from a recent population based survey. Ethn Dis 3:404–412

Garrow JS 1988 Obesity and related diseases. Churchill Livingstone, Edinburgh

Gifford RW, Alderman MH, Chobanian AV et al 1993 The 5th report of the Joint National Committee on Detection, Evaluation and Treatment of High Blood Pressure (JNCV). Arch Intern Med 153:154–183

Hagley KE 1990 Chronic non-communicable diseases and their impact on Caribbean women. West Indian Med J 39:4–11

Harris JE 1993 Global dimensions of the African diaspora, 2nd edn. Howard University Press, Washington DC

Hoyos MD 1993 Understanding obesity in the Caribbean. Postgrad Doctor (Caribbean) 9:130–136

Litvak J, Ruiz L, Restrepo H, McAlister A 1987 The growing non-communicable disease burden, a challenge for the countries of the Americas. Bull Pan Am Health Org 21:156–171

Shaper AG 1996 Obesity and cardiovascular disease. In: The origins and consequences of obesity. Wiley, Chichester (Ciba Found Symp 201) p 90–107

Stamler J, Berkson M, Dyer A et al 1975 Relationship of multiple variables to blood pressure. Findings from four Chicago epidemiologic studies. In: Oglesby PMD (ed) Epidemiology and control of hypertension. Year Book Medical Publishers, Chicago, IL, p 307–358

Weigle DS 1994 Appetite and the regulation of body composition. FASEB J 8:302–310

Willett W 1990 Nutritional epidemiology. Oxford University Press, Oxford, p 217–244

WHO 1990 Diet, nutrition and the prevention of chronic diseases. World Health Organization, Geneva (Technical Report Series 797)

DISCUSSION

Fraser: I have a comment on the origins of Afro-Caribbeans. Although Rainford Wilks suggested that virtually all Afro-Caribbeans originated from the Bight of Benin, they also originated from Gambia, which is located on the southern side of Senegal. The ethnicity of peoples originating from this region is different from those from the Bight of Benin because caravan routes across central West Africa through Timbuktu brought many different populations into the Gambian area. We have blood pressure and body mass index (BMI) data for this population going back as far as 1970, which demonstrate the increase in both measurements over this period. However, the blood pressure data of 1974, which were obtained using the World Health Organization 160/95 mmHg criteria, gave a slightly higher prevalence, although there was a much lower proportion of subjects treated.

Ferro-Luzzi: I was interested in Rainford Wilks' comment that there was a decrease in BMI in the older age groups of both sexes. Could you tell me what was the mean age of this older age group?

Wilks: I don't know the mean age, but the oldest people in this age category were 74 years old.

Ferro-Luzzi: There are problems with using BMI as an indicator of overweight in elderly people because of the well-known difficulties of measuring their true heights. I also have another, related point. In rural populations in Senegal, Zimbabwe and Mali we found that the BMI of older men was lower than at younger ages, which is in agreement with your results, but the BMI of women showed a definite increase with age, which does not agree with your results. On the other hand, in studies conducted on rural populations in Ethiopia and India we found that the BMI of women decreased from the age of 30 years onwards. We do not have an explanation for these observations, but we tend to believe that the diverse trends in BMI of women with age might reflect their social status. Could this explanation be applied to your sample of women in rural Cameroon?

Wilks: I don't know. What is the mean life expectancy for women in Ethiopia?

Ferro-Luzzi: I am not certain because the age assessment is poor in Ethiopia but it is likely to be low. Ethiopia has a high proportion of adults with low BMIs: the mean BMI of the rural population I'm studying is about $18\,\mathrm{kg/m^2}$.

McKeigue: One should bear in mind that the cross-sectional relationships between BMI and age may be cohort effects, i.e. that there is a cohort of women born later who will be more obese throughout their lifetime. It doesn't mean that people actually lose weight after the age of 30, those older women may have been thin throughout their entire lifetime.

Ravussin: Price et al (1993) have shown a dramatic increase in obesity among Pima Indians born after World War II when compared to those born before the war. This increase appeared to be associated with increased exposure to western customs and diet following 1945. Another factor which may explain part of the decrease in BMI in older populations is the increasing prevalences of other diseases that influence body weight, such as cancer and non-insulin-dependent diabetes mellitus (NIDDM).

Prentice: I hope to leave this symposium with a greater understanding of the slope of the relationships between BMI (or body fat, waist/hip circumference ratio or whatever measure of obesity we have) and disease, against different genetic, racial and environmental backgrounds. Your results are the first steps in this direction. The second part of your hypothesis was that most of the variance in hypertension could be explained by obesity, and you showed us some striking relationships between the two. However, to really test this hypothesis we need to find out whether the prevalence of hypertension is the same in these populations in a given band of BMI. In other words, after adjusting for BMI is there the same prevalence of hypertension?

Wilks: We have not looked at that. Our statistician, Dan McGee, has presented us with another difficulty in that blood pressure has to be introduced into the model. We found that the measurements of blood pressure did not vary because of the intervention of treatment. Therefore, his point was that it would be difficult to demonstrate the exact role of obesity in this multifactorial disease across these sites using blood pressure because blood pressure was not a reflection of hypertension.

However, we rely on blood pressure measurements, even though they do not reflect hypertension, because just looking at untreated hypertensive patients would give us an extremely small sample size and we would be unable to answer those kind of questions. A similar situation occurs when looking at the same population across a BMI gradient. I suspect that there would be smaller differences in blood pressure because if the aetiology is multifactorial, then presumably such differences will be greater between countries than within the same country.

Fraser: If we look at our recognition, our treatment and our control of blood pressure across the three Caribbean sites, we observe that in Barbados a higher percentage of people are diagnosed and treated. Therefore, there is a higher level of intervention which results in exactly the same blood pressure levels.

Shaper: At least within the UK, this may say something about our ability to treat hypertension. The blood pressure levels of treated hypertensives are the about the same as those of untreated controls. However, the former group presumably had a much higher blood pressure prior to treatment. Nevertheless, when looking at mean blood pressures, I wouldn't worry too much about whether they were treated or untreated, because the values are going to be roughly the same.

Blundell: It would be interesting to find out how much the pharmacological treatment of hypertension interferes with the relationship between obesity and energy balance. Beta blockers cause a decrease in basal metabolic rate and this effect could give rise to a long-term positive energy balance, which would result in weight gain.

Fraser: Methyldopa, which is used widely in St. Lucia, has a similar effect.

McKeigue: I would like to discuss how to handle data sets in which a large per cent of people with hypertension have been treated. The method of looking at treatment-adjusted medians can be applied to multivariate analyses, and we have described statistical methods of doing this. However, when we've used those methods, the answers do not differ significantly from those obtained using the mean blood pressure (White et al 1994). We also have some data from our survey in the UK on whether the slope of the relationship between obesity and blood pressure is steeper in some high risk populations than in others (Chaturvedi et al 1993). We compared Afro-Caribbean and European adults, and we found that the slope of the relationship between blood pressure and BMI is steeper in Afro-Caribbean populations, at least in men (Poulter et al 1984, Sever et al 1980). This is consistent with other data on the epidemiology of hypertension in people of Black African descent, which have shown that the rise in blood pressure with age is steeper in populations of Black African descent, and the only populations where that is not the case are rural populations studied in the 1960s in Kenya and southern Africa. That is, in these lean populations there was no hypertension and no rise in blood pressure with age. Therefore, we can probably formulate the susceptibility to hypertension in Black populations as being an exaggerated susceptibility to the rise in blood pressure that occurs with weight gain.

Shaper: And the involvement of other factors.

McKeigue: The existence of these other factors that are important as determinants of increased susceptibility in Black populations remains to be established.

Ferro-Luzzi: Is anything known about the effect of salt intake on blood pressure in these populations?

Wilks: We have some data on salt intake in these populations. It is consistent with the gradient of BMI and blood pressure.

Shaper: Are you assuming that it has an independent effect?

Wilks: Yes.

Heymsfield: This is just a minor technical note. It's difficult to measure blood pressure in obese people. There are a number of biases built into the measurement, particularly if you use the same cuff size in large populations, because you can obtain erroneous blood pressure measurements in relation to body weight.

Wilks: I can assure you that this was taken into consideration. The standard approach in our studies was to measure the mid–upper arm circumference and use the appropriate cuff size.

Blundell: I would like to draw your attention to another consequence of obesity, and that is the consequence arising from negative cultural pressure. All of these societies, with the exception of the USA, have a fairly relaxed approach towards fat people. Only in the USA is there an aggressive cultural attitude towards obesity. One of the consequences of this negative attitude would be to coerce individuals to try to diet. Since dieting is a stressful process, which would be expected to influence neuroendocrine profiles, the cultural attitude towards obesity could play a role in the physiological aspects of obesity.

Wilks: I'm not aware of any data in Jamaica or in the African communities on the attitude towards obesity. It wasn't measured in this particular study.

Blundell: The anthropological studies suggest that in most societies, obesity is prized rather than castigated.

Astrup: What do you mean by dieting?

Blundell: Trying to reduce food intake in order to lose body weight.

Astrup: But weight reduction is the most effective way of reducing blood pressure, so if dieting is successful blood pressure is decreased. A failure of these efforts may cause weight fluctuations, but there is still no evidence that it causes hypertension.

Blundell: If that is the case, then dieting is an important variable in these communities because it may contribute to the changes that accompany obesity.

Allison: I am aware only of some anecdotal studies of preferences for various body shapes in Africa. The anthropological studies have been summarized by Brown & Konner (1987), but these are also quasi-anecdotal. Not a single culture has been found that values obesity. What many developing societies value, according to Brown & Konner, was described as plumpness, which is different. Obesity may still be spurned in other countries, which could lead to various stresses.

Ferro-Luzzi: In my experience, there are populations, especially African ones, that will deliberately overeat for cultural reasons. After harvest both men and women place a loose bracelet above the elbow, which monitors their progress in the post-harvest weight gain. The person who gains weight the quickest (i.e. has the tightest bracelet) wins this traditional contest. In other African countries, young girls are fattened to help them find a husband.

Allison: At least by American standards, I would call these women that come out of those fattening huts as plump and not as obese.

Björntorp: Some of us believe that the relationship between obesity and hypertension is mediated by insulin resistance. Groop et al (1993) have found a polymorphism in the glycogen synthase gene that is closely linked to insulin resistance and development of diabetes. They have found that this polymorphism is prevalent in hypertensives, which illustrates that a genetic component is involved.

Bouchard: The glycogen synthase gene is probably not closely linked to insulin resistance and diabetes. It was shown to be associated with insulin resistance in at least one study but in this study it accounted only for a very small number of the diabetes cases (Groop et al 1993, Orho et al 1995).

Hitman: A mutation in the glycogen synthase gene which leads to NIDDM has yet to be identified despite disease-associated polymorphisms being described (Groop et al 1993, Bjorbaek et al 1994). A possibility is that the association between NIDDM and the glycogen synthase gene is spurious or that the disease-associated polymorphism is in linkage disequilibrium with another gene in close proximity to the glycogen synthase gene.

Björntorp: The defect is in an intron. It is prevalent in the Finnish population.

Bouchard: Yes, but it is not responsible for most cases of obesity, if any at all. Moreover, obesity is not necessarily a cause of hypertension or NIDDM. There are plenty of diabetics and hypertensives who have a normal body mass. In other words, for obese persons to develop hypertension or diabetes, they likely need to be susceptible or prone to these disorders. I also believe that it is rather unlikely that a genetic component will be identified by population studies because there is so much genetic variation even within populations. We first need to identify, by careful molecular studies, these genes that increase the susceptibility to, rather than being the specific cause of, those disorders in the presence of obesity. Once we have these genes, then we may be able to establish when obesity or visceral obesity becomes a risk factor for the development of hypertension or diabetes.

References

Bjorbaek C, Echwald SM, Hubricht P et al 1994 Genetic variants in promoters and coding regions of the muscle glycogen synthase and the insulin-responsive GLUT4 genes in NIDDM. Diabetes 43:976–983

Brown PJ, Konner M 1987 An anthropological perspective on obesity. Ann N Y Acad Sci 499:29–46

Chaturvedi N, McKeigue PM, Marmot MG 1993 Resting and ambulatory blood pressure differences in Afro-Caribbeans and Europeans. Hypertension 22:90–96

Groop LC, Kankuri M, Schalin-Jäntti C et al 1993 Association between polymorphism of the glycogen synthase gene and non-insulin-dependent diabetes mellitus. New Engl J Med 328:10–14

Orho M, Nikula-Ijäs P, Schalin-Jäntti C, Permutt MA, Groop LC 1995 Isolation and characterization of the human muscle glycogen synthase gene. Diabetes 44:1099–1105

Poulter N, Khaw KT, Hopwood BE et al 1984 Blood pressure and its correlates in an African tribe in urban and rural environments. J Epidemiol Community Health 38:181–185

Price RA, Charles MA, Pettitt DJ, Knowler WC 1993 Obesity in Pima Indians: large increases among post-World War II birth cohorts. Am J Phys Anthropol 92:473–479

Sever PS, Gordon D, Peart WS, Beighton P 1980 Blood pressure and its correlates in urban and tribal Africa. Lancet II:60–64

White IR, Chaturvedi N, McKeigue PM 1994 Median analysis of blood pressure for a sample including treated hypertensives. Stat Med 13:1635–1641

Metabolic consequences of obesity and body fat pattern: lessons from migrant studies

Paul M. McKeigue

Department of Epidemiology and Population Sciences, London School of Hygiene and Tropical Medicine, Keppel Street, London WC1E 7HT, UK

Abstract. Prevalence of non-insulin-dependent diabetes mellitus and mortality from coronary heart disease are higher in people of South Asian (Indian, Pakistani and Bangladeshi) descent living in urban societies than in other ethnic groups. The high prevalence of diabetes is one manifestation of a pattern of metabolic disturbances related to central obesity and insulin resistance, which includes raised plasma very low density lipoprotein triglyceride and low plasma high density lipoprotein-cholesterol. Average waist/hip circumference ratios are higher in South Asians than in Europeans of similar body mass index: in this respect South Asians differ from other populations such as Pima Indians where high prevalence of non-insulin-dependent diabetes mellitus occurs in association with generalized obesity. The high rates of coronary heart disease in South Asians are most easily explained by the effects of this central obesity/insulin resistance syndrome, although ethnic differences in fasting lipids are unlikely to account fully for the excess risk. In Afro-Caribbean migrants, the prevalence of diabetes is almost as high as in South Asians but the lipid disturbances characteristic of the insulin resistance syndrome do not occur to the same extent. This may account for the low rates of coronary heart disease in this group.

1996 The origins and consequences of obesity. Wiley, Chichester (Ciba Foundation Symposium 201) p 54–67

Diabetes in South Asians

In people of South Asian (Indian, Pakistani and Bangladeshi) descent living in urban societies, the prevalence of non-insulin-dependent diabetes is far higher than in Europeans. Table 1 summarizes the results of surveys in South Asian populations which have used glucose tolerance tests and World Health Organization criteria. The prevalence of 19% in our own survey of South Asian men and women aged 40–69 years in the UK (McKeigue et al 1991) is remarkably consistent with surveys in other overseas South Asian populations (Miller et al 1989, Zimmet et al 1983, Omar et al

54

TABLE 1   Prevalence of non-insulin-dependent diabetes in South Asians

Country	Year of study	Age of subjects	Prevalence (%)	Reference
Overseas				
Trinidad	1977	35–69	21	Miller et al 1989
Fiji	1983	35–64	25	Zimmet et al 1983
South Africa	1985	30+	22	Omar et al 1985
Singapore	1990	40–69	25	Hughes et al 1990b
Mauritius	1990	35–64	20	Dowse et al 1990
England	1991	40–69	19	McKeigue et al 1991
India				
Karnataka (urban)	1985	45–64	29	Ramachandran et al 1988
Madras (urban)	1992	45–64	18	Ramachandran et al 1992
Tamil Nadu (rural)	1992	45–64	3	Ramachandran et al 1992

1985, Hughes et al 1990a, Dowse et al 1990) and in urban India (Ramachandran et al 1988, 1992). For comparison, in this age group the prevalence of diabetes in men and women of European descent in the UK is about 4% (McKeigue et al 1991). In a recent survey of a rural Indian population (Ramachandran et al 1992), prevalence was 3% in the age group 40–64 years, which is similar to that in Europeans in the UK.

Coronary heart disease in South Asians

From the 1950s onwards, reports began to appear of unusually high rates of coronary heart disease (CHD) in South Asians overseas compared with other groups in the same countries (Danaraj et al 1959, Adelstein 1963, Sorokin 1975). Recent mortality data for South Asians overseas (Hughes et al 1990b, Tuomilehto et al 1984, Miller et al 1989, Steinberg et al 1988, Office of Population Censuses and Surveys 1990) are summarized in Table 2. In comparison with high risk populations such as Europeans in South Africa or the UK, the relative risk for CHD mortality associated with South Asian origin is about 1.4 (Steinberg et al 1988, Office of Population Censuses and Surveys 1990), and in comparison with relatively low risk groups, such as Chinese in Singapore (Hughes et al 1990b) or Africans in Trinidad (Miller et al 1989), the relative risk is about 3.0. In England and Wales high coronary mortality is common in Hindus originating from Gujarat in western India, in Sikhs originating from Punjab in northern India, and in Muslims from Pakistan and Bangladesh (Balarajan et al 1984, McKeigue & Marmot 1988). Reliable population-based coronary mortality data from South Asia are not available, but in two northern Indian cities the prevalence of Minnesota-coded major Q waves on electrocardiograms has been reported to be at least as high as in European populations (Sarvotham & Berry 1968, Chadha et al 1990). In contrast, very low prevalence rates have been recorded in rural India (Dewan et al 1974, Jajoo et al 1988).

The consistency of the high CHD risk in urban South Asian populations around the world, affecting both sexes and with early onset in men, suggests a common underlying cause. Surveys comparing risk factors in South Asians and other groups have shown that the high coronary disease rates in South Asians are not explained by differences in smoking, hypertension, plasma cholesterol or haemostatic activity (Miller et al 1988, McKeigue et al 1988). Most South Asian patients with coronary disease are not diabetic (Hughes et al 1989), and glucose intolerance alone cannot explain more than a small proportion of the excess coronary risk in South Asian people (Miller et al 1989).

Insulin resistance and central obesity in South Asians

In a study comparing Bangladeshi migrants to east London with native Europeans, we identified a pattern of intercorrelated metabolic disturbances in Bangladeshi men and women: high prevalence of non-insulin-dependent diabetes, high levels of insulin and triglyceride after a glucose load, and low levels of high density lipoprotein–cholesterol (HDL–C) (McKeigue et al 1988). This pattern corresponds to the insulin resistance syndrome described by others (Reaven 1988, DeFronzo & Ferrannini 1991). The occurrence of this syndrome in South Asians was confirmed in a larger study of Indian and Pakistani subjects in west London: the Southall Study (Table 3) (McKeigue et al 1991). At 2 h after a glucose load mean insulin levels were about twice as high in South Asians as in Europeans.

South Asian men and women have a more central distribution of body fat than Europeans, with thicker trunk skinfolds and markedly higher mean waist/hip circumference ratios (WHRs) for a given level of body mass index (BMI). This ethnic difference in WHR is equivalent to about two-thirds of one standard deviation in men and about one standard deviation in women (McKeigue et al

TABLE 2   Mortality from coronary heart disease in South Asians overseas

Country	Year of study	Groups contrasted	Age of subjects	Mortality ratio	Reference
Singapore	1980–1986	South Asian/ Chinese	30–69	3.8	Hughes et al 1990a
Fiji	1980	South Asian/ Melanesian	40–59	3.0	Tuomilehto et al 1984
Trinidad	1977 1986	South Asian/ African	35–69	2.4	Miller et al 1989
South Africa	1985	South Asian/ European	35–74	1.4	Steinberg et al 1988
England	1979–1983	South Asian/ European	20–69	1.4	Office of Population Censuses and Surveys 1990

TABLE 3 Mean levels of coronary risk factors in South Asians and Europeans in the Southhall Study (data from McKeigue et al 1991)

Population	BMI (kg/m²)	WHR	Median systolic blood pressure (mmHg)	Diabetes prevalence (%)	2 b insulin (mU/l)	Total cholesterol (mmol/l)	HDL–cholesterol (mmol/l)	2 b triglyceride (mmol/l)
Men								
European	25.9	0.94	121	5	19	6.1	1.25	1.39
South Asian	25.7	0.98	126	20	41	6.0	1.16	1.72
Afro-Caribbean	26.3	0.94	128	15	22	5.9	1.37	0.99
Women								
European	25.2	0.76	120	2	21	6.3	1.58	1.01
South Asian	27.0	0.85	126	16	44	6.0	1.38	1.27

BMI, body mass index; HDL, high density lipoprotein; WHR, waist/hip circumference ratio.

1991). In both South Asians and Europeans we found that glucose intolerance and 2 h insulin were more strongly associated with WHR than with BMI (McKeigue et al 1992), although the ethnic differences in diabetes prevalence and insulin levels were not fully accounted for by WHR (McKeigue et al 1991). Average BMI and insulin levels are much lower in rural Indians than in urban Indian populations (Snehalatha et al 1994) or migrants to England (Bhatnagar et al 1995). This is consistent with the urban/rural differences in prevalence of diabetes and CHD that have been described (Sarvotham & Berry 1968, Dewan et al 1974, Ramachandran et al 1992). The tendency for South Asians to accumulate intra-abdominal fat without necessarily developing generalized obesity contrasts with other populations at high risk of diabetes, such as Pima Indians (Knowler et al 1981) and Nauruans (Zimmet et al 1977), in whom average BMIs are considerably higher than in populations of European origin. The occurrence of metabolic disturbances associated with insulin resistance in people of South Asian descent in widely different environments, even several generations after migration, suggests that some genetic predisposition to develop insulin resistance exists in this group. The ability to store fat in intra-abdominal depots and to rely on lipid rather than glucose as fuel for muscle may have been an advantage in times of unreliable food supply.

Relationship of lipid disturbances to central obesity

In the Southall Study WHR was correlated more strongly with plasma triglyceride than with any other metabolic variable. A clue to the possible mechanism of this association may lie in the response of plasma triglyceride levels to glucose challenge. Between fasting and 2 h after a glucose load, the average change in plasma triglyceride was -1% in South Asian men and -6% in European men (McKeigue et al 1991). In both ethnic groups the change in plasma triglyceride levels was directly correlated with WHR: men with central obesity have high fasting triglyceride levels which fall less in response to a glucose load. The most likely mechanism of this effect is that the rise in insulin levels suppresses lipolysis of fat to non-esterified fatty acids (NEFA), which are the main substrate for hepatic triglyceride synthesis. We found that the level of 2 h plasma NEFA was correlated with both WHR and plasma triglyceride levels. This association is consistent with the results of two studies which have shown that the rate of decline of NEFA in response to insulin infusion is closely related to elevation of very low density lipoprotein (VLDL) triglyceride levels (Yki-Jarvinen & Taskinen 1988) and to central obesity (Coon et al 1992). It is likely that the relationship between central obesity and triglyceride levels is mediated through effects on the supply of NEFA to the liver. Raised triglyceride levels in turn may lower plasma HDL-C levels and cause changes in the composition and size of particles in the low density lipoprotein (LDL) fraction (Austin et al 1990).

Relationship to coronary heart disease in South Asians

Baseline data from the Southall Study show strong cross-sectional associations of electrocardiographic Q waves in South Asian men with glucose intolerance, elevated insulin and triglyceride levels (McKeigue et al 1993). Confirmation that this accounts for the high CHD risk will depend on prospective studies. We can test hypotheses about the mechanism of increased CHD risk by studying the distribution of risk factors in different South Asian groups. If the hypothesis that the insulin resistance syndrome underlies the high CHD risk in South Asians is correct, then the disturbances which cause CHD must be consistently present in all the groups originating from South Asia who share the high CHD risk. Table 4 summarizes the results of comparisons between these groups. Although systolic and diastolic blood pressures are correlated with insulin levels in South Asians, as in other populations, it is only in Sikhs and Hindus of Punjabi origin that average blood pressures are higher than in Europeans (McKeigue et al 1991). The average HDL–C level is lower in Hindu and Muslim South Asian men than in the native British population, but in Sikh men the average HDL–C level is no lower than in native British men (McKeigue et al 1991). It follows that the increased CHD risk in South Asians cannot be mediated mainly through blood pressure or HDL–C. Common to all South Asian populations at high risk of CHD are central obesity, hyperinsulinaemia, high diabetes prevalence and raised triglyceride levels after a glucose load (McKeigue et al 1988, 1991). The increased CHD risk may be mediated through some disturbance of lipoprotein metabolism related to increased synthesis of VLDL triglyceride. Control of obesity and increased physical activity are likely to be the most effective means of reducing the risk of CHD in South Asians if the insulin resistance hypothesis is correct.

Epidemiology of diabetes and coronary heart disease in Afro-Caribbeans

Table 5 summarizes surveys that have compared the prevalence of non-insulin-dependent diabetes in Afro-Caribbeans or African-Americans with Europeans: the ratio of diabetes prevalence in people of African descent to that in Europeans was 1.8

TABLE 4   Which features of the insulin resistance syndrome are common to all the South Asian groups who share high coronary heart disease risk?

Common to all South Asian populations at risk	*Not common to all South Asian populations at risk*
Central obesity	High blood pressure (not Muslims)
Hyperinsulinaemia	Low HDL–C (not Sikhs)
High diabetes prevalence	High fasting triglyceride
High post-glucose triglyceride levels	

HDL–C, high density lipoprotein–cholesterol.

TABLE 5 Diabetes prevalence by World Health Organization criteria in people of African and European descent

Country of study	Year of study	Sex	Age	Prevalence (%) in those of European descent	Prevalence (%) in those of African descent	Reference
Trinidad	1978	male and female	35–69	6	12	Beckles et al 1986
USA	1980	male and female	40–64	10	18	Harris et al 1987
UK (Southall)	1989	male	40–64	5	14	McKeigue et al 1991
UK (Brent)	1991	male	40–64	7	13	Chaturvedi et al
		female	40–64	4	18	1993

in the USA (Harris et al 1987), 2.4 in Trinidad (Beckles et al 1986) and about 3.0 in the UK (McKeigue et al 1991, Chaturvedi et al 1993). In contrast to the high CHD mortality of South Asians overseas, in England and Wales in 1979–1983 the relative risk of CHD mortality was 0.45 in Caribbean-born men and 0.76 in Caribbean-born women compared with the national average (Office of Population Censuses and Surveys 1990). Although CHD mortality is low, mortality from stroke and hypertension is twice as high in Afro-Caribbeans as in the general population (Office of Population Censuses and Surveys 1990). Mortality from stroke and hypertensive end-organ damage is high in African-Americans also, and when groups of similar socioeconomic status are compared, mortality from CHD is lower in men of Black African descent than in those of European descent. In the Charleston Heart Study, the relative risk of death from CHD in Blacks compared with Caucasians was 0.56 in men of low socioeconomic status and 0.69 in those of high socioeconomic status (Keil et al 1992). This dissociation between high prevalence of diabetes and hypertension and relatively low CHD mortality rates in Afro-Caribbean and African-American people has never been explained.

Insulin, lipids and body fat pattern in Afro-Caribbeans

In the Southall Study the prevalence of non-insulin-dependent diabetes in Afro-Caribbean men was almost as high as in South Asian men but serum insulin levels were similar in Afro-Caribbean and European men (McKeigue et al 1991) (Table 3). Afro-Caribbean men have lower plasma triglyceride and higher HDL–C levels than European men: in these respects Afro-Caribbean men resemble European women. Table 1 shows that at 2 h after a glucose load plasma triglyceride levels are nearly 30% lower in Afro-Caribbean than in European men. These differences in

TABLE 6 Brent study: fasting triglyceride and high density lipoprotein–cholesterol (HDL–C) in men by ethnicity and glucose tolerance (data from Chaturvedi et al 1994)

Population	Triglyceride (mmol/l)	HDL-C (mmol/l)
European		
normoglycaemic	1.49[a]	1.36[b]
glucose intolerant	1.89	1.25
Afro-Caribbean		
normoglycaemic	1.36	1.52
glucose intolerant	1.22[c]	1.51[d]

[a]Comparison with European glucose intolerant $P < 0.05$; comparison with Afro-Caribbean normoglycaemic $P < 0.001$.
[b]Comparison with European glucose intolerant $P < 0.05$; comparison with Afro-Caribbean normoglycaemic $P < 0.001$.
[c]Comparison with Afro-Caribbean normoglycaemic not significant; comparison with European glucose intolerant $P < 0.001$.
[d]Comparison with Afro-Caribbean normoglycaemic not significant; comparison with European glucose intolerant $P < 0.05$.

triglyceride and HDL–C levels have been found consistently in studies comparing Afro-Caribbean and African-American men with men of European descent (Slack et al 1977, Morrison et al 1981, Chaturvedi et al 1993). In a subsequent study in Brent we found that the relatively favourable lipid pattern of Afro-Caribbean compared with European men was maintained even in those with glucose intolerance (Table 6).

In contrast to South Asians, there is no evidence that Afro-Caribbean people tend to have a more central pattern of obesity than Europeans. Mean WHRs are no higher in Afro-Caribbean than in European men, although glucose intolerance is associated with higher WHRs in Afro-Caribbeans just as much as in Europeans or South Asians (Table 7) (McKeigue et al 1991). The mean for waist/thigh circumference ratio, an alternative measure of body fat distribution, is markedly lower in Afro-Caribbeans than in either of the two other ethnic groups. This emphasizes the limitations of relying on one anthropometric index such as WHR to compare body fat pattern in groups with different physique. In any case it is clear that the high prevalence of non-insulin-dependent diabetes in Afro-Caribbeans is not part of a generalized syndrome of metabolic disturbances associated with central obesity, as it is in South Asians. The differences in triglyceride and HDL–C levels between Afro-Caribbean and European men are in the opposite direction to the differences that we would predict from the hypothesis that non-insulin-dependent diabetes is but one manifestation of an insulin resistance syndrome. The favourable lipoprotein pattern in Afro-Caribbean men may be one reason for the low CHD mortality despite high prevalence of diabetes and hypertension in this group.

Acknowledgements

The Southall Study was supported by the UK Medical Research Council and the British Heart Foundation.

TABLE 7 Southall Study: mean obseity indices in men by ethnicity and glucose tolerance

Population	Sample size	BMI (kg/m²)	WHR	WTR
European				
normoglycaemic	1395	25.7	0.93	1.60
glucose intolerant	111	28.2	0.99	1.71
South Asian				
normoglycaemic	1056	25.4	0.97	1.65
glucose intolerant	352	26.5	1.00	1.71
Afro-Caribbean				
normoglycaemic	158	25.8	0.93	1.52
glucose intolerant	48	28.2	0.98	1.60

BMI, body mass index; WHR, waist/hip circumference ratio; WTR, waist/thigh circumference ratio.

References

Adelstein AM 1963 Some aspects of cardiovascular mortality in South Africa. Br J Prev Soc Med 17:29–40

Austin MA, King MC, Vranizan KM, Krauss RM 1990 Atherogenic lipoprotein phenotype: a proposed genetic marker for coronary heart disease risk. Circulation 82:495–506

Balarajan R, Adelstein AM, Bulusu L, Shukla V 1984 Patterns of mortality among migrants to England and Wales from the Indian subcontinent. Br Med J 289:1185–1187

Beckles GLA, Miller GJ, Kirkwood BR, Alexis SD, Carson DC, Byam NTA 1986 High total and cardiovascular disease mortality in adults of Indian descent in Trinidad, unexplained by major coronary risk factors. Lancet I:1298–1301

Bhatnagar D, Anand IS, Durrington PN et al 1995 Coronary risk factors in people from the Indian subcontinent living in west London and their siblings in India. Lancet 345:405–409

Chadha SL, Radhakrishnan S, Ramachandran K, Kaul U, Gopinath N 1990 Epidemiological study of coronary heart disease in urban population of Delhi. Indian J Med Res 92:424–430

Chaturvedi N, McKeigue PM, Marmot MG 1993 Resting and ambulatory blood pressure differences in Afro-Caribbean and Europeans. Hypertension 22:90–96

Chaturvedi N, McKeigue PM, Marmot MG 1994 Relationship of glucose intolerance to coronary risk in Afro-Caribbean compared with Europeans. Diabetologia 37:765–772

Coon PJ, Rogus EM, Goldberg AP 1992 Time course of plasma free fatty acid concentrations in response to insulin: effect of obesity and physical fitness. Metabolism 41:711–716

Danaraj TJ, Acker MS, Danaraj W, Ong WH, Yam TB 1959 Ethnic group differences in coronary heart disease in Singapore: an analysis of necropsy records. Am Heart J 58:516–526

DeFronzo RA, Ferrannini E 1991 Insulin resistance: a multifaceted syndrome responsible for NIDDM, obesity, hypertension, dyslipidemia, and atherosclerotic cardiovascular disease. Diabetes Care 14:173–194

Dewan BD, Malhotra KC, Gupta SP 1974 Epidemiological study of coronary heart disease in a rural community in Haryana. Indian Heart J 26:68–78

Dowse GK, Gareeboo H, Zimmet P et al 1990 High prevalence of NIDDM and impaired glucose tolerance in Indian, Creole and Chinese Mauritians. Diabetes 39:390–396

Harris MI, Hadden WC, Knowler WC, Bennett PH 1987 Prevalence of diabetes and impaired glucose tolerance and plasma glucose levels in U.S. population aged 20–74 yr. Diabetes 36:523–534

Hughes LO, Cruickshank JK, Wright J, Raftery EB 1989 Disturbances of insulin in British Asian and white men surviving myocardial infarction. Br Med J 299:537–541

Hughes K, Yeo PPB, Lun KC et al 1990a Cardiovascular diseases in Chinese, Malays and Indians in Singapore. II. Differences in risk factor levels. J Epidemiol Community Health 44:29–35

Hughes K, Lun KC, Yeo PPB 1990b Cardiovascular diseases in Chinese, Malays and Indians in Singapore. I. Differences in mortality. J Epidemiol Community Health 44:24–28

Jajoo UN, Kalantri SP, Gupta OP, Jain AP, Gupta K 1988 The prevalence of coronary heart disease in rural population from central India. J Assoc Physicians India 36:689–693

Keil JE, Sutherland SE, Knapp RG, Tyroler HA 1992 Does equal socioeconomic status in black and white men mean equal risk of mortality? Am J Public Health 82:1133–1136

Knowler WC, Pettitt DJ, Savage PJ, Bennett PH 1981 Diabetes incidence in Pima Indians: contributions of obesity and parental diabetes. Am J Epidemiol 113:144–156

McKeigue PM, Marmot MG 1988 Mortality from coronary heart disease in Asian communities in London. Br Med J 297:903

McKeigue PM, Marmot MG, Court YDS, Cottier DE, Rahman S, Riemersma RA 1988 Diabetes, hyperinsulinaemia and coronary risk factors in Bangladeshis in east London. Br Heart J 60:390–396

McKeigue PM, Shah B, Marmot MG 1991 Relation of central obesity and insulin resistance with high diabetes prevalence and cardiovascular risk in South Asians. Lancet 337:382–386

McKeigue PM, Pierpoint T, Ferrie JE, Marmot MG 1992 Relationship of glucose intolerance and hyperinsulinaemia to body fat pattern in South Asians and Europeans. Diabetologia 35:785–791

McKeigue PM, Ferrie JE, Pierpoint T, Marmot MG 1993 Association of early-onset coronary heart disease in South Asian men with glucose intolerance and hyperinsulinemia. Circulation 87:152–161

Miller GJ, Kotecha S, Wilkinson WH et al 1988 Dietary and other characteristics relevant for coronary heart disease in men of Indian, West Indian and European descent in London. Atherosclerosis 70:63–72

Miller GJ, Beckles GLA, Maude GH et al 1989 Ethnicity and other characteristics predictive of coronary heart disease in a developing country: principal results of the St James survey, Trinidad. Int J Epidemiol 18:808–817

Morrison JA, Khoury P, Mellies M, Kelly K, Horvitz R, Glueck CJ 1981 Lipid and lipoprotein distributions in black adults. The Cincinnati Lipid Research Clinic's Princeton School Study. JAMA 245:939–942

Office of Population Censuses and Surveys 1990 Mortality and geography: a review in the mid-1980s. The Registrar-General's decennial supplement for England and Wales. HMSO, London

Omar MAK, Seedat MA, Dyer RB, Rajput MC, Motala AA, Joubert SM 1985 The prevalence of diabetes mellitus in a large group of South African Indians. S Afr Med J 67:924–926

Ramachandran A, Jali MV, Mohan V, Snehalatha C, Viswanathan M 1988 High prevalence of diabetes in an urban population in south India. Br Med J 297:587–590

Ramachandran A, Snehalatha C, Dharmaraj D, Viswanathan M 1992 Prevalence of glucose intolerance in Asian Indians: urban–rural difference and significance of upper-body adiposity. Diabetes Care 15:1348–1355

Reaven GM 1988 Role of insulin resistance in human disease. Diabetes 37:1595–1607

Sarvotham SG, Berry JN 1968 Prevalence of coronary heart disease in an urban population in northern India. Circulation 37:939–953

Slack J, Noble N, Meade TW, North WRS 1977 Lipid and lipoprotein concentrations in 1604 men and women in working populations in north-west London. Br Med J 2:353–356

Snehalatha C, Ramachandran A, Vijay V, Viswanathan M 1994 Differences in plasma insulin responses in urban and rural Indians: a study in southern Indians. Diabetic Med 11:445–448

Sorokin M 1975 Hospital morbidity in the Fiji islands with special reference to the saccharine disease. S Afr Med J 49:1481–1485

Steinberg W J, Balfe DL, Kustner HG 1988 Decline in the ischaemic heart disease mortality rates of South Africans 1968–1985. S Afr Med J 74:547–550

Tuomilehto J, Ram P, Eseroma R, Taylor R, Zimmet P 1984 Cardiovascular diseases in Fiji: analysis of mortality, morbidity and risk factors. Bull WHO 62:133–143

Yki-Jarvinen H, Taskinen M-R 1988 Interrelationships among insulin's antilipolytic and glucoregulatory effects and plasma triglycerides in nondiabetic and diabetic patients with endogenous hypertriglyceridemia. Diabetes 37:1271–1278

Zimmet P, Taft P, Guinea A, Guthrie W, Thoma K 1977 The high prevalence of diabetes on a Central Pacific island. Diabetologia 13:111–115

Zimmet P, Taylor R, Ram P et al 1983 Prevalence of diabetes and impaired glucose tolerance in the biracial (Melanesian and Indian) population of Fiji: a rural–urban comparison. Am J Epidemiol 118:673–688

DISCUSSION

Garrow: The object of the Vermont overfeeding experiment was to take young men without family or personal histories of either obesity or diabetes, overfeed them and see what happened to their insulin sensitivity (Sims et al 1973). The result was that it decreased, and furthermore, when the subjects lost weight it increased to its former level. This is the strongest evidence we have that an increase in fat mass causes insulin insensitivity, and that this is restorable on weight loss.

McKeigue: I agree, but the mechanism of the relationship between central obesity and insulin resistance is not known.

Bray: The Vermont study also examined the relationship between diet and insulin response, and showed that diet was an important factor in controlling the response to insulin. What corrections did you make in your study for the dietary differences between these groups of subjects?

McKeigue: We have no data on the diet of Afro-Caribbean people in the UK, but we have studied the diet of South Asians and Europeans in that cohort (Sevak et al 1994). We found that there weren't large differences in the percentage of energy obtained from fats and carbohydrates — the percentage of energy from fats is slightly lower in the South Asians and the ratio of polyunsaturates to saturates is slightly higher. There was no relationship between diet and plasma insulin levels, even when contrasting those in the top quartile for insulin levels with those in the bottom quartile.

Heitmann: To understand the mechanism between a high central obesity level and insulin levels, we may have to adopt the total body fat mass approach. For instance,

Lundgren et al (1989) showed that the prediction of the 12-year incidence of diabetes in middle-aged women using the BMI is much lower than when using the waist/hip circumference ratio (WHR). However, the incidence prediction was even greater when using the body fat mass. There was a threefold stronger prediction of total mortality from the body fat mass compared to that from the body mass index (BMI), and a twofold stronger prediction from the body fat mass compared to that from the WHR. This suggests that total fat deposits as well as central fat deposits are important.

McKeigue: We also have skinfold data on that cohort (McKeigue et al 1991, 1992). The skinfold measurements excluding those of the trunk are lower in South Asians than in Europeans. Therefore, the difference in WHR between the two groups may be a difference in fat distribution rather than in adiposity. Without direct measurements of body fat mass by underwater weighing it's difficult to be sure that there aren't some differences in adiposity between those groups. However, in that same data set, the cross-sectional relationship with diabetes is stronger for WHRs than for any combination of skinfold measurements.

Swinburn: I'm sure that there are differences in total adiposity, with Asians being fatter at any given BMI. A BMI of $25\,kg/m^2$ is probably overweight for a South Asian but normal for a European (Wang et al 1994).

York: The literature indicates that visceral fat is a health risk factor (Bouchard et al 1993). Is there any information regarding the relative distribution of central fat in these two different populations, as opposed to visceral and subcutaneous fat?

McKeigue: We have no data as yet using computed axial tomography scans, although we're trying to do such a study now. The skinfold data and measurements of the sagittal abdominal diameter in the supine position, which is a measurement of visceral fat, show the same pattern as the WHR measurements, i.e. markedly higher values in South Asians. The differences in trunk skinfolds are not as large as the differences in sagittal abdominal diameter.

Bouchard: I would be cautious here as with any prediction. You cannot predict the amount of visceral fat in a given individual from any anthropometric measurement. The standard error of estimating visceral fat from sagittal diameter or waist circumference is about $25\,cm^2$. If a group has an average visceral fat area of $100\,cm^2$, for example, then the 95% confidence interval values will range between 50 and $150\,cm^2$ (Després et al 1991). The prediction does not work well for a given individual, although it is better on a group basis.

Björntorp: Kvist et al (1988) have suggested that measurements of the volume of visceral fat, rather than the surface area, produces a stronger relationship.

I have another point and then a question. I was interested to see that the level of triglycerides during glucose tolerance was decreased by a lesser extent in subjects with visceral obesity. This might be due to the observation that the anti-lipolytic effect of insulin is smaller in visceral fat than in other fat depots.

The question is that the more we look at psychosocial and socioeconomic factors, the stronger the relationship seems to be between such factors and the WHR. Have you looked at this in the populations that you have studied?

McKeigue: We have not found any relationships between socioeconomic or psychosocial factors and central obesity in this data set. This may be because our measures are too insensitive.

Hitman: You showed that the insulin levels in Afro-Caribbeans was intermediate between those of Caucasians and South Asians. I would like to raise the concept of genetic admixture. It is possible that you have obtained these intermediate values because you have studied Afro-Caribbeans who have an admixture of Caucasian and African genes.

James: The issue of the genetic background of these populations, and the extent to which genetic analyses of the Afro-Caribbeans can effectively measure this admixture of genes was discussed at a joint British Medical Research Council/Caribbean Council for Medical Research conference in June/July this year in Jamaica: the conclusion was that there was a 25% admixture of Caucasian genes in the Afro-Caribbeans in the West Indies.

McFarlane-Anderson: We have estimated that the admixture in both Jamaica and Chicago is about 25% (Forrester et al 1996).

Bouchard: But it varies from about 10% to 50% in the USA, depending on geographical location and communities.

Hitman: We need to know more about the African data before we can discuss admixture effectively. Levitt et al (1993) showed that that there was a moderately high prevalence of diabetes in South Africa. Furthermore, studies of insulin action in Black Americans suggests two variants of non-insulin-dependent diabetes mellitus: one with normal insulin sensitivity and one with insulin resistance (Banerji & Lebovitz 1992).

Allison: Walker published some studies from Africa showing that among obese African women, there was relatively low incidence of sequelae such as diabetes in South Africa (Walker et al 1989, 1990, 1991). However, in terms of the admixture question, I don't know about in South Africa, but MacLean et al (1974) looked at admixture among Afro-Americans and the ponderal index, which is related to BMI. They failed to find a significant association, although they did find an association with blood pressure. We're trying to replicate some of those studies in our lab using the same measurements of admixture but with more sophisticated body composition techniques.

McKeigue: We have a large population of West African migrants in London and one or two other cities which have arrived more recently than the Caribbean migrants. There were about 50 West Africans in our survey, and their blood pressure and insulin levels did not differ significantly from those who migrated to the Caribbean (Chaturvedi et al 1993).

References

Banerji MA, Lebovitz HE 1992 Insulin action in Black Americans with NIDDM. Diabetes Care 15:1295–1302
Bouchard C, Després J-P, Mauriége P 1993 Genetic and non-genetic determinants of regional fat distribution. Endocr Rev 14:72–93

Chaturvedi N, McKeigue PM, Marmot MG 1993 Resting and ambulatory blood pressure differences in Afro-Caribbeans and Europeans. Hypertension 22:90–96

Després JP, Prud'homme D, Pouliot MC, Tremblay A, Bouchard C 1991 Estimation of deep abdominal adipose tissue accumulation from simple anthropometric measurements in men. Am J Clin Nutr 54:471–477

Forrester T, McFarlane-Anderson N, Bennett F et al 1996 Angiotensinogen and blood pressure among Blacks: findings from a community survey in Jamaica. J Hypertens 14:315–321

Kvist H, Chowdhury B, Grangärd U, Tylén U, Sjöström L 1988 Total and visceral adipose tissue volumes derived from measurements with computed tomography in adult men and women: predictive equations. Am J Clin Nutr 48:1351–1361

Levitt NS, Katzenellenbogen JM, Bradshaw D, Hoffman MN, Bonnici F 1993 The prevalence and identification of risk factors for NIDDM in urban Africans in Cape town, South Africa. Diabetes Care 16:601–607

Lundgren H, Bengtsson C, Blohme G, Lapidus L, Sjöström L 1989 Adiposity and adipose tissue distribution in relation to incidence of diabetes in women: results from a prospective population study in Gothenburg, Sweden. Int J Obes 13:413–423

MacLean CJ, Adams MS, Leyshon WC et al 1974 Genetic studies on hybrid populations. III. Blood pressure in an American Black community. Am J Hum Genet 26:614–626

McKeigue PM, Shah B, Marmot MG 1991 Relation of central obesity and insulin resistance with high diabetes prevalence and cardiovascular risk in South Asians. Lancet 337:382–386

McKeigue PM, Pierpoint T, Ferrie JE, Marmot MG 1992 Relationship of glucose intolerance and hyperinsulinaemia to body fat pattern in South Asians and Europeans. Diabetologia 35:785–791

Sevak L, McKeigue PM, Marmot MG 1994 Relation of hyperinsulinemia to dietary intake in South Asian and European men. Am J Clin Nutr 59:1069–1074

Sims EAH, Danforth E Jr, Horton ES, Bray GA, Glennon JA, Salans LB 1973 Endocrine and metabolic effects of experimental obesity in man. Rec Prog Horm Res 29:457–496

Walker ARP, Walker BF, Walker AJ, Vorster HH 1989 Low frequency of adverse sequelae of obesity in South African rural Black women. Int J Vitam Nutr Res 59:224–228

Walker ARP, Walker BF, Manetsi B, Tsotetsi NG, Walker AJ 1990 Obesity in Black women in Soweto, south Africa: minimal effects on hypertension, hyperlipidaemia and hyperglycaemia. J Royal Soc Health 110:101–103

Walker ARP, Walker BF, Manetsi B, Molefe O, Walker AJ, Vorster HH 1991 Obesity in indigent elderly rural African women: effects on hypertension, hyperlipidaemia and hyperglycaemia. Int J Vitam Nutr Res 61:244–250

Wang J, Thorton JC, Russell M, Burastero S, Heymsfield S, Pierson RN 1994 Asians have lower body mass index (BMI) but higher percent body fat than do whites: comparisons of anthropometric measurements. Am J Clin Nutr 60:23–28

Diabetes

Per Björntorp

Department of Heart and Lung Diseases, University of Göteborg, Sahlgren's Hospital, S-413 45 Göteborg, Sweden

Abstract. A relationship exists between obesity and non-insulin-dependent diabetes mellitus. Central, abdominal obesity carries a particularly high risk that is most likely associated with enlargement of visceral fat deposits. A multiple endocrine perturbation is associated with visceral obesity. This consists of a hypersensitive hypothalamic-pituitary-adrenal (HPA) axis, with resulting excess of cortisol secretion upon stimulation. Growth hormone levels in both sexes are diminished and testosterone concentrations in men are lower than normal. In women a moderate hyperandrogenism is often present. The elevated sensitivity of the HPA axis may be a primary event, followed by adrenal androgen production in women and by interaction at several levels, with inhibition of both the growth hormone and pituitary-gonadal axes. Together, these endocrine perturbations seem to be able to centralize body fat to visceral depots because of a high density of steroid hormone receptors. The endocrine perturbations are most likely followed by insulin resistance. Elevated cortisol levels, deficiencies in sex-specific steroid hormones and excess androgens result in insulin resistance. The endocrine abnormalities in visceral obesity are followed by insulin resistance, both directly and indirectly via contribution of excess free fatty acids from centralized body fat depots. The hyperactivity of the HPA axis may be due to frequent challenges and it is amplified by a deficient feedback inhibition. A depressive, helplessness reaction to stress may be involved. Such stress factors may be found in socioeconomic and psychosocial handicaps, as suggested by results of population studies. This hypothesis is strongly supported by the reproduction of an identical condition in non-human primates that react with a depressive reaction upon psychosocial types of stressors. The perturbations of the HPA axis may thus be in the centre of the syndrome. Studies of this axis in established non-insulin-dependent diabetes mellitus suggest similar perturbations, but the information is not conclusive.

1996 The origins and consequences of obesity. Wiley, Chichester (Ciba Foundation Symposium 201) p 68–89

The relationship between obesity and non-insulin-dependent diabetes mellitus (NIDDM) may now be considered established. The development of NIDDM is generally thought to be a combination of insulin resistance and an insufficiency of the β-cell function to produce compensatorily elevated insulin levels to overcome the peripheral insulin resistance. Although obesity may be associated with a weak β-cell function, it is mainly the insulin resistance that has been the focus of recent research.

Clinical and epidemiological studies of insulin resistance in central obesity

Recent studies have shown that obesity localized to central depots is more prone to develop insulin resistance than peripheral obesity (Kissebah & Krakower 1994, Björntorp 1993). The localization of the defect in central obesity at the tissue level has been studied in detail by Kissebah & Krakower (1994). These investigators have shown that muscular insulin sensitivity, as assessed by clamp measurements, is severely diminished, and that hepatic glucose output shows a diminished inhibitory response to insulin, particularly at submaximal insulin levels (but not to the extent that is seen in NIDDM). Hepatic clearance of insulin is also decreased. Therefore, combined deteriorations in peripheral insulin sensitivity, including insulin resistance of hepatic glucose production and leakage of insulin through the liver, have been demonstrated.

Central obesity in these studies is measured by the waist/hip circumference ratio (WHR). Epidemiological studies have shown that centralization of body fat is a more powerful predictor of NIDDM than obesity, which is defined conventionally using the body mass index (BMI) (Ohlsson et al 1985).

Later studies have focused more precisely on this problem. The WHR is a composite measurement: it does not just measure adipose tissue distribution. Measurements of visceral fat mass by computed tomography scans have shown that in Japanese-Americans visceral fat mass has a stronger predictive power for the development of NIDDM than other measured body fat compartments (Bergstrom et al 1990). Furthermore, the abdominal sagittal diameter, a close approximation of visceral fat mass (Kvist et al 1988), indicates the statistical strength of this adipose tissue depot to predict disease (Seidell et al 1994).

The unique statistical power of the WHR to predict the development of several prevalent diseases (Björntorp 1992a), including NIDDM (Ohlsson et al 1985), suggests that a component other than visceral fat may contribute to the observed associations. WHR is a rather poor measurement of visceral fat mass (Kvist et al 1988), particularly in lean subjects. A small hip circumference would also result in an elevated WHR. The hip circumference includes large muscle masses in the gluteal region, so it may be considered that the WHR contains information on the status of muscle tissue. Muscle tissue is a major determinant of peripheral insulin sensitivity (De Fronzo 1992), and may therefore contribute to the insulin resistance observed with an elevated WHR in both quantitative and qualitative terms. This should be studied in further detail.

Pathogenetic considerations

The statistical relationships between central obesity and either the WHR or the perturbations of the peripheral effects on insulin are striking in both cross-sectional, case-control studies, and population studies, where a high risk for the development of NIDDM has also been found.

The question then is how this statistical relationship may be explained.

A pathogenetic role of visceral adipose tissue?

In principle, the statistical findings may indicate a cause–effect relationship or that the associations are causally unrelated, so that visceral fat accumulation and insulin resistance are parallel phenomena that are both caused by a third factor. A cause–effect relationship has been suggested (Björntorp 1990), with free fatty acids (FFA) as the mediating trigger mechanism. Visceral fat has a rapid turnover and a high sensitivity for lipolytic stimuli. With excess visceral fat, portal FFA would then be expected to be elevated, particularly in situations when lipolysis is turned on, such as in starvation and stress. There are several known effects of FFA on the liver. First, gluconeogenesis seems to be driven by FFA, and may therefore show signs of insulin resistance. This might be amplified by the apparent insensitivity for the antilipolytic effect of insulin on visceral adipocytes. In other words, elevation of insulin secretion may have less inhibitory effects on lipolysis from visceral depots than from other depots, and therefore leave a higher concentration of FFA in the portal vein uninhibited. Furthermore, FFA seem to be the driving mechanism for hepatic synthesis and secretion of very low density lipoproteins. In addition, FFA inhibit insulin uptake in hepatocytes, and may contribute to the decreased hepatic clearance of insulin in the liver in visceral obesity. This would then contribute to peripheral hyperinsulinaemia (for review with detailed references, see Björntorp 1990). Furthermore, it cannot be excluded that portal FFA contribute to systemic FFA concentrations where enlarged visceral depots are at hand (Björntorp 1994).

Visceral adipose tissue may therefore contribute to: the creation of hepatic and muscular insulin resistance, via FFA in the portal vein; fasting hyperglycaemia, via poorly inhibited hepatic gluconeogenesis; hypertriglyceridaemia; and elevated peripheral insulin concentrations. These are most of the abnormalities seen as a cluster in syndrome X (Reaven 1988) or metabolic syndrome (Björntorp 1993).

Although this evidence seems compelling, the information is mainly obtained from studies in rats. Direct studies in humans are difficult and complicated because of the topographic anatomy of the portal vein. Recent indirect evidence, however, has strengthened the hypothesis that portal FFA trigger the above-mentioned abnormalities. By utilizing density measurements of the liver, which are indirect measurements of lipid contents, it has been shown that visceral fat mass and peripheral insulin resistance are related to hepatic triglyceride contents (Banerji et al 1995, Goto et al 1995). This seems to provide links between visceral fat mass, hepatic triglyceride contents and peripheral insulin resistance. The latter relationship has previously been observed in direct determinations of hepatic triglyceride contents (Kral et al 1977). A logical chain of events is that elevated levels of portal FFA in visceral obesity lead to hepatic triglyceride accumulation, with its presumed consequences as discussed above. However, this does not explain why the levels of visceral fat mass become elevated in visceral obesity: if anything, the elevated lipolytic sensitivity of visceral depots would lead to a diminution of visceral fat mass.

An alternative hypothesis is that a third factor is responsible for both visceral fat accumulation and insulin resistance. Recent evidence suggests that such a factor might be a multiple endocrine abnormality seen in visceral obesity. This consists of elevated cortisol and androgen (in women) secretions and diminished concentrations of growth hormone and sex-specific steroid hormones (for review, see Björntorp 1993).

Endocrine regulation of body fat distribution

It is well known that visceral fat accumulation follows an excess of cortisol in clinical conditions such as Cushing's syndrome. Furthermore, deficiency of both growth hormone and testosterone in ageing men, and oestrogen/progesterone in menopausal women, is paralleled by increased visceral fat masses, reversible partially or totally by appropriate replacement therapy (for review and detailed references, see Björntorp 1993). Cortisol in the presence of insulin seems to stimulate lipid-accumulating metabolic pathways, whereas the sex steroid hormones and growth hormones exert opposite effects, i.e. they inhibit lipid accumulation and stimulate lipid mobilization. These effects are more pronounced in adipose tissue regions that have a high density of steroid hormone receptors, where visceral adipocytes seem to occupy a leading position. Furthermore, because visceral adipose tissue seems to have a rich blood flow and a dense innervation, endocrine changes resulting in effects on adipose tissue metabolism would be more pronounced in visceral depots than in other fat depots (for review and detailed references, see Björntorp 1993).

Results of clinical, interventional, cellular and molecular studies are compatible with the interpretation that the endocrine perturbations associated with visceral obesity may direct storage fat preferentially to visceral fat depots. It is plausible that upon stimulation, these enlarged depots mobilize excess FFA which induce hepatic mechanisms that lead to metabolic perturbations.

Endocrine regulation of insulin sensitivity

The endocrine abnormalities trigger peripheral and hepatic insulin resistance. These are well-known effects of cortisol. Recent studies have shown that deficiencies of sex-specific steroid hormones, testosterone in men and oestrogen in women, may contribute to insulin resistance. Moderately hypogonadal men are insulin resistant, which is markedly improved by replacement with testosterone. Postmenopausal women are also frequently insulin resistant (for review, see Björntorp 1993). Intervention studies have resulted in marked improvements in the diabetic condition of insulin-resistant women who have NIDDM (B. Andersson, T. Ljung, L. Hahn, L. Å. Mattsson, P. Björntorp, unpublished results 1995). However, it does not necessarily follow that non-diabetic, insulin-resistant, menopausal, visceral obese women would react with an improved insulin sensitivity. This has not yet been tested. Furthermore, it is not clear whether the insulin resistance in non-diabetic, menopausal, visceral obese women is due primarily to hyperandrogenicity, a robust phenomenon in these women, or to oestrogen deficiency. Testosterone deficiency in male rats and oestrogen deficiency in female rats is followed by marked insulin resistance, which is reversible after adding testosterone and oestrogen, respectively. The mechanisms involved seem to be a combination of inhibitory effects on the translocation of glucose transporters and on glycogen synthase activity (Rincon et al 1996). Excess testosterone in both male and female rats is also followed by insulin resistance, and here, in addition to the mechanisms described above, the delivery of insulin through capillary transport appears to be diminished (for review, see Björntorp 1995).

The effects of growth hormone from this aspect are not entirely clear. Excess growth hormone is known to be followed by insulin resistance, and growth hormone is a diabetogenic hormone. On the other hand, growth hormone-deficient humans are also insulin resistant (Bengtsson et al 1993). The effects of physiological substitution with growth hormone, both in quantitative terms and as far as mode of administration are concerned, have currently not been carefully studied.

In summary, the endocrine perturbations of visceral obesity are most likely followed by insulin resistance. This presumption is based on clinical, interventional and experimental studies. It can, however, not be excluded that some of these effects are mediated secondarily via the release of FFA from visceral and/or peripheral depots, because cortisol has a permissive effect on lipolysis. This does, however, require a high level of growth hormone because without growth hormone, cortisol inhibits lipolysis (M. Ottosson, personal communication 1995). Growth hormone levels are low in individuals with visceral obesity (Bengtsson et al 1993).

Summary of peripheral effects of the endocrine perturbations in visceral obesity

As briefly reviewed above there is considerable evidence that the combined endocrine perturbations in visceral obesity — elevated levels of cortisol, androgens (women) and insulin, and low levels of sex-specific hormones and growth hormone — may at least contribute both to visceral fat accumulation and peripheral insulin resistance. It is therefore conceivable that the endocrine abnormalities may be diabetogenic via the induction of insulin resistance.

Origin of the endocrine perturbations

The multiple character of the endocrine perturbations suggests a central origin. The elevated cortisol secretion seems to stem from a hypersensitive hypothalamic-pituitary-adrenal (HPA) axis. Several laboratories have observed increased levels of adrenocorticotrophic hormone (ACTH), β-endorphin and/or cortisol when this axis is challenged at different levels. The administration of ACTH results in an elevated secretion of cortisol and, in women, an increased androgen concentration in the circulation (Mårin et al 1992, Pasquali et al 1993, Vague et al 1970). Corticotrophin-releasing hormone (CRH) or arginine vasopressin (AVP) induce the secretion of higher than normal levels of ACTH and cortisol (Pasquali et al 1993, 1996), and physical or mental laboratory stress tests result in elevated cortisol levels (Mårin et al 1992, Moyer et al 1994). This indicates a hyper-responsivity of the HPA axis upon stimulations at central regulatory sites of mental and physical stress, acting via hypothalamic centres, and at the levels of the pituitary and adrenals.

There is considerable evidence that this type of reaction is followed by inhibition of other pituitary/peripheral endocrine axes by CRH and/or cortisol (Chrousos & Gold 1992). An elevated response to challenge of the HPA axis would then be followed not only by increased secretions of adrenal hormones (cortisol and androgens), but also by an inhibition of the secretion of growth hormone and sex steroid hormone. It is therefore likely that the hypersensitivity of the HPA axis is a central perturbation not only for the endocrine abnormalities, but also for the peripheral regulation of body fat distribution and insulin sensitivity as reviewed above.

The regulation of the hypothalamic-pituitary-adrenal axis

The HPA axis is regulated by several rather complex mechanisms. There is evidence that even the most proximal parts of the regulatory chain, the stress centres, are hyper-reactive, so it would seem logical to examine the origin of the hypersensitivity of the HPA axis at this level. If the origin is to be found in central mechanisms, one would presumably find secondary consequences at more distal points of regulation. For example, hormonal receptors might be affected, and the endocrine glands might be hypertrophied as a consequence of being repeatedly overstimulated.

There is some evidence available along these lines. An important regulatory mechanism of the HPA axis is the feedback inhibition exerted by glucocorticoid receptors in the brain and pituitary (Sapolsky et al 1986). This can be tested by administration of exogenous glucocorticoids and measuring the resulting inhibition of cortisol secretion. By using smaller than conventional (1 mg) of dexamethasone we have recently been able to show a diminished inhibition of cortisol concentrations in the circulation (Ljung et al 1996), suggesting a down-regulation of central, regulatory glucocorticoid receptors. Recent experiments have revealed that the glucocorticoid receptors in adipose tissue show a deficient function, parallel to the glucocorticoid receptor effects in the CNS, regulating the HPA axis (M. Ottosson, unpublished observations 1995). This might be a primary, genetically determined abnormality, or a secondary consequence of over-secretion of cortisol, which by itself seems to down-regulate or even destroy central glucocorticoid receptors (Sapolsky et al 1986).

The diurnal concentration curves of ACTH and cortisol provide important information on the status of the HPA axis. During steady-state, non-stressed conditions the cortisol secretion pattern does not seem to be altered. The levels of ACTH are actually low, as are the levels of growth hormone (Ljung et al 1996). These results may be interpreted to mean that the secretion of CRH in the non-stressed, resting condition is actually low, producing lower than normal ACTH secretions. This assumption is supported by the observation of low CRH levels in the cerebrospinal fluid under non-stressed conditions (Strömbom et al 1996). The ability of lower than normal ACTH concentrations to uphold an unchanged cortisol secretion suggests a sensitive adrenal responsiveness to ACTH, either at the ACTH receptor level or simply by a hypertrophy of the gland. These suggestions are supported by the observations of an abnormally elevated cortisol secretion after challenge with ACTH (Mårin et al 1992, Pasquali et al 1993).

The data available may thus so far be interpreted to mean that at rest the ACTH levels are low, but there are signs of hyper-responsive adrenals. However, upon challenges proximal to the hypophysis, ACTH production becomes higher than normal. Activated and resting conditions of the HPA axis then seem different. This is a finding which seems to be in general agreement with animal data on conditions with a hypersensitive HPA axis after stress (Dallman 1993).

The currently available information at the level of the pituitary is very limited. Challenges with CRH and AVP have only been performed with maximal doses (Pasquali et al 1993, 1996). This tells little about the sensitivity of the CRH receptor in the pituitary, which may be down-regulated with diminished responses to submaximal levels of CRH. However, the increased responses to high levels of CRH and AVP suggest a high capacity of the CRH receptor to mediate secretory responses. The low levels of CRH in cerebrospinal fluid are uncertain, in terms of the levels at the actual active site of CRH in the appropriate central region, but would suggest that the CRH-secreting mechanisms are relatively inactive in the resting condition.

At present the data available seem, very tentatively, to be best interpreted in the following way. In the resting condition the HPA axis has a lower than normal activity at the pituitary level, and perhaps also at the level of the CRH secretory mechanisms. Upon challenges, however, the activity is abnormally elevated at both the pituitary and adrenal levels. This is caused or amplified by a down-regulation of central, inhibitory glucocorticoid receptors.

This rather speculative interpretation seems to be compatible with an origin of the HPA axis perturbations in the CNS. It seems possible that frequent, central, stimulatory signals to the HPA axis cause an elevated capacity and/or sensitivity of HPA responses at the pituitary and/or adrenal levels by down-regulation of central glucocorticoid receptors in combination with adrenal hypersensitivity and/or potential hypertrophy. In the resting state the axis would be expected to show lower than normal activity in humans, which is analogous to observations in the rat. This low activity is presumably found at the level of proximal CRH releasing mechanisms because the results suggest that the levels of ACTH and CRH are low in the resting state.

This should be seen in the light of the evidence of a hyper-responsiveness to standardized laboratory stress tests. The challenges from the stress centres in the brain might, at the current state of knowledge, be the primary factors that produce the observed adaptations of the HPA axis. This does not exclude primary regulatory faults of the HPA axis at the gene level; for example, those that influence the regulation of the axis via the glucocorticoid receptors or the ACTH and CRH receptors.

Central mechanisms

The secretion of CRH is regulated by a complex system in the brain. Both serotonin and adrenergic receptors are involved (McEwen et al 1993). The serotonergic neurons seem at present to be of particular interest for a number of reasons. The HPA axis abnormalities (McEwen et al 1993) and several other characteristics of subjects with visceral obesity suggest serotonergic involvements. Traits of depression and anxiety have been observed in both women and men (Lapidus et al 1989, Rosmond et al 1996a). Recent data suggest surprisingly strong relationships between somatic variables such as the WHR and fasting insulin with Beck's depression scale as well as equally detailed measurements of anxiety from questionnaires. These data have been obtained from men selected from WHR measurements without obvious symptoms of clinical psychiatric disease (Ljung et al 1996). Interestingly, depression as well as anxiety conditions are characterized not only by a hyperactive HPA axis (Carrol 1982, Graeff 1993), but also by a pathological serotonin metabolism and binding in the brain in studies employing positron emission tomography scans (Ågren et al 1993). Furthermore, drugs blocking serotonin re-uptake, elevating serotonin in the serotonin receptor clefts, have proven very efficient in the treatment of these conditions.

Obese subjects, in general, have lower than normal 5-hydroxyindolacetic acid (5-HIAA) levels in their cerebrospinal fluid (Strömbom et al 1996). A large body of animal data from several species have demonstrated that low serotonin levels are followed by increased food ingestion (for review, see Fuller et al 1992). Furthermore, serotonin agonists and re-uptake inhibitors are effective in humans (for review, see Blundell & Hill 1987). This is therefore an additional piece of evidence suggesting involvement of the serotonergic nervous system in visceral obesity. Of particular interest is the finding of a correlation between 5-HIAA and CRH in the cerebrospinal fluid of visceral obese subjects, suggesting a tight coupling between the serotonergic system and the HPA axis (Strömbom et al 1996). Furthermore, carbohydrate craving, a specific symptom of central serotonin deficiency (Conn & Sanders-Bush 1987), was found to be inversely related to 5-HIAA concentrations only in visceral obese subjects (Strömbom et al 1996).

Alcohol intake and smoking are followed by activation of the HPA axis, probably due to central mechanisms, at least partly mediated via serotonergic neurons (Eriksson & Humble 1990). There are several reports indicating that smoking and a high intake of alcohol are followed by visceral fat distribution (for review, see Kissebah & Krakower 1994).

In summary, psychiatric traits, carbohydrate craving, associations between serotonergic neurons or serotonin metabolites in the cerebrospinal fluid with the HPA axis activity, alcohol consumption and smoking are all characteristics of visceral obese subjects and, therefore, strongly suggest the involvement of the serotonergic nervous system in this condition.

Psychological aspects

It seems possible that psychological factors might provide a background to the phenomena reported above. Reactions to stress may be followed by either a fight-or-flight reaction, stimulating mainly the catecholaminergic system, or a depressive, defeatist, helplessness type of response. The latter is characterized endocrinologically by a hyperactivity of the HPA axis as well as decreased sex steroid hormone secretions. Furthermore, depressive and anxiety reactions are also associated (Henry & Stephens 1977). It does not seem far-fetched to consider that the use of stimulants, such as alcohol and tobacco, would be a consequence of such a reaction. Therefore, a depressive reaction to stress would be an interesting background candidate for the pathogenesis of the syndrome of visceral obesity. The sensitization to standardized stress tests (Mårin et al 1992, Moyer et al 1994) might be considered as another piece of evidence in this direction.

There are several environmental factors in modern society that expose individuals to stress reactions. The response may vary, depending on coping abilities, and result in a depressive, helplessness reaction in susceptible individuals. We have searched for such factors in several studies based on randomly selected middle-aged populations. The independent variables in these studies are the BMI and the WHR, which have been adjusted to analyse the associations with various socioeconomic and psychosocial factors.

Various socioeconomic factors in men — a low education, physical type of work, a low social class, being out of work and problems at work — have been found to be associated with the WHR, independent of the BMI, alcohol and smoking. Interestingly, the BMI shows no such relationships (Larsson et al 1989, Rosmond et al 1996b). There is a different picture for women (Lapidus et al 1989), probably as a result of examining subjects born in the early 20th century when there were marked differences in the working conditions between men and women. This is currently being re-examined in a cohort of women born in the 1940s.

Psychosocial factors have been similarly examined. In men there were strikingly strong relationships between the WHR and living alone or being divorced. Furthermore, men with an elevated WHR had few leisure activities except for watching television (Rosmond et al 1996b). These relationships were again independent of BMI, alcohol and smoking, and suggest that a poor psychosocial environment may be associated with a central distribution of body fat. Interestingly, BMI, adjusted for WHR, alcohol and smoking was associated with living with a partner (except in the most obese quintile), and a more favourable psychosocial adaptation, in other words a totally different picture (Rosmond et al 1996b). The data in women are less complete, but again suggest that differences exist between the sexes. Women with elevated WHR (adjusted for BMI) have characteristics suggesting executive type of personalities, in combination with hyperandrogenicity as well as smoking and alcohol habits (Lapidus et al 1989). It seems highly likely that the WHR or visceral obesity are associated with different socioeconomic, psychosocial and personality characteristics in men and women. This is currently being investigated.

In summary, the above observations suggest that men with centralized body fat stores, even without obesity, are related to poor socioeconomic and psychosocial conditions. Depressive and anxiety traits, as well as alcohol and smoking, are statistical associates both in men and women. We have therefore speculated (Björntorp 1988a,b, 1992b, 1993) that such factors may be of importance for the induction of a stress reaction of a depressive, helplessness type, with activation of the HPA axis and its somatic consequences.

This hypothesis is strongly supported by recent work in non-human primates. Upon experimental change of social hierarchy, monkeys who cannot defend a high rank position develop a depressive stress reaction. This mild experimental intervention is reminiscent of humans striving to climb the socioeconomic ladder, where many meet a failure. The failing monkeys develop enlarged adrenals, a hyperactive HPA axis with a mild defect in the glucocorticoid receptor brake, amenorrhea, visceral fat accumulation, insulin resistance, elevated blood pressure and plasma lipids as well as coronary atherosclerosis and impaired glucose tolerance (Shively et al 1987, Jayo et al 1993). The similarity with the human syndrome of visceral obesity is quite striking; in fact, in all variables measured in parallel, the conditions are identical. This lends strong support to our suggestion that psychosocial and socioeconomic stress factors, leading to a depressive reaction, perhaps amplified by associated alcohol and smoking habits, may in fact be primary factors in the pathogenesis of the syndrome of visceral obesity (Björntorp 1988a,b, 1992b, 1993).

The hypothalamic-pituitary-adrenal axis in established non-insulin-dependent diabetes mellitus

The above attempts to synthetize accumulated evidence suggest that the activity of the HPA axis may be a critical factor in the development of visceral obesity and insulin resistance, the two most powerful predictors of NIDDM currently known. If this were correct, one would suspect to find abnormalities in the HPA axis in established NIDDM. There are a number of such reports (Hudson et al 1984, Cameron et al 1987, Vermes et al 1985, Tsigos et al 1993, Surwit & Feinglos 1983, Surwit et al 1986), suggesting that this is indeed the case. However, several of these studies suffer from not dividing insulin-dependent diabetes mellitus and NIDDM, not controlling for the perturbed glucose homeostasis or analysing only single hormone tests. A few studies suggest, however, that the activity of the HPA axis is indeed elevated, either by measurements of cortisol output, diurnal hormone curves or dexamethasone inhibition tests (Hudson et al 1984, Cameron et al 1987, Vermes et al 1985). The difficulties encountered by the abnormal glucose homeostasis in established

NIDDM, which may secondarily cause endocrine perturbations, indicate that the information from the prediabetic condition of visceral obesity is more valuable.

References

Ågren H, Reibring L, Hartvig P et al 1993 Monoamine metabolism in human prefrontal cortex and basal ganglia. PET studies using [β-^{11}C]1-5-hydroxytryptophan and [β-^{11}C]L-DOPA in healthy volunteers and patients with unipolar major depression. Depression 1:71–81

Banerji MA, Buckley C, Chaiken RL, Gordon D, Lebovitz HE, Kral JG 1995 Liver fat, serum triglycerides and visceral adipose tissue in insulin-sensitive and insulin-resistant Black men with NIDDM. Int J Obes 19:846–850

Bengtsson B-Å, Edén S, Lönn L et al 1993 Treatment of adults with growth hormone (GH) deficiency with recombinant human GH. J Clin Endocrinol Metab 76:309–317

Bergstrom RW, Newell-Morris LL, Leonetti DL, Shuman WP, Wahl PW, Fujimoto WY 1990 Association of elevated fasting C-peptide level and increased intra-abdominal fat distribution with the development of NIDDM in Japanese–American men. Diabetes 39:104–111

Björntorp P 1988a Abdominal obesity and the development of noninsulin dependent diabetes mellitus. Diabetes Metab Rev 4:615–622

Björntorp P 1988b Possible mechanisms relating fat distribution and metabolism. In: Bouchard C, Johnston F (eds) Fat distribution during growth and later health outcomes. Alan R Liss, New York, p 175–191

Björntorp P 1990 'Portal' adipose tissue as a generator of risk factors for cardiovascular disease and diabetes. Arteriosclerosis 10:493–496

Björntorp P 1991 Adipose tissue distribution and function. Int J Obes 15:67–81

Björntorp P 1992a Abdominal fat distribution and disease: an overview of epidemiological data. Ann Med 24:15–18

Björntorp P 1992b Psychosocial factors and fat distribution. In: Ailhaud G, Guy-Grand B, Lafontan M, Ricquier D (eds) Obesity in Europe 91. John Libbey, London, p 377-387

Björntorp P 1993 Visceral obesity: a 'civilization syndrome'. Obesity Res 1:206–222

Björntorp P 1994 Fatty acids, hyperinsulinemia, and insulin resistance: which comes first? Curr Opin Lipidol 5:166–174

Björntorp P 1995 Insulin resistance: the consequence of a neuroendocrine disturbance? Int J Obes (suppl 1) 19:6S–10S

Blundell JE, Hill AJ 1987 Serotonergic modulation of the pattern of eating and the profile of hunger-satiety in humans. Int J Obes (suppl 3) 11:141S–155S

Cameron OG, Thomas B, Tiongco D, Hariharan M, Gaeden JF 1987 Hypercortisolism in diabetes mellitus. Diabetes Care 10:662–663

Carrol BJ 1982 The dexamethasone suppression test for melancholia. Br J Psychiatry 140:292–304

Chrousos G, Gold P 1992 The concept of stress and stress system disorders. JAMA 267:1244–1252

Conn PJ, Sanders-Bush E 1987 Central serotonin receptors effector systems, physiological roles and regulation. Psychopharmacol 92:267–277

Dallman MF 1993 Stress update: adaptation of the hypothalamic-pituitary-adrenal axis to chronic stress. Trends Endocrinol Metab 4:62–69

De Fronzo RA 1992 Pathogenesis of type 2 (non-insulin dependent) diabetes mellitus: a balanced overview. Diabetologia 35:389–397

Eriksson E, Humble M 1990 Serotonin in psychiatric pathophysiology. In: Pohl R, Gershon S (eds) Progress in basic and clinical pharmacology series, vol 3: Biological basis of psychiatric treatment. Karger, Basel, p 66–119

Fuller RW 1992 The involvement of serotonin in regulation of pituitary–adrenal function. Front Neuroendocrinol 13:250–270

Goto T, Onuma T, Takebe K, Kral JG 1995 The influence of fatty liver on insulin clearance and insulin resistance in non-diabetic Japanese subjects. Int J Obes 19:841–845

Graeff FG 1993 Role of 5-HT in defensive behavior and anxiety. Rev Neurosci 4:181–211

Henry JP, Stephens PM 1977 Stress, health, and the social environment. A sociobiological approach to medicine. Springfield, New York

Hudson JL, Hudson MG, Rotschild AJ, Vignati L, Schatzberg AF, Melby JC 1984 Abnormal results of dexamethasone suppression tests in non-depressed patients with diabetes mellitus. Arch Gen Psychiatry 41:1086–1089

Jayo JM, Shively CA, Kaplan JR, Manuck SB 1993 Effects of exercise and stress on body fat distribution in male Cynomolgus monkeys. Int J Obes 17:597–604

Kissebah AH, Krakower GR 1994 Regional adiposity and morbidity. Physiol Rev 74:761–811

Kral JG, Lundholm K, Sjöström L, Björntorp P, Scherstén T 1977 Hepatic lipid metabolism in severe human obesity. Metabolism 26:1025–1031

Kvist H, Chowdhury B, Grangård U, Tylén U, Sjöström L 1988 Total and visceral adipose tissue volumes derived from measurements with computed tomography in adult men and women: predictive equations. Am J Clin Nutr 48:1351–1361

Lapidus L, Bengtsson C, Hällström T, Björntorp P 1989 Obesity, adipose tissue distribution and health in women. Results from a population study in Gothenburg, Sweden. Appetite 12:25–35

Larsson B, Seidell J, Svärdsudd K et al 1989 Obesity, adipose tissue distribution and health in men. The study of men born in 1913. Appetite 13:37–44

Ljung T, Andersson B, Björntorp P, Mårin P 1996 Inhibition of cortisol secretion by dexamethasone in relation to body fat distribution, a dose-response study. Obesity Res 4:277–282

Mårin P, Darin N, Amemeiya T, Andersson B, Jern S, Björntorp P 1992 Cortisol secretion in relation to body fat distribution in obese premenopausal women. Metabolism 41:882–886

Mårin P, Kvist H, Lindstedt G, Sjöström L, Björntorp P 1993 Low concentrations of insulin-like growth factor-l in abdominal obesity. Int J Obes 17:83–89

McEwen BS, Cameron H, Chao HM et al 1993 Adrenal steroids and plasticity of hippocampal neurons: toward an understanding of underlying cellular and molecular mechanisms. Cell Mol Neurobiol 13:457–482

Moyer AE, Rodin J, Grilo CH, Cummings N, Larsson LM, Rebuffé-Scrive M 1994 Stress-induced cortisol response and fat distribution in women. Obesity Res 2:255–262

Ohlsson L, Larsson B, Svärdsudd K et al 1985 The influence of body fat distribution on the incidence of diabetes mellitus. Diabetes 34:1055–1058

Pasquali R, Cantobelli S, Casimirri F et al 1993 The hypothalamic-pituitary-adrenal axis in obese women with different patterns of body fat distribution. J Clin Endocrinol Metab 77:341–346

Pasquali R, Anconetani B, Chattat R et al 1996 The hypothalamic-pituitary-adrenal axis activity and its relationship to the autonomic nervous system in women with visceral and subcutaneous obesity. Effects of the corticotropin-releasing factor arginine vasopressin test and of stress. Metabolism 45:351–356

Reaven GH 1988 Role of insulin resistance in human disease. Diabetes 37:1595–1607

Rincon J, Holmäng A, Wahlström EO et al 1995 Mechanisms behind insulin resistance in rat skeletal muscle following oophorectomy and additional testosterone treatment. Diabetes 45:615–621

Rosmond R, Lapidus L, Mårin P, Björntorp P 1996a Mental distress, obesity and body fat distribution in middle-aged men. Obesity Res 4:245–252

Rosmond R, Lapidus L, Björntorp P 1996b The influence of occupational and social factors on obesity and body fat distribution in middle-aged men. Int J Obes 20:599–607

Sapolsky RM, Krey LC, McEwen BS 1986 The neuroendocrinology of stress and aging: the glucocorticoid cascade hypothesis. Endocr Rev 7:289–301

Seidell JC, Andres R, Sorkin JD, Muller DC 1994 The sagittal waist diameter and mortality in men: the Baltimore Longitudinal Study on Aging. Int J Obes 18:61–67

Shively C, Clarkson FB, Miller C, Weingand KW 1987 Body fat distribution as a risk factor for coronary artery atherosclerosis in female Cynomolgus monkeys. Arteriosclerosis 7:226–231

Strömbom U, Krotkiewski K, Blennow K, Mansson JE, Ekman R, Björntorp P 1996 The concentrations of monoamine metabolites and neuropeptides in the cerebrospinal fluid of obese women with different body fat distribution. Int J Obes 20:361–368

Surwit RS, Feinglos NM 1983 The effect of relaxation on glucose tolerance in non-insulin dependent diabetes mellitus. Diabetes Care 7:203–204

Surwit RS, McCubbin JA, Kuhn JA, McGee CM, Gerstenfeld D, Feinglos MN 1986 Alprazolam reduces stress hyperglycemia in ob/ob mice. Psychosom Med 48:278–282

Tsigos C, Young RJ, White A 1993 Diabetic neuropathy is associated with increased activity of the hypothalamic-pituitary-adrenal axis. J Clin Endocrinol Metab 76:554–558

Vague J, Vague P, Boyer J, Cloix M 1970 Anthropometry of obesity, diabetes, adrenal, and beta-cell functions. In: Rodriques RR, Vallance-Owen J (eds) Diabetes. Excerpta Medica, Amsterdam, p 517–525

Vermes J, Steinmetz E, Schooal J, Van der Ween EA, Tilders FJH 1985 Increased levels of immunoreactive β-endorphin and corticotropin in noninsulin dependent diabetes mellitus. Lancet II:725–726

DISCUSSION

Astrup: Corticotrophin-releasing factor (CRF) stimulates sympathetic nervous system activity. You showed that CRF could be a mediator of some of the abnormalities in the periphery, such as insulin resistance. What is the current status on that?

Björntorp: The sympathetic nervous system axis and the cortisol axis are closely connected, so it's difficult to stimulate one without stimulating the other. We haven't yet looked at the sympathetic nervous system in detail, but we have observed that men with elevated waist/hip circumference ratios (WHRs) have a different haemodynamic reaction to stress. Men with high WHRs have more peripheral resistance than normal men, who respond with an elevated heart rate and less peripheral resistance (Jern et al 1992).

Garrow: The Vermont experimental overfeeding study was done 30 years ago on 19 young men (Sims et al 1973), so it's high time that we do another one to find out whether the changes in hormonal sensitivity come before or after the deposition of adipose tissue.

Bouchard: We have repeated the Vermont overfeeding study with 24 subjects (Bouchard et al 1990) and looked at almost all the variables that Per Björntorp has discussed. We found similar correlations between abdominal visceral fat and total fat mass gain, but they were only low level correlations. However, in our study, the surplus of energy was clamped, so that everyone was overfed by the same amount (1000 kcal/day). Perhaps this was a critical factor. The results were certainly different from the Vermont overfeeding study.

Shetty: Keys et al (1950) have done re-feeding studies. When they re-fed semi-starved subjects, they were able to show that those who received the largest amount of energy had the largest increase both in fat gain and in waist circumference.

Björntorp: But it is necessary to separate people with central and peripheral obesity.

York: Have there been any studies where people with central obesity have been starved to see if the overactivity of the hypothalamic-pituitary-adrenal (HPA) axis is retained?

Björntorp: No. At first sight this seems to be the obvious logical control experiment to do, but I'm not sure that this is meaningful because the sympathetic system of many reduced subjects is affected as if they were starving, so this would not represent a good control.

Bray: There are difficulties in measuring the activity of the sympathetic nervous system. We used the R–R interval variability in the electrocardiogram to measure sympathetic activity in a group of subjects with timed respiration. We found that there was an increase in sympathetic activity using spectral analysis with upper central obesities, that is subjects with high WHRs and increased visceral fat. Therefore, a component of that sympathetic nervous system may play a role in the development of central obesity.

Ravussin: A few recent studies have shown a striking positive relationship between obesity and the activity of the sympathetic nervous system. When direct measurements of sympathetic nervous system activity are performed by microneurography, one finds that muscle sympathetic nerve activity is directly correlated with per cent body fat (Spraul et al 1993, Jones et al 1996, Scherrer et al 1994). Furthermore, we found that the higher level of sympathetic nervous system activity in males is mostly due to a more central distribution of body fat (Jones et al 1996). There is now, therefore, increasing evidence that obesity is associated with higher and not lower sympathetic nervous system activity.

Astrup: Jones et al (1996) have shown that the activity of the sympathetic nervous system, measured by direct nerve recordings, increases with increasing abdominal obesity in males. In contrast, females have lower levels of activity with increasing body fat.

James: That raises the issue of cause and effect. We've been implying that as the abdominal fat increases, the sympathetic nervous system activity increases, but we are always talking about cross-sectional analyses rather than data before and after weight change.

Björntorp: I would like to take the opportunity to ask Arne Astrup what is the current situation on the measurements of energy expenditure in upper- and lower-body obesity?

Astrup: The situation is confusing at the moment. It seems that subjects with upper-body obesity have a slightly higher resting metabolic rate after differences in fat-free mass and total fat mass have been taken into account. The higher metabolic rate could be the result of a higher level of sympathetic nervous system activity.

McKeigue: There are many clamp studies which show that euglycaemic insulin infusions cause an increase in muscle sympathetic nerve activity, measured by microelectrode recordings (Anderson et al 1992, Berne et al 1992). This appears to be a direct effect of insulin on the CNS, independent of hyperglycaemia. As far as we know, the function of that is to counteract the insulin-mediated vasodilation that would otherwise result in hypotension.

A Finnish group have published a paper showing that people with central obesity have a much larger decrease in cortisol levels after a glucose load than people without central obesity (Hautanen & Adlercreutz 1993). They suggested that the direction of causation could be the other way round, i.e. that in people with central adiposity the central fat is full of cortisol receptors which use up the cortisol more quickly. Therefore, the whole HPA axis is switched towards being overactive because it has to maintain the levels of cortisol.

Björntorp: It is not known which starts first. In my opinion, it is more likely that the overactivity of the HPA axis is the primary event, and we have evidence to support this (Björntorp 1993).

Stunkard: The field of psychiatry has been interested for a long time in stress, and more recently in CRF. A factor that inhibits CRF has just been discovered, and it may be possible to use it to help sort these problems out (Redei et al 1995). Blocking the activity of CRF with this inhibitory factor may allow us to intervene between the stressor and the target organ.

Björntorp: That's a nice idea. There are, however, difficulties with inhibiting the HPA axis. At present we are trying to do this in different ways.

Hitman: You mentioned that one explanation for your findings could be that glucocorticoid receptor activity is lower than normal. Familial glucocorticoid deficiency is due to at least four different mutations of the glucocorticoid receptor gene, and it is associated with hypertension. Do you know of any data on the levels of visceral fat in this syndrome? One may expect it to be increased.

Björntorp: No, I haven't thought of that.

Bouchard: We have studied one of the glucocorticoid receptor gene mutations. We found that there was a significant relationship between the mutation and amount of visceral fat, but only in individuals of normal weight. When people were obese, the effect of the polymorphism seemed to be overridden (Buemann et al 1996). The mutation lies outside the promoter region and it is not in the exons.

Björntorp: I hope I didn't imply that this is necessarily a genetic effect.

James: You have implied that sustained stress entrains a CRF process, which leads to a sequence of changes resulting in visceral fat accumulation, and this accumulation then causes a series of secondary effects. I'm not quite clear where the concordant peripheral glucocorticoid receptor changes lie in that pathway. How does this relate to the central fattening process?

Björntorp: There is a balance between cortisol production and receptor density. In Cushing's syndrome there is a high level of cortisol and the glucocorticoid receptors are down-regulated, but there are still elevated glucocorticoid effects on the periphery. I imagine that the situation is the same in visceral obesity but not so dramatic.

James: So you don't necessarily believe that this is a familial condition with a particular predisposition to deposit visceral fat, but that there may be a familial condition of extreme stress in families which leads to that?

Björntorp: The genes could act at any level above or from the glucocorticoid receptor to peripheral tissues.

Campfield: One recent advance has been the identification of leptin (the *Ob* protein) and the demonstration of its interesting biological activity (Campfield et al 1996, Halaas et al 1995, Pellymounter et al 1995, Rentsch et al 1995, Stephens et al 1995, Weigle et al 1995). Have you looked for leptin mRNA in the adipose tissues of those with upper-body obesity?

Björntorp: No I haven't. As far as I understand it, leptin is involved with obesity, defined as elevated total fat mass, and visceral fat distribution is probably regulated differently.

Campfield: We don't know this. We know that obese people as a group have high levels of leptin. We don't know whether there are differences in the amount of leptin between the upper and lower body.

Hitman: There's some literature demonstrating that there's an increased expression of leptin in visceral fat, as against subcutaneous fat, so the expression of *Ob* in these tissues may be differentially regulated.

Campfield: Yes. But what I'm asking is what do *in vitro* manipulations of explanted tissue do to the levels of leptin mRNA? Of course the measurements of leptin mRNA may be uninformative and we may need to look for differences in the levels of leptin.

Ravussin: In collaboration with J. M. Friedman's lab, we found that plasma leptin levels are tightly correlated with per cent body fat in more than 45 subjects including Caucasians and Pima Indians ($r = 0.86$, Maffei et al 1995). Because of this tight correlation, one can propose, perhaps facetiously, that it is possible to measure body fat in people just by measuring plasma leptin levels. The strong correlation between obesity and plasma leptin levels has been recently confirmed by Considine et al (1996).

Campfield: But in the scattergram there are a few interesting people who have a high BMI and a low level of leptin, and vice versa. Leptin levels increase linearly and then reach a plateau, which I believe has been described by Friedmann's group (Maffei et al 1995) as well as Jose Caro's group (Considine et al 1996).

I'm also concerned that we are attributing the reason for increased visceral fat only to stress. The HPA axis can be overactive for a variety of reasons. There may be a predisposition to have a higher or lower activity in this system in response to different perturbations of the whole system. We shouldn't necessarily imply that everybody that has increased visceral fat is under some kind of psychological stress.

Björntorp: Stress is one factor, but I agree that other factors are probably involved. For example, we have recently looked in more detail at the tendency towards depression in relation to WHR and HPA axis measurements, and there are surprisingly strong positive correlations. Alcohol, smoking and anxiety are also involved and there are most likely other background factors.

Hitman: We're talking about an interaction between genetic susceptibility and the environment. There is a strong environmental component, but it is possible that a disease-associated mutation in the glucocorticoid receptor might exist, which, in the face of stress, causes the overactivity of the HPA axis and hence obesity.

Bouchard: I agree that stress could be a factor and that other factors are also involved. In our overfeeding study, we observed an increase in visceral fat following overfeeding. Even though there was six times more variance for the visceral fat increase between pairs of identical twins than within pairs, members of the same pair were not perfectly similar in response (Bouchard et al 1990). One could argue that those who gained more visceral fat were more stressed by the overfeeding. However, this is unlikely. We certainly did not see any evidence for this in their behaviour.

Hitman: There could be a genetic variant that is common in the population, which in the absence of the required environmental factor would not lead to excess visceral fat deposition.

Shaper: Could visceral fat be deposited without the gene variant?

Hitman: It depends to what extent. If a gene variant is present in 15% of the population, for example, then it is possible that everyone deposits visceral fat if they have the gene variant plus exposure to the environmental factor. On the other hand, there may be a variant that protects against the deposition of visceral fat in the face of other environmental factors. Lastly, there may be some cases in which the excess deposition of visceral fat is entirely environmentally or genetically determined; but I would predict this would not be the common cause.

York: I would like to return to the cause–effect relationship and draw peoples' attention to some relevant studies in animals, which may or may not be reasonable models for humans. However, most of these results suggest that the increase in the activity of the HPA axis occurs later on in these animal syndromes and that it is probably secondary to the development of obesity. For example, in obese Zucker rats exposed to stress the increased activity of the HPA axis is evident by the high secretion of corticosterone. In addition, there is a change in the diurnal rhythm of glucocorticoid secretion, which occurs fairly late in the development of the syndrome when obesity is fairly well pronounced. The rat studies also show that obesity is not dependent on the levels of glucocorticoids. It may not be appropriate to look only at abnormalities of the glucocorticoid receptors because there is now evidence from studies of the obese rat that the glucocorticoid receptor protein accumulates in the nucleus (Jenson et al 1996). This is probably not due to a defect in the receptor protein itself, but there may be an abnormality in the regulation of the receptor recycling system that will not be picked up by a genetic analysis of the glucocorticoid receptor.

Björntorp: In non-obese Sprague–Dawley rats subjected to stress, fat accumulates in the mesenteric region (Rebuffé-Scrive et al 1992), so these observations are not just confined to obese rats. In addition, studies in non-human primates show that psychosocial stress is followed by identical changes, not only in the accumulation of visceral fat, but also in the endocrine and metabolic perturbations we see in our subjects with visceral fat accumulation. This is strong evidence that stress is involved (Jayo et al 1993). I have been told that the Zucker rat is stress sensitive, what is the distribution of fat in these rats?

York: Fat is distributed everywhere. Brindley et al (1981) showed that rats fed on a high fat diet have an increased level of HPA activity in response to stress, which may be relevant to human obesity.

James: This HPA effect was not observed when they were overfed with carbohydrate.

Blundell: Are we talking about responsivity to stress involving a greater intrinsic sensitivity, or a greater preponderance of stress in the environment applied to the individual? In the experiments with monkeys, you placed an alpha male lower down in the hierarchy. These are probably normal animals without any strong internal anxiety. The stress is applied from the outside and the monkeys respond with all the characteristics of the visceral fat syndrome. It would be useful to clarify for human obesity whether or not we're talking about individuals with visceral obesity who have a high intrinsic anxiety or who experience a greater preponderance of life stressor events. There are two models: (1) the chronic burden, i.e. that such people simply do have more stressful events in their lives; or (2) the critical threshold, i.e. that they are exposed to only one or two extremely stressful events that produce dramatic effects. Obese people do report that they experience a high level of uncomfortable life events (hassles) that cause them anxiety. Therefore, it would be useful to differentiate between the potency of the externally applied stressor and the sensitivity of the internal physiological system which mediates anxiety.

Björntorp: Yes, this is important. We are now taking advice on how to ask obese persons questions about the stress that they experience (in other words, perceived stress), and we are also trying to map personality types.

Ferro-Luzzi: Stress may be important as a risk factor for obesity, but I am intrigued by the fact that many people are seemingly under a lot of stress but do not become obese. Why is this?

Björntorp: It is possible that such people can cope efficiently with the environment.

Stunkard: We have been talking mostly about the response to stress. It's worth bearing in mind the efforts to quantify stressors, such as those by Sarason et al (1978).

Björntorp: Two of the strongest factors associated with WHRs in men are living alone and divorce. Twenty per cent of the men in the first WHR quintile are divorced and this figure increases to 40% in the fifth quintile (Rosmond et al 1996).

Campfield: The effect of various anti-depressant medications on people has been studied. Some people eat more when they are stressed, and some people eat less. Studies with tricyclic anti-depressants turn out to be a mixed bag — some people increase food intake on medication, whereas others decrease their food intake. One has to ask how does one use food to deal with stress, and how does stress lead to changes in feeding behaviour? There will not be a uniform response among all people who accumulate visceral fat. An individual's history of stress effects on food intake, drug response or feeding responses to intervention may allow us to design an interesting study.

McKeigue: The epidemiology of the central obesity and insulin resistance syndrome in South Asians is not explained by psychosocial factors. There is an absence of any class gradient among any of the metabolic variables that we've looked at in the South Asian populations (McKeigue et al 1989). This isn't only seen in recent migrants. The South Asian population in the UK are mostly first-generation migrants who have only been in the UK since the 1960s, but other overseas South Asian populations (in Trinidad, Fiji, South Africa and Singapore) have settled in those areas since the mid-nineteenth century. I cannot construct any psychosocial explanation that encompasses such different populations in such different environments.

Shetty: But even rural to urban migration within a country is a major stress event. For instance when the Punjabis migrated into urban regions, they must have been subjected to enormous stress.

Björntorp: You cannot come up with a socioeconomic explanation of your results, but have you looked at perceived stress? I would also intuitively think that the active factors most likely vary in different populations.

James: In other words, stress may involve one's perception of how one can cope with change, so how can you be confident that this is not involved in your study?

McKeigue: We asked questions based on Karasek's questionnaire, which measures job demands and job stress (Karasek et al 1981), and the responses were not related to central adiposity. Questions about control over work are almost identical to, although perhaps a more refined measure of, occupational class.

Shaper: There seems to be a remarkably biased attitude to what constitutes stress in different societies. It seems as though societies undergoing civil war or famine, for example, are subjected to stresses that are somehow different to the sophisticated stresses that affect civil servants. There is no evidence that those grossly stressed societies develop more visceral fat.

Roberts: How important is stress in genetically susceptible people relative to other factors such as diet and exercise?

Blundell: This question cannot be answered until we develop the tools to examine the issues properly. Simply hoping to pick up effects with general surveys won't work because the tools are not sufficiently sensitive. There is another issue here that may be important in thinking about stress and obesity. People who suffer high levels of stress or tension (which we can call anxiety) frequently take medication in the form of minor tranquillizers to reduce their anxiety. These drugs, called anxiolytics, have the potential to cause weight gain. Indeed, it is known among animal researchers that one of the most effective ways to induce a rat to eat is to give an injection of chlordiazepoxide (diazepam). There also exists a number of clinical studies indicating a relationship between anxiolytic medication and weight gain. This may well constitute a form of iatrogenic-induced obesity.

Björntorp: If the activity of the HPA axis is a crucial factor, then it will be important to develop simple diagnostic tests. We have developed a dexamethasone inhibition test that you can do at home on salivary cortisoles, and we are studying its associations with respect to different socioeconomic factors on a new population.

Fraser: We have attempted to define and evaluate stress in terms of ambitions and goals, and the inability of people to achieve them. We have a multiple input index that is valid in several populations. Paul McKeigue's study of migrant populations may be a manifestation of that, in that the migrants may have very major goals and cannot achieve them in their new societies. We have incorporated a modified Dressler questionnaire in the International Study of Hypertension in Blacks (ICSHIB) (Dressler et al 1988), in the hope that we will be able to generate data relating stress to central obesity.

Garrow: I have a small factual question for Per Björntorp. The proportion of visceral fat increases with age. Does this confound any of the other factors that have been reported as being associated with visceral fat?

Björntorp: No. We always control for this.

Bray: Can you explain the gender-specific differences in insulin resistance in terms of testosterone?

Björntorp: Hyperandrogenous women are insulin resistant, and there have also been some studies of men who have taken high doses of androgen-like steroids and become insulin resistant. Insulin resistance also occurs in men when their testosterone level is too low, but this is not the case for women: they do not become insulin resistant even when their testosterone level is zero. This suggests that there are gender-specific windows above or below which insulin resistance develops. It's possible that different mechanisms are operating on either side of the window because above the window there seem to be more effects on glucose transport and below the window there are more effects on glycogen synthase.

McKeigue: It may be difficult to determine whether these gender-specific differences are really effects of testosterone. The relationship between androgen levels and insulin resistance in women is in large part attributable to polycystic ovary syndrome. There's some evidence that the primary lesion may be insulin resistance, and the ovarian dysfunction and excess testosterone are secondary to the effects of insulin on the ovary. As for the relationship between the effects of testosterone and insulin resistance in men, other mechanisms may be involved, such as peripheral oestrogen production in adipose tissue and the anabolic effect of giving testosterone to men, which depletes fat reserves.

Björntorp: When we give female rats small amounts of testosterone to make them hyperandrogenic they become insulin resistant (Holmäng et al 1990). Also if transsexual women are given testosterone they become insulin resistant (Polderman et al 1994). Therefore, this represents one pathway to insulin resistance, although I cannot exclude the possibility that there are other ways.

Heymsfield: How can you explain the observation that increased cortisol secretion in upper-body obesity occurs even though some manifestations of Cushing's syndrome — such as osteoporosis, hirsuitism and moon facies — are missing?

Björntorp: The levels of cortisol might not be high enough.

References

Anderson EA, Balon TW, Hoffman RP, Sinkey CA, Mark AL 1992 Insulin increases sympathetic activity but not blood pressure in borderline hypertensive humans. Hypertension 19:621–627

Berne C, Fagius J, Pollare T, Hjemdahl P 1992 The sympathetic response to euglycaemic hyperinsulinaemia. Evidence from microelectrode nerve recordings in healthy subjects. Diabetologia 35:873–879

Björntorp P 1993 Visceral obesity: a 'civilization syndrome'. Obes Res 1:206–222

Bouchard C, Tremblay A, Després JP et al 1990 The response to long-term overfeeding in identical twins. New Engl J Med 322:1477–1482

Brindley DN, Cooling J, Glenny HP et al 1981 Effects of chronic modification of dietary fat and carbohydrate on the insulin, corticosterone and metabolic responses of rats fed acutely with glucose, fructose or ethanol. Biochem J 200:275–283

Buemann B, Vohl MC, Chagnon M et al 1996 Abdominal visceral fat is associated with a BclII restriction fragment length polymorphism at the glucocorticoid receptor gene locus, submitted

Campfield LA, Smith FJ, Rosenbaum M, Hirsch J 1996 Human eating: evidence for a physiological basis using a modified paradigm. Neurosci Biobehav Rev 20:133–137

Considine RV, Sinha MK, Heiman ML et al 1996 Serum immunoreactive leptin concentrations in normal-weight and obese humans. N Engl J Med 334:292–295

Dressler WW, Grell GAC, Gallagher PN, Viteri FE 1988 Blood pressure and social class in a Jamaican community. Am J Public Health 78:714–716

Halaas JL, Gajiwala KS, Maffei M et al 1995 Weight-reducing effects of the plasma protein encoded by the obese gene. Science 269:543–546

Hautanen A, Adlercreutz H 1993 Altered adrenocorticotropin and cortisol secretion in abdominal obesity: implications for the insulin resistance syndrome. J Intern Med 234:461–469

Holmäng A, Svedberg J, Jennische E, Björntorp P 1990 Effects of testosterone on muscle insulin sensitivity and morphology in female rats. Am J Physiol 259:555E–560E

Jayo JM, Shively CA, Kaplan JR, Manuck SB 1993 Effects of exercise and stress on body fat distribution in male Cynomolgus monkeys. Int J Obes 17:597–604

Jenson M, Kilroy G, York DA, Braymer HD 1996 Abnormal regulation of hepatic glucocorticoid receptor mRNA and receptor protein distribution in the obese Zucker rat. Obesity Res, in press

Jern S, Bergbrant A, Björntorp P, Hansson L 1992 Relation of central hemodynamics to obesity and body fat distribution. Hypertension 19:520–527

Jones PP, Snitker S, Skinner JS, Ravussin E 1996 Gender differences in muscle sympathetic nerve activity: effect of body fat distribution. Am J Physiol Endocrinol Metab 33:363E–366E

Karasek R, Baker D, Marxer F, Ahlbom A, Theorell T 1981 Job decision latitude, job demands and cardiovascular disease: a prospective study of Swedish men. Am J Public Health 71:694–705

Keys A, Brozek J, Henschell A, Mickelsen O, Taylor HL 1950 The biology of human starvation. University of Minnesota Press, Minneapolis, MN

Maffei M, Halaas J, Ravussin E et al 1995 Leptin levels in human and rodent: measurement of plasma leptin and ob mRNA in obese and weight-reduced subjects. Nat Med 1:1155–1161

McKeigue PM, Miller GJ, Marmot MG 1989 Coronary heart disease in south Asians overseas: a review. J Clin Epidemiol 42:597–609

Pelleymounter M, Cullen M, Baker M et al 1995 Effects of the obese gene product on body weight regulation in ob/ob mice. Science 269:540–543

Polderman KH, Gooren LJG, Asscheman H, Bakker A, Heine RJ 1994 Induction of insulin resistance by androgens and oestrogens. J Clin Endocrinol Metab 79:265–271

Rebuffé-Scrive M, Walsh UA, McEwan BS, Rodin J 1992 Effect of chronic stress and exogenous glucocorticoids on regional fat distribution and metabolism. Physiol Behav 52:583–590

Redei E, Hildebrand H, Aird F 1995 Corticotropin release-inhibiting factor is preprothyrotropin-releasing hormone 178–199. Endocrinology 136:3557–3563

Rentsch J, Levens N, Chiesi M 1995 Recombinant *ob* gene product reduces food intake in fasted mice. Biochem Biophys Res Commun 214:131–136

Rosmond R, Lapidus L, Björntorp P 1996 The influence of occupational and social factors on obesity and body fat distribution in middle-aged men. Int J Obes 20:599–607

Sarason IG, Johnson JH, Siegel JM 1978 Assessing the impact of life changes: development of the Life Experiences Survey. J Consult Clin Psychol 46:932–946.

Scherrer U, Randin D, Tappy L, Vollenweider P, Jéquier E, Nicod P 1994 Body fat and sympathetic nerve activity in healthy subjects. Circulation 89:2634–2640

Sims EAH, Danforth E Jr, Horton ES, Bray GA, Glennon JA, Salans LB 1973 Endocrine and metabolic effects of experimental obesity in man. Rec Prog Horm Res 29:457–496

Spraul M, Ravussin E, Fontvieille AM, Rising R, Larson DE, Anderson EA 1993 Reduced sympathetic nervous activity: a potential mechanism predisposing to body weight gain. J Clin Invest 92:1730–1735

Stephens TW, Basinski M, Bristow PK et al 1995 The role of neuropeptide Y in the antiobesity action of the obese gene product. Nature 377:530–532

Weigle DS, Bukowski TR, Foster DC et al 1995 Recombinant OB protein reduces feeding and body weight in the *ob/ob* mouse. J Clin Invest 96:2065–2070

Obesity and cardiovascular disease

A. G. Shaper

Department of Primary Care and Population Sciences, Royal Free Hospital School of Medicine, Rowland Hill Street, London NW3 2PF, UK

Abstract. The strong and consistent relationship observed between body weight and blood pressure develops early in life, and overweight/obesity[1] in adult life is a good predictor of hypertension. Weight reduction leads to a decrease in blood pressure and prevention of weight increase lowers the incidence of hypertension, but obesity is not necessarily the direct cause of raised blood pressure. Obesity is not established as an independent risk factor for stroke beyond its association with other risk factors. Obesity is a relatively weak risk factor for coronary heart disease (CHD) but it is closely associated with almost all other coronary risk factors. Thus, becoming obese on a Western high fat diet, with development of excess central fat, promotes atherogenesis through a wide range of biochemical and hormonal parameters, including insulin sensitivity. The obesity–CHD relationship is further confused by the weight loss associated with smoking and smoking-related disease, and is confounded by risk factors that accompany the development and maintenance of obesity. Weight loss in middle-aged populations does not apparently lower CHD incidence, possibly because of lack of specificity in methods of weight reduction. Irrespective of the mechanisms involved, early prevention of atherogenic weight gain in young adulthood is an important public health goal towards the control of hypertension and CHD.

1996 The origins and consequences of obesity. Wiley, Chichester (Ciba Foundation Symposium 201) p 90–107

Obesity, blood pressure and hypertension

A vast amount of evidence confirms that a strong relationship exists between body weight and blood pressure. In the Intersalt Study of 10 000 men and women aged 20–59 years drawn from 52 centres in 32 countries, the body mass index (BMI) was strongly, positively and independently associated with systolic blood pressure in individual subjects in all age groups, and the effect was also strong across countries. However, within the centres sodium (positively), potassium (negatively) and alcohol (positively) intakes were also independently and significantly related to blood pressure (Dyer & Elliott 1989, Dyer et al 1994).

---

[1]In this paper the terms overweight and obesity are used interchangeably, unless a specific definition is indicated (as in the British Regional Heart Study data). The justification for not using a standard definition of obesity, such as a body mass index of more than 30 kg/m[2] will be apparent throughout the paper and in the conclusion.

The critical question is whether the rise in blood pressure in most populations with increasing age is due predominantly to increasing body weight in those populations. In 34 000 Caucasian men and women in Chicago, within each of five relative weight groups from <100% to ≥135%, blood pressure increased with increasing age. However, at every age level there was an increase in blood pressure with increasing relative weight (Fig. 1). The data suggest an age–blood pressure relationship even in the absence of obesity, suggesting that factors other than body weight, such as micronutrient intake (Pan et al 1986), are involved.

Literature describing exotic populations with low blood pressure which does not rise with age and the impact of rural–urban migration on the blood pressure of these populations suggests that the major determinants of blood pressure are increased body weight, increased sodium intake and decreased potassium intake, with some contribution from alcohol (Poulter & Sever 1994). The National Health and Nutrition Examination Surveys (NHANES) II data show clearly that the higher prevalence of hypertension in North American Blacks cannot be attributed to obesity alone, and also emphasize the greater relative risk of hypertension in younger obese subjects compared with older subjects (Van Itallie 1985). Obesity is an excellent predictor of hypertension, and a number of longitudinal studies confirm that men reporting a diagnosis of hypertension in adult life were heavier in their youth than those who remained normotensive (Havlik et al 1983). This again suggests that weight per se may not be critical but that there are factors common to both weight gain and increasing blood pressure which may have their major impact in early adult life. The large number of trials showing that weight reduction leads to reduction in blood pressure provides some support for the causal role of obesity in hypertension and this effect seems to relate more closely to weight loss than to dietary sodium restriction (Tuck et al 1981). Several studies suggest that weight control may reduce the incidence of hypertension in those with high to normal blood pressure but in almost all of these studies intervention involves other aspects of diet and lifestyle (Stamler et al 1989), although calorie reduction appears to be more effective than sodium restriction (Trials of Hypertension Prevention Collaborative Research Group 1992).

Therefore, there is an intimate but inadequately explained relationship between increasing body weight and increasing blood pressure. How one becomes fat, i.e. the various pathways to overweight, may be more critical than just being fat, and there is a complex interplay between nutrients, particularly sodium and potassium, that supersedes the effects of any single factor (Reusser & McCarron 1994). There is no convincing evidence to support the hypotheses relating saturated, monounsaturated or polyunsaturated fats to blood pressure (Morris & Sacks 1994), although the dietary composition will determine the metabolic characteristics of central fat, with consequences for atherosclerosis unrelated to blood pressure.

Obesity and stroke

Most studies of the association between obesity and stroke have found little if any adverse effect. The search for causality is confounded by the close association

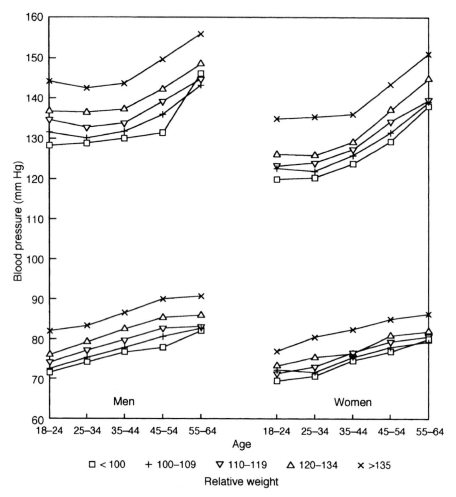

FIG. 1.   Relationship between age and mean blood pressure in five relative weight groups. Chicago Heart Association Detection Project 1967–1973 (Pan et al 1986).

between obesity and other risk factors for stroke, although the Framingham Study has suggested that obesity is an independent risk factor given a long enough period of exposure (Hubert et al 1983). There is currently an opinion that the role of obesity may have been underestimated because the standard multivariate analysis controls for the mechanisms by which obesity protractedly exerts its influence. In the Whitehall Study of British male civil servants aged 40–64 followed for at least 15 years with no adjustments for blood pressure, blood lipids or diabetes, increasing quartiles of BMI were associated with increasing risk of fatal stroke, the effect being most marked in those who had never smoked (Shinton et al 1991).

Because the effects of obesity may be gradual in development, a lifelong history of obesity may be more important in the assessment of stroke risk than current weight in middle age. In studies of American college alumni, the more obese students had an increased risk of stroke in later years compared with their leaner colleagues (Paffenbarger & Wing 1971). Shinton et al (1995) found no relationship between stroke events and current BMI but there was an increased risk of stroke in the top quartile of both maximum reported BMI and BMI at age 21 years with odds ratios of 2.25 and 2.13, respectively. The risk was most marked in those who had never smoked.

Trends in stroke

Throughout the industrialized world, stroke mortality rates have been declining over the past several decades. This decline has been accompanied by an increase in mean BMI and self-reported diabetes mellitus, and there is strong evidence from studies in Minnesota and Finland that much of the fall in mortality can be explained by changes in blood pressure, serum total cholesterol and cigarette smoking (McGovern et al 1992, Vartiainen et al 1995), and some of the increase in BMI (about 25% in men and 17% in women) has been attributed to giving up smoking (Flegal et al 1995).

Consequently, obesity contributes to stroke through its effects on blood pressure, blood lipids and diabetes, and also through its inverse relationship with physical activity (Wannamethee & Shaper 1989). These associations do not negate the importance of obesity in the risk of stroke because obesity is intimately involved in the progress of all these factors to levels that constitute risk for stroke.

Obesity and coronary heart disease

In most western societies obesity carries a twofold risk of coronary heart disease (CHD), both in men and in women. However, as for stroke, obesity is closely associated with increased levels of blood pressure and serum total cholesterol, and once these have been adjusted for in multivariate analysis, obesity no longer has an independent effect in predicting CHD. However, to adjust for factors that are among the mechanisms by which obesity brings about vascular disease seems illogical in trying to establish aetiology. In addition, many studies fail to take into account the effect of cigarette smoking on reducing body weight and increasing vascular disease.

In the Seven Countries Study, middle-aged men in Yugoslavia, Finland, Italy, the Netherlands, Greece, USA and Japan were surveyed between 1958 and 1970 with follow-up to the present day for mortality only (Keys 1980). The marked differences between the cohorts in incidence rates of CHD were not significantly related to differences in average BMI or total skinfold thickness. In none of these populations was BMI or fatness significantly associated with CHD incidence or mortality. In addition, the lack of a relationship between BMI and CHD mortality is evidenced by the association of a progressive decline in mortality rates for CHD in many western countries with a progressive increase in the prevalence of obesity. Obesity per se would not appear to be a necessary cause of CHD, but some pathways to obesity and some patterns of obesity are almost certainly more atherogenic than others.

Body mass index and other risk factors

There are well-established relationships between BMI and age, socioeconomic status, smoking, physical activity and alcohol intake. BMI is also strongly associated with blood lipid levels (Thelle et al 1983). Serum total cholesterol increases with increasing BMI until about 28 kg/m² but thereafter it shows no further increase. The relationship between BMI and high density lipoprotein–cholesterol is negative and linear, and the relationship between BMI and triglycerides is positive and linear (Fig. 2). These data help to explain the early fall in triglycerides that is associated with weight loss and the difficulties encountered in reducing serum total cholesterol by weight reduction in very obese subjects.

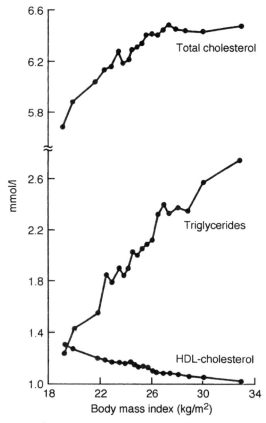

FIG. 2.   The relationship between body mass index (kg/m²) and total cholesterol, high density lipo-protein–cholesterol and triglycerides, all in mmol/l in middle-aged British men (Thelle et al 1983).

TABLE 1 Body mass index (BMI, kg/m^2) and percentage distribution of cardiovascular risk factors in middle-aged men (British Regional Heart Study)

BMI group	n	SBP[a]	Cholesterol[a]	HDL-C[b]	Triglycerides[a]	Glucose[c]	Uric acid[a]	Haematocrit[d]
<20.0	268	12.3	6.4	7.4	2.4	9.0	7.1	23.9
20.0–21.9	703	12.0	11.2	10.8	5.0	8.5	10.2	26.9
22.0–23.9	1549	15.5	16.7	15.9	13.9	8.7	13.0	29.4
24.0–25.9	2080	20.4	20.0	18.2	19.3	9.1	17.6	30.8
26.0–27.9	1638	24.3	23.6	23.5	24.9	10.2	24.7	34.0
28.0–29.9	858	29.2	22.3	29.8	30.3	11.4	30.3	33.8
30.0–31.9	387	32.0	25.5	34.4	37.2	13.3	38.5	40.6
>32.0	249	51.8	24.2	36.8	36.7	17.3	36.1	43.0

[a]Per cent in top quintile. SBP, systolic blood pressure.
[b]Per cent in lowest quintile. HDL-C, high density lipoprotein-cholesterol.
[c]Per cent in top decile.
[d]Per cent greater than 46%.

Data from the Framingham Offspring Study suggest that the prevalence of risk factors for cardiovascular disease rises rapidly from BMIs greater than 20 kg/m^2 (Garrison & Kannel 1993). This claim is strongly supported by the British Regional Heart Study (BRHS) data, which show a progressive change in most risk factors from BMI < 20 kg/m^2 through to BMI ≥ 32 kg/m^2 (Table 1).

Human experimental evidence indicates that weight gain on the usual American diet is directly responsible for the changes observed in a wide range of biochemical and hormonal factors which are characteristic of insulin insensitivity (Sims et al 1973). It is suggested that the fundamental metabolic defect following from central obesity may be reduced sensitivity to insulin, from which all other metabolic disturbances associated with obesity are derived. The BRHS data, which reflect spontaneous rather than experimental obesity, show strong positive relationships between BMI and insulin levels. The mean insulin concentration increases steadily from a BMI of < 20 kg/m^2 and the percentage of high levels (top decile) increases sixfold over the range of BMI (Table 2). Conversely, with increasing deciles of serum insulin concentration, the mean BMI and the percentage of men with obesity (≥ 28 kg/m^2) also increase progressively (Table 3). It is posited that CHD is also an expression of insulin resistance arising from central obesity because: the risk of CHD is doubled in those with diabetes; diabetes is linked with many risk factors common to CHD; and non-insulin-dependent diabetes mellitus (NIDDM) is due to insulin insensitivity.

Serum insulin and coronary heart disease

In 12 years of follow-up in the BRHS men, a non-linear relation was observed between non-fasting serum insulin concentrations and major CHD events (Fig. 3), with an almost twofold increase in the age-adjusted relative risk of heart attack in the 10th decile of the serum insulin distribution ($\geq 35.3\,\mathrm{mU/l}$) relative to the other nine deciles combined (relative risk 1.7, 95% confidence interval 1.3–2.2). After adjustment for a wide range of biological and lifestyle risk factors for CHD, the relative risk was attenuated but remained significant (relative risk 2.1, 95% confidence interval 1.4–3.1).

Although the data are consistent with the hypothesis that a high level of serum insulin is atherogenic, the strikingly non-linear form of the association and the attenuation on multivariate analysis suggest that insulin is not a necessary factor in the development of CHD and that it may well accompany or follow changes that have taken place in other biochemical variables. Hyperinsulinism may merely be a marker for common aetiological factors in the development of both CHD and NIDDM (Perry et al 1995).

In many developing countries in Africa and Asia, NIDDM is common and strongly linked with obesity, but in such populations CHD is rare. This suggests that insulin resistance and glucose intolerance are not necessary for the development of atherosclerosis and CHD. We are back to the issue of pathways to obesity. Becoming

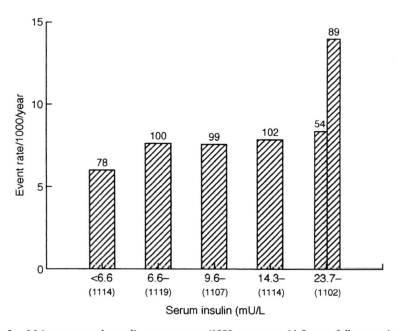

FIG. 3.   Major coronary heart disease event rate/1000 per year at 11.5 years follow-up, in the first to fourth quintiles of serum insulin concentration and in the ninth and 10th deciles, in middle-aged British men. Number of events above each bar and number of men in each group in parentheses below each bar (Perry et al 1995).

TABLE 2 Body mass index (BMI) and serum insulin concentration (mU/l, geometric mean) and percentage of each BMI group with levels in the top decile of the ranked insulin distribution (British Regional Heart Study)

BMI group	Serum insulin concentration	% Top decile
>20.0	8.3	4.4
20.0–21.9	8.8	4.3
22.0–23.9	10.6	5.5
24.0–25.9	12.3	8.2
26.0–27.9	14.0	11.9
28.0–29.9	16.1	16.9
30.0–31.9	19.7	23.1
>32.0	23.3	29.7

fat on a high carbohydrate diet with consequent low mean blood cholesterol may result in insulin insensitivity and diabetes, but the internal biochemical environment may still not be appropriate for the development of atherosclerosis and CHD.

Body weight and mortality

Extreme obesity increases the risk of mortality, particularly from CHD, although there is still argument as to the precise level of obesity that should be labelled as hazardous

TABLE 3 Serum insulin distribution (mU/l, deciles), mean body mass index (BMI, kg/m^2) and percentage obesity (BMI ⩾ 28 kg/m^2) in middle-aged men (British Regional Heart Study)

Serum insulin	Mean BMI	% Obese
1	23.5	5.8
2	24.3	9.9
3	25.0	11.1
4	25.1	14.3
5	25.7	19.1
6	25.7	18.0
7	25.9	22.9
8	26.1	26.1
9	26.4	25.6
10	27.4	38.9

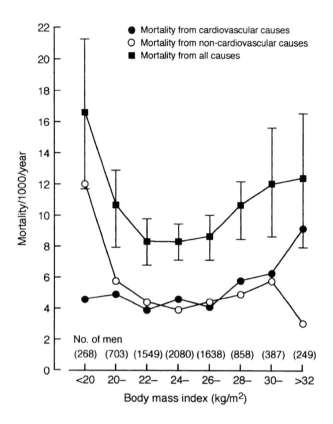

FIG. 4. Mortality from all causes and from cardiovascular and non-cardiovascular causes in middle-aged British men according to body mass index during nine years follow-up. Vertical bars indicate 95% confidence intervals for total mortality (Wannamethee & Shaper 1989).

(Kushner 1993). Because most of the risk factors for CHD rise progressively from low body weight to high body weight (Table 1), the question as to which level of BMI or other measure of body weight/fatness is associated in the short-term with death or an increased risk of a major cardiovascular event seems irrelevant. In a western society, increasing weight means increasing risk of pathology, although the rate and intensity of the process will differ considerably between individuals and populations. A recent editorial in the *New England Journal of Medicine* asks "Within the range of 'normal' weights, is it better to be thinner", and answers categorically, "No, within the broad range of BMIs under 27 there is very little relation between body weight and mortality" (Byers 1995). In the light of our knowledge of the progressive increase in risk factor levels as BMI increases, this conclusion and the assumptions that may flow from it, must be regarded as seriously misleading. It may be true for mortality and for major cardiovascular events; it is not true for the risk of disease or the risk of mortality.

In the BRHS, after nine years follow-up there was a significant U-shaped relation between BMI and total mortality (Fig. 4) with the very lean men (<20 kg/m^2) having the highest mortality (Wannamethee & Shaper 1989). This increased mortality was largely attributable to non-cardiovascular causes and in particular to smoking-related deaths. There was little difference in mortality from non-cardiovascular causes among the other BMI groups. For cardiovascular deaths there was a significant tendency for mortality to increase with increasing BMI. The U-shaped relation between BMI and mortality was most pronounced in the oldest men (55–59 years). The raised mortality in obese men ($\geqslant 28$ kg/m^2; the top fifth of the BMI distribution) was due largely to cardiovascular causes and was seen most clearly in the oldest age group, suggesting that the impact of obesity on cardiovascular health takes its major toll with advancing years.

Smoking

In the BRHS, as in other studies, there was a strong inverse association between BMI and cigarette smoking, with smoking making a major contribution to increased mortality in lean men (<20 kg/m^2). In men who had never smoked, lean men had the lowest mortality, and in the remaining men, there was a significant tendency for mortality to increase with increasing BMI, suggesting that when smoking does not confound the issue, increasing BMI is associated with increasing mortality (Wannamethee & Shaper 1989).

Women

The Nurses' Health Study (USA) has shown, in the optimal analysis in women who had never smoked and had recently had stable weight, that the lowest mortality was among the leanest women (BMI <19.0 kg/m^2), who, incidentally, were at least 15% below the average USA weight for middle-aged women (Manson et al 1995). Mortality did not increase substantially up to a BMI of 27 kg/m^2, although trends were apparent for CHD and cancer among women at average weights and among those who were mildly overweight. A BMI of 22 kg/m^2 or more at age 18 years was associated with a significant elevation in subsequent mortality from cardiovascular disease, and weight gain after 18 years had to be more than 10 kg to increase subsequent mortality due to cardiovascular disease or cancer.

Weight change and the risk of heart attack

Most national health authorities recommend weight reduction in the population as a measure towards the reduction of cardiovascular mortality on the assumption that the relationship between BMI and cardiovascular disease is reversible. However, the evidence that weight loss per se decreases CHD events is much less certain than its known effect of reducing cardiovascular risk factors such as blood pressure and blood lipids (Goldstein 1992).

In recent studies from the USA, both weight gain and weight loss have been associated with increased risk of cardiovascular mortality (Lee & Paffenbarger 1992, Pamuk et al 1993, Higgins et al 1993). In the BRHS men free from doctor-diagnosed CHD, weight change was determined during the first five years of follow-up, and fatal and non-fatal heart attacks recorded over the subsequent 6.5 years (Walker et al 1995). Men who gained 4–10% body weight and those with stable weight had the lowest rates of heart attack (Fig. 5). Men who lost weight had an increased risk of heart attack, which after adjustment for a wide range of risk factors was similar to the risk in the stable group. Thus, there was no increased risk of heart attack but there was no benefit. The men who gained > 10% body weight had a significantly increased risk of heart attack. Men who were initially overweight (BMI 25.0–27.9 kg/m^2) or obese (BMI $\geq$ 28 kg/m^2) showed no benefit from weight loss. A small amount of weight gain (4–10%) in the overweight or obese men was associated with decreased risk, whereas considerable weight gain (> 10%) was associated with increased risk.

These findings are similar to those of the Harvard Alumni Study (Lee & Paffenbarger 1992), the NHANES I study (Pamuk et al 1993) and the Framingham Study (Higgins et al 1993). In the Framingham Study, those who lost weight showed improvements in blood pressure and blood cholesterol levels but they also showed an association with continued smoking and an increased prevalence and incidence of cardiovascular disease, diabetes mellitus, other diseases and higher death rates.

None of these studies have information on the proportion of men losing weight who did so intentionally, but it appears that the most marked weight loss took place in those who were initially obese, in those with a recall of a doctor diagnosis of hypertension and diabetes, and in those who had the highest levels of measured blood pressure and cholesterol. A pessimistic conclusion would be that obesity leads to changes which are irreversible and that prevention of obesity is the only answer. A more optimistic hypothesis is that weight reduction per se is not sufficient and that it must be specifically linked to measures likely to reduce blood cholesterol and blood pressure, with cessation of smoking and with increased physical activity.

Weight cycling

It has been suggested that cycles of weight loss followed by weight gain increase the risk of diabetes, hypertension, hyperlipidaemia and CHD, and in the Framingham Study those whose body weight fluctuated often or greatly had higher risk of CHD and death than persons with relatively stable body weight (Lissner 1991). However, in the Honolulu Heart Programme involving middle-aged Japanese-American men, those who had large fluctuations in weight or a weight loss of 4.5 kg or more (or both) were found to have a higher prevalence of CHD, diabetes mellitus and hypertensive disease than those whose weight was more stable (Iribarren et al 1995). They were heavier at baseline, more likely to be heavy drinkers who had either stopped smoking

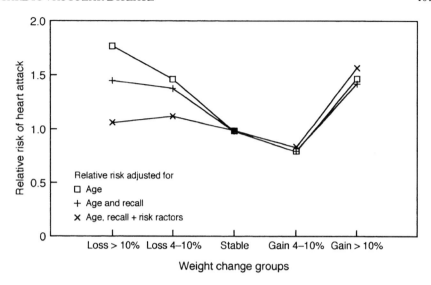

FIG. 5. Relative risk of heart attack (fatal and non-fatal) in middle-aged British men by weight change over five years, adjusted sequentially for: (i) age; (ii) age and recall of a doctor diagnosis of hypertension or diabetes; and (iii) age, recall and other risk factors (body mass index, smoking status at screening and, five years later, systolic blood pressure, serum total cholesterol, forced expiratory volume in 1 s and social class) (Walker et al 1995).

(with weight fluctuation) or they continued smoking (with weight loss). Among men who had never smoked, there was no association between weight loss and variation in weight with death from cardiovascular causes. The authors concluded that the health hazards of weight loss and variation may not be applicable to otherwise healthy people.

Distribution of body fat

It is now well established that those with visceral obesity (deep abdominal fat) are at highest risk of cardiovascular disease (Larsson et al 1992), so that estimates of risk based on BMI or other crude measures alone will underestimate risk associated with specific types of obesity. Magnetic resonance imaging and spectroscopy now provide non-invasive methods for mapping the distribution and composition of adipose tissue. It seems clear that different patterns of diet and physical activity lead to fat accumulations in different sites, with differing metabolic and hormonal correlates and differing disease outcomes.

Conclusion

In western societies, increasing body weight from about $20 \, \text{kg/m}^2$ upwards is associated with increasing levels of risk factors for cardiovascular disease and with increasing risk of cardiovascular morbidity and mortality. Levels of BMI currently regarded as acceptable may not be biologically normal. The concept of a risk-free zone until a BMI of 27 or 28 kg/m^2 is reached is misleading and the ideal BMI is likely to be nearer 20–22 kg/m^2. Health targets that focus on reducing the proportion of those with BMI over 30 kg/m^2 are likely to be of little or no value.

How individuals and societies become fat may be critical. Some pathways to obesity and some patterns of obesity are almost certainly more atherogenic than others. Atherogenic weight gain in early adulthood that is maintained or increased in middle age is likely to constitute the greatest hazard to health. The specific prevention of atherogenic weight gain in youth and early adulthood may be a most rewarding public health policy.

Acknowledgements

The British Regional Heart Study is a British Heart Foundation Research Group and is also supported by the Department of Health and The Stroke Association.

References

Byers T 1995 Body weight and mortality. N Engl J Med 333:723–724

Dyer AR, Elliott P 1989 The INTERSALT study: relation of body mass index to blood pressure. J Hum Hypertens 3:299–308

Dyer AR, Elliott P, Shipley M, Stamler R, Stamler J 1994 Body mass index and association of sodium and potassium with blood pressure in INTERSALT. Hypertension 23:729–736

Flegal KM, Troiano RP, Pamuk ER, Kuczmarski RJ, Campbell SM 1995 The influence of smoking cessation on the prevalence of overweight in the United States. N Engl J Med 333:1165–1170

Garrison RJ, Kannel WB 1993 A new approach for estimating healthy body weights. Int J Obes 17:417–423

Goldstein DJ 1992 Beneficial health effects of modest weight loss. Int J Obes 16:397–415

Havlik RJ, Hubert HB, Fabsitz RR, Feinleib M 1983 Weight and hypertension. Ann Intern Med 98:855–859

Higgins M, D'Agostino R, Kannel W, Cobb J 1993 Benefits and adverse effects of weight loss: observations from the Framingham study. Ann Intern Med 119:758–763

Hubert HB, Feinleib M, McNamara PM, Castelli WP 1983 Obesity as an independent risk factor for cardiovascular disease: a 26-year follow-up of participants in the Framingham Heart Study. Circulation 67:968–977

Iribarren C, Sharp DS, Burchfiel CM, Petrovitch H 1995 Association of weight loss and weight fluctuation with mortality among Japanese-American men. N Engl J Med 333:686–692

Keys A (ed) 1980 Seven countries: a multivariate analysis of death and coronary heart disease. Harvard University Press, Cambridge, MA

Kushner RF 1993 Body weight and mortality. Nutr Rev 51:127–136

Larsson B, Bengtsson C, Björntorp P et al 1992 Is abdominal body fat distribution a major explanation for the sex difference in the incidence of myocardial infarction? Am J Epidemiol 135:266–273

Lee IM, Paffenbarger RS 1992 Change in body weight and longevity. JAMA 268:2045–2049

Lissner L, Odell PM, D'Agostino RB et al 1991 Variability of body weight and health outcomes in the Framingham population. N Engl J Med 324:1839–1844

Manson JE, Willett WC, Stampfer MJ et al 1995 Body weight and mortality among women. N Engl J Med 333:677–685

McGovern PG, Burke GL, Sprafka JM, Xue S, Folsom AR, Blackburn H 1992 Trends in mortality, morbidity and risk factor levels from 1960 through 1990. The Minnesota Heart Study. JAMA 268:753–759

Morris MC, Sacks FM 1994 Dietary fats and blood pressure. In: Swales JD (ed) Textbook of hypertension. Blackwell Scientific, Oxford, p 605–618

Paffenbarger RS, Wing AL 1971 Chronic disease in former college students. 11. Early precursors of nonfatal stroke. Am J Epidemiol 94:524–530

Pamuk ER, Williamson DF, Serdula MK, Madans J, Byers TE 1993 Weight loss and subsequent death in a cohort of United States adults. Ann Intern Med 119:744–748

Pan W-H, Nanas S, Dyer A et al 1986 The role of weight in the positive association between age and blood pressure. Am J Epidemiol 24:612–623

Perry IJ, Wannamethee SG, Whincup PH, Shaper AG, Walker MK, Alberti KGMM 1996 Serum insulin and incident coronary heart disease in middle-aged British men. Am J Epidemiol 144:224–234

Poulter, Sever PS 1994 Low blood pressure populations and the impact of rural–urban migration. In: Swales JD (ed) Textbook of hypertension. Blackwell Scientific, Oxford, p 22–36

Reusser ME, McCarron DA 1994 Micronutrient effects on blood pressure regulation. Nutr Rev 52:367–375

Shinton R, Shipley M, Rose G 1991 Overweight and stroke in the Whitehall study. J Epidemiol Community Health 45:138–142

Shinton R, Sagar G, Beevers G 1995 Body fat and stroke: unmasking the hazards of overweight and obesity. J Epidemiol Community Health 49:259–264

Sims EAH, Danforth E Jr, Horton ES, Bray GA, Glennon JA, Salans LB 1973 Endocrine and metabolic effects of experimental obesity in man. Recent Prog Horm Res 29:457–496

Stamler R, Stamler J, Gosch FC et al 1989 Primary prevention of hypertension by nutritional-hygienic means: final report of a randomized controlled trial. JAMA 262:1801–1807

Thelle DS, Shaper AG, Whitehead TP, Bullock DG, Ashby D, Patel I 1983 Blood lipids in middle-aged British men. Br Heart J 49:205–213

Trials of Hypertension Prevention Collaborative Research Group 1992 The effects of non-pharmacologic interventions on blood pressure of persons with high normal levels: results of the Trials of Hypertension Prevention. JAMA 267:1213–1220

Tuck ML, Sowers J, Dornfeld L, Kledzik G, Maxwell M 1981 The effect of weight reduction on blood pressure, plasma renin activity and plasma aldosterone levels in obese patients. N Engl J Med 304:930–933

Van Itallie TB 1985 The problem of obesity: health implications of overweight and obesity in the United States. Ann Intern Med 103:983–988

Vartiainen E, Sarti C, Tuomilehto J, Kuulasmaa K 1995 Do changes in cardiovascular risk factors explain changes in mortality from stroke in Finland? Br Med J 310:901–904

Walker M, Wannamethee G, Whincup PH, Shaper AG 1995 Weight change and risk of heart attack in middle-aged British men. Int J Epidemiol 24:694–703

Wannamethee G, Shaper AG 1989 Body weight and mortality in middle-aged British men: impact of smoking. Br Med J 299:1497–1502

DISCUSSION

Bray: The data from the Nurses' Health Study show that the increase in body mass index (BMI) only becomes significant at a BMI of 27–29 kg/m². However, the increase, on both a population basis and a resource basis, is too small, and is therefore unapproachable in a practical sense and may not even be important in a clinical or biological sense. The increase in BMI from 20 to 25 or 27 kg/m^2 is of such a small magnitude, unless there is weight gain. Weight gain and fat distribution are two separate issues, and fat distribution may be the overriding issue.

Shaper: You used the word 'resource', and so you must have certain practical thoughts in your mind about what ought to be done in a population in which, using the definitions I've used, about 80% of the population will be overweight. We're not looking at whether a particular level is statistically significant in terms of risk or mortality, we're looking at the risk factors that are gradually increasing in these individuals. In our society we see that the risk levels start to increase early on and they are progressive. Unless we aim at a population average BMI of about 22 or 23 kg/m^2, we are going to continue to experience high levels of cardiovascular disease. I'm not suggesting that we should attempt to persuade everybody to reach that level; that would be an impossible task. However, I'm talking about future targets.

Astrup: You presented a balanced view of the relationship between weight loss and mortality. Most studies have not taken into account the cause of the weight loss, i.e. whether it's intentional or unintentional, or whether it results from a pre-existing disease. However, the Williamson et al (1995) study claimed to be the first study that distinguished between unintended and intended weight loss. They showed that even modest weight loss among obese women was associated with a pronounced decrease in mortality from cancer and cardiovascular disease. Also, the Swedish obesity study by Sjöström, although there is no mortality data available yet, shows that the incidence of hypertension, diabetes and coronary heart disease (CHD) is significantly lower in the weight loss intervention group (L. Sjöström, unpublished results 1995).

Heymsfield: The most important BMI measurement is the integrated lifetime BMI because duration is a critical factor in cardiovascular risk. The 25-year follow-up of the Framingham Study showed that obesity was an independent risk factor for coronary disease after controlling for lipids, smoking and blood pressure (Hubert et al 1983). This was apparent only after 25 years of follow-up.

Shaper: I agree. The longer these studies continue, the more interesting the data become. This is true for stroke as well as for CHD.

Hitman: One has to be careful when making inferences about different BMIs from epidemiological studies showing increments of risk. We have learnt many lessons from the cholesterol data, where there is a U-shaped curve and an increment of risk that increases from about 5 mmol/l onwards. However, we have learnt that it is important to look at other risk factors and the intervention trials. There is little point in intervening at intermediate cholesterol levels in the absence of any other risk factors for ischaemic heart disease. For example, take the case of a woman with a cholesterol level of 7.5 mmol/l who is pre-menopausal, a non-smoker, not hypertensive or diabetic, and has a family history of longevity. Many clinicians would suggest that intervention with drug therapy in this case is not necessary. Alternatively, take the case of a woman with a cholesterol level of 6 mmol/l on an optimal diet and who has ischaemic heart disease. There is little doubt from the intervention trials that this person should be treated with drugs to aim at a cholesterol level below 5.2 mmol/l. Consequently, it is would be dangerous to assume that one should intervene at all levels of increased BMI without regard to associated risk factors.

Garrow: In the Nurses' Health Study the first data point at which the 95% confidence interval does not go down to 1.00 is in the group 27–28.9 kg/m². However, the previous data points have increased steadily. When all the smokers and people with unstable weights are excluded, there are only 531 deaths (compared to the initial 4726 deaths). Therefore, the power to detect this change is decreased by the smaller number of deaths. Also, if the smokers are excluded, increased mortality at lower weights is eliminated. If we can be sure that there aren't increased risks at lower weights, we can advocate lower levels with a clearer conscience. The observation that the 25–27 kg/m² category error bar still touches 1.00 is not a good enough reason for advocating that it's the ideal weight to be.

Allison: We are not yet certain that there is no increase in mortality at lower BMI values. There are a number of limitations in the argument that the increase in mortality is strictly monotonic over BMI. For example, the argument that it's due to smoking holds up in the Nurses' Health Study, but this is only a single study. Gerry Shaper presented data from the British Regional Heart Study in which there was a sharp increase in mortality in the lowest BMI category of those who had never smoked. Why did you ask us to ignore this?

Shaper: Because there were only three cases in that group, two of which had cancer and the other was an alcoholic.

Allison: But there are other studies that have controlled for smoking and have not revealed a marked difference in the shape of the curve at lower BMI values (Troiano et al 1996). The data in the Nurses' Health Study are limited to Caucasian women aged between 30–55. June Stevens and colleagues analysed data from the American Cancer Society, which was the largest study of Black men and women ever performed (Plankey et al 1995, Kolodziejczyk et al 1995). They excluded those who had never smoked from the data sets and found that there was either no relationship between BMI and mortality or a U-shaped relationship. Also, the Nurses' Health Study did not examine the effect of age on these relationships, so they may change over time. Therefore, we cannot necessarily accept that there is no increase in mortality in the lower BMI categories.

Garrow: But in the Nurses' Health Study the y-axis was labelled age-adjusted relative risk.

Allison: That's not the same as determining whether the relationships change with age.

McKeigue: As epidemiologists we have some responsibility for having misled everyone with these U-shaped and J-shaped curves relating mortality to body weight and associated variables such as blood pressure, plasma cholesterol or insulin. In the past we have underestimated the degree of confounding by co-morbidity that is present in these data sets. The J-shaped or U-shaped relationships are observed consistently in older populations with high proportions of smokers, and they are not observed in younger, non-smoking populations that are followed through into middle age. This is exactly what one would expect if the J-shaped relationship is due to confounding by co-morbidity. Adjusting for smoking is not sufficient to control for this confounding effect. Smoking is only one of the factors that causes weight loss and it is associated with increased mortality. The argument about J-shaped curves has been present in studies of blood pressure for even longer than those of BMI. Glynn et al (1995) have demonstrated that a positive linear relationship exists between blood pressure and mortality, even in data from the elderly, when the analysis is carefully controlled for confounding by co-morbidity. The same would probably apply to many of the BMI data sets. Most of the studies that show J-shaped curves have not made serious attempts to control for the effects of co-morbidity.

Rissanen: After controlling for this kind of morbidity bias, much of the remaining confounding effect derives from socioeconomic factors. For example, the relation of BMI and mortality among Finns is almost linear in upper social classes but J-shaped in lower classes (A. Rissanen, unpublished results 1995).

Campfield: In my opinion these studies are useful, but are they relevant at the level of the individual? The results of epidemiological studies can only be used as guidelines, and they should not be used to make public health policy statements. I would like to know how the results of epidemiological studies affect how intervention trials should be performed, and how individuals should be counselled about their weight change and relative risk.

Prentice: Although Gerry Shaper's brief was to address only heart disease, in my opinion it is a somewhat sterile argument to talk about the cost of obesity just on the basis of CHD. We need to make a more holistic judgement of what the cost is to the individual. We know that most obese people are not worried about dying a couple of years early, that is not what really impinges on them, it is the other psychosocial and morbidity factors. In terms of the costs of the obesity epidemic to the health services, I doubt whether CHD is the most important issue.

Shaper: In the last few minutes, I would like to summarize my views on the discussion that has taken place. Firstly, my allotted task at this symposium was to talk about obesity, overweight and cardiovascular disease, and that's what I've done. Cardiovascular disease is probably one of the major causes of mortality and morbidity, so it is not unreasonable to make some extrapolations from that to total mortality and morbidity.

I haven't seen the Williamson data, but I agree with Arne Astrup that the issue of planned weight loss is critical. There have been few studies of intentional weight loss and we need to know whether these studies intended only to reduce weight or whether they intended to lower blood lipid levels as well. When I presented our data showing that there did not appear to be any benefit from unintentional weight loss, I did not suggest that losing weight was not beneficial in any way, I was merely looking for evidence that one could present to the public that it was of major benefit. Weight loss is beneficial but it is clear that it is confounded by many other factors.

Graham Hitman likened these studies to those of cholesterol. It is apparent that the level of cholesterol is also confounded by other factors, such as pre-existing disease. When pre-existing disease is taken into account, there is a linear relationship between cholesterol levels and the risk of cardiovascular disease. A linear relationship may also be observed for BMI in the absence of confounding factors.

Concerning the point about individuals and populations, I'm not suggesting that every individual who is overweight has a high risk of an obesity-related disease. I am asking, in a population model, what is primarily responsible for the major cardiovascular epidemics? Is obesity, with a high saturated fat intake and high blood cholesterol, a major factor? Is atherogenic central obesity a key issue? I'm beginning to think that it is, because the epidemiological studies over the last 20 years have shown that obesity itself isn't that important, rather it is the other factors that are associated with it and these will depend upon which nutritional pathway has led to obesity.

References

Glynn RJ, Field TS, Rosner B, Hebert PR, Taylor JO, Hennekens CH 1995 Evidence for a positive linear relation between blood pressure and mortality in elderly people. Lancet 345:825–829

Hubert HB, Feinleib M, McNamara PM, Castelli WP 1983 Obesity as an independent risk factor for cardiovascular disease: a 26-year follow-up of participants in the Framingham Heart Study. Circulation 7:968–977

Kolodziejczyk M, Stevens J, Plankey M 1995 The BMI–mortality relationship in African-American men aged 30–64. Obesity Res (suppl 3) 3:405S

Plankey MW, Stevens J, Palesch YY, Rust PF, O'Neil PM, Williamson DR 1995 The impact of education and smoking on the BMI–mortality relationship in white and African-American women. Obesity Res (suppl 3) 3:386S

Troiano RP, Frongillo EA, Sobal J, Levitsky DA 1996 The relationship between body weight and mortality: a quantitative analysis of combined information from existing studies. Int J Obes 20:63–75

Williamson DF, Pamuk E, Thun M, Flanders D, Byers T, Heath C 1995 Prospective study of intentional weight loss and mortality in never-smoking overweight US white women aged 40–64 years. Am J Epidemiol 141:1128–1141

Genetics of obesity in humans: current issues

Claude Bouchard

Physical Activity Sciences Laboratory, Laval University, Sainte-Foy, Québec G1K 7P4, Canada

Abstract. During the last decade, we have begun to understand some of the reasons why people become obese as assessed by excess body mass for height or excess total body fat content. Obesity frequently aggregates in families. However, this familial resemblance is caused not only by genetic effects but also by lifestyle, and environmental and cultural factors. Thus the genetic heritability of the obesity phenotypes accounts for up to 50% of the age- and gender-adjusted phenotypic variances. These results have been confirmed by overfeeding and negative energy balance studies. The effects of single segregating genes can be detected only under the correct experimental conditions. Most scientists in the area believe that these genes can be identified and that the DNA mutations associated with human obesities will be uncovered. Indeed, association and linkage studies, quantitative trait loci and positional cloning research strategies, and transgenic mouse models are sufficiently promising to suggest that these aims can be achieved. A review of the evidence reported thus far reveals that there are already four loci with strong evidence of linkage with obesity phenotypes in humans.

1996 The origins and consequences of obesity. Wiley, Chichester (Ciba Foundation Symposium 201) p 108–117

Scientists involved in the study of the causes of human obesity have become optimistic about the possibility of identifying the genes associated with the predisposition to this disease. There are good reasons to believe that this new enthusiasm is justified. Our growing understanding of the human genome, the high degree of homology between humans and common laboratory mammal models for a large number of genes and chromosomal regions, and the availability of a variety of technologies and tools to study and manipulate DNA in the laboratory are among the most important reasons for the present level of hope in the obesity research community. The genes associated with an increased susceptibility to gain weight and becoming obese will be eventually identified and characterized. However, the difficulties that will have to be overcome along this path should not be underestimated. There is still a long way to go because human obesity is not a simple entity.

Genetics, body mass and body fat

Most studies have used the body mass index (BMI) as the phenotype of interest. In a report published by the Carnegie Institute of Washington in 1923, C. B. Davenport described the first comprehensive attempt to understand the role of inheritance in human body mass for stature. Among his findings, normal weight parents will sometimes have children that become obese in adult life. He also observed the converse: obese parents frequently have children that have a normal weight when they become adults. However, his study demonstrated quite convincingly that BMI values were more similar among family members than among unrelated persons. Seventy years later, we know a little more about the familial aggregation of obesity but the progress made has not been breathtaking.

Heritability levels

The level of heritability has been considered in a large number of twin, adoption and family studies. The level of heritability is simply the fraction of the population variation in a trait (e.g. BMI) that can be explained by genetic transmission. Results obtained by a number of investigators indicate that the heritability level estimates depend on how the study was conducted and on the kinds of relatives upon which it is based. For instance, studies conducted with identical twins and fraternal twins or identical twins reared apart have yielded the highest heritability levels, with values clustering around 70% of the variation in BMI.

In contrast, the adoption studies have generated the lowest heritability estimates, i.e. up to about 30%. The family studies have generally found levels of heritability intermediate between the twin and the adoption study reports. A few investigations have included all or most of these kinds of relatives in the same analysis. Using analytical techniques developed to use all the information and maximum likelihood procedures, these studies have concluded that the true heritability estimate for BMI in large sample sizes was 25–40%. Recent surveys undertaken in Sweden and the USA with the collaboration of severely obese and morbidly obese subjects, together with information obtained on their parents, siblings and spouses, suggest that the genetic contribution to obesity may indeed be around 25–40% of the individual differences in BMI (Bouchard 1994).

The single gene hypothesis

Several studies based on familial data have reported that a single major gene for high body mass was segregating from the parents to their children. However, three studies did not find support for Mendelian transmission unless age and/or gender variations in the major gene were taken into account. From this small body of data, the trend seems to be for a major recessive gene accounting for about 20–25% of the variance (but with age-associated effects) with a gene frequency of about 0.2 (Price 1994, Bouchard 1994).

One can therefore estimate that the homozygotes for the putative recessive gene may represent about 5%, and in some cases up to 9%, of the population. These results must be viewed with great caution as they are based only on the unmeasured genotype approach and the genes that could be responsible for this effect have not yet been identified.

The risk of becoming obese

A number of studies have reported that obese children frequently had obese parents. Thus, in about 30% of the cases, both parents of obese children are obese, with a range in frequency of about 5–45%. It has also been estimated that about 25–35% of the obese cases occur in families with normal weight parents despite the fact that the risk of becoming obese is higher if the person had obese parents.

It is commonly observed that severely or morbidly obese persons are on the average about $10 \, \text{kg/m}^2$ heavier than their parents, brothers and sisters. These obese subjects are clearly much heavier than their obese relatives of the previous generation. Moreover, the prevalence of obesity is increasing from generation to generation in almost all populations that have been studied so far. However, we still have not established the level of risk (the so-called λ_R value) for a first-degree relative of an overweight, a moderately obese or a severely obese person in comparison to the population prevalence of the condition.

Response to experimental overfeeding

It is generally recognized that there are some individuals who are prone to excessive accumulation of fat and for whom losing weight represents a continuous battle. On the other hand, there are others who seem relatively well protected against such a menace. Differences in the sensitivity of individuals to gain fat when chronically exposed to positive energy balance and the dependence or independence of such differences on the genotype have been studied in order to examine whether genetic factors are involved. If the answer to both questions is affirmative then one can conclude that there is a significant genotype–environment interaction effect. The results of a complex experiment suggest that such an effect exists for total body fat and fat topography.

We studied 12 pairs of male identical twins who consumed a caloric surplus of 4.2 MJ per day, six days per week, for 100 days (Bouchard et al 1990). We observed significant increases in body weight and fat mass after the 353 MJ overfeeding protocol, and that there were considerable interindividual differences in the adaptation to excess calories. This variation was not randomly distributed, as indicated by the significant intrapair resemblance in response. For instance, there was at least threefold more variance in response between pairs than within pairs for gains in body weight and fat mass. These data demonstrate that some individuals are more at risk than others to gain fat (high responders) when surplus energy intake is set at the same level for everyone and when all subjects are confined to a sedentary lifestyle. The intra-identical twin pair response to the standardized caloric surplus suggests that the amount of fat stored is likely influenced by the genotype. However, the intrapair resemblance in the amount of weight or fat mass gained reached only about 0.50 as shown by the intraclass coefficients computed with the changes in these phenotypes with overfeeding. In other words, non-genetic factors were responsible for the intrapair variation in body mass and body fat gains.

Response to negative energy balance

Seven pairs of young adult male identical twins completed a negative energy balance protocol during which they exercised on cycle ergometers twice a day, nine out of 10 days, over a period of 93 days while being kept on a constant daily energy and nutrient intake (Bouchard et al 1994). The mean total energy deficit caused by exercise above the estimated energy cost of body weight maintenance reached 244 MJ. Baseline energy intake was estimated over a period of 17 days preceding the negative energy balance protocol. Mean body weight loss was 5.0 kg and it was entirely accounted for by the loss of fat mass. Fat-free mass was unchanged. Body energy losses reached 191 MJ, which represented about 78% of the estimated energy deficit. Decreases in metabolic rates and in the energy expenditure of activity not associated with the cycle ergometer protocol must have occurred to explain the difference between the estimated energy deficit and the body energy losses. Intrapair resemblance was observed for the changes in body weight, fat mass, per cent fat, body energy content and sum of 10 skinfolds. Even though there were large individual differences in response to the negative energy balance and exercise protocol, subjects with the same genotype were more alike in responses than subjects with different genotypes, particularly for body fat and body energy losses.

The main purpose of the study was to establish whether there were individual differences in response to negative energy balance solely produced by endurance exercise and to demonstrate whether these differences in response were greater between genotypes than for a given genotype. Changes in body mass, body fat and body energy content were characterized by more heterogeneity between twin pairs than within pairs. These results are remarkably similar to those that we reported earlier for body mass, body fat and body energy gains with 12 pairs of twins subjected to a 100-day overfeeding protocol (Bouchard et al 1990).

Single gene effects

We developed a summary of the human obesity gene map at the time of the October 1995 meeting of the North American Association for the Study of Obesity (Bouchard & Pérusse 1996). Support for a role of a gene in human obesity or variation in body fat content can currently be obtained from six lines of evidence:

(1) Mendelian disorders;
(2) single gene rodent models;

(3) quantitative trait loci (QTL) from crossbreeding experiments;
(4) transgenic and knock-out models;
(5) association studies;
(6) linkage studies.

This review addresses only the issue of excess body mass for height (BMI) or body fat content (per cent fat, fat mass, sum of a number of skinfolds) and does not deal with fat distribution phenotypes. More information can be found in previous reviews on these topics (Bouchard 1994, 1995a,b, Pérusse & Bouchard 1996).

The evidence drawn from these lines of clinical and experimental research can be summarized as follows. (1) Twelve loci linked to Mendelian disorders exhibiting obesity as one clinical feature are known. (2) Six loci causing obesity in rodent models of the disease have been recognized. (3) Eight chromosomal regions where QTL, identified by crossbreeding experiments with informative strains of mice, have been defined. (4) Ten candidate genes exhibiting a statistical association with BMI or body fat have been reported. (5) Nine loci found to be linked to a relevant phenotype are known and in four cases the evidence for linkage is rather strong. The latter are mapped to 2p25, 6p21.3, 7q33 and 20q12–13.11. (6) A number of studies have concluded that there is no association or linkage with a given marker or gene.

Table 1 lists those genes, loci or markers for which the evidence of an association or a linkage with obesity, BMI or body fat content is more robust. The list includes the loci from single gene rodent models, QTL from crossbreeding experiments, Mendelian disorders exhibiting obesity as one of the clinical features, and genes supported by robust evidence from association and linkage studies conducted on human populations. Four chromosomal arms (2p, 6p, 7q and 20q) are of particular interest because strong evidence for linkage with a marker in each of these regions has been reported. However, to date, no study has replicated the linkage for any of the four chromosomal areas. Other regions of considerable interest include 1p, 3p, 11p, 15q and possibly Xq. The compendium of markers and genes related to obesity or body fat is likely to grow significantly in the coming years.

Complexity of human obesity

Obesity is a complex multifactorial trait evolving under the interactive influences of dozens of effectors from the social, behavioural, physiological, metabolic, cellular and molecular domains. Segregation of the genes is not easily detected in familial or pedigree studies and whatever the influence of the genotype on the aetiology, it is generally attenuated or exacerbated by non-genetic factors.

In this context, the distinction between 'necessary' genes and 'susceptibility' genes is particularly relevant (Greenberg 1993). For instance, there are several examples of necessary loci resulting in obesity; that is, carriers of the deficient alleles have the disease (such as in Prader-Willi syndrome). However, they represent only a small fraction of the obese population. In contrast, a susceptibility gene is defined as one

TABLE 1 A summary of the human and rodent (human homologous regions) potentially associated or linked with obesity or body fat

Human chromosome	Locus
1p36–32	mouse Do1
1p35–31	mouse Db
1p35–31	rat Fa
1q31–32	D1S202
2p24–23	ApoB
2p25[a]	ACP1[a]
3p21	mouse Do2
3p13–12	BBS3
4p16.3	ACH
4q21	mouse Fat
5p14–12	mouse Do3
5q11–13	mouse Mob4
6p21	BF
6p21	GLO1
6p21.3[a]	TNFα[a]
7q31	mouse Ob
7q22–36	mouse Mob2
7q33[a]	KEL[a]
8q22–23	Cohen syndrome
9pter-32	mouse Do1
10q21–26	mouse Mob1
11p15.1	mouse Tubby
11p14-ter	mouse Mob1
11q13	BBS1
13q14.1–14.2	ESD
14q13–32	mouse Mob3
15q11.2–12	PWS
15q22.3–23	BBS4
16p13–11	mouse Mob1
16q21	BBS2
20	NZB QTL
20q11	PPCD
20q12–13.11[a]	ADA[a]
20q13	mouse Yellow
22q11	P1
Xq21	Choroideraemia
Xq21.1–22	WTS
Xq25–27	SGBS
Xq26–27	BFLS

[a]Loci showing the strongest evidence of linkage in human studies.
Weak associations or linkages are not included. Data from Bouchard & Pérusse (1996).

that increases susceptibility or risk for the disease but is not necessary for disease expression. An allele at a susceptibility loci may make it more likely that the carrier will become affected, but the presence of that allele is not sufficient by itself to explain the occurrence of the disease. It merely lowers the threshold for a person to develop the disease.

In addition, it is likely that body fat content is also modulated over the lifetime of a person by a variety of gene–environment interaction effects. These effects result from the fact that sensitivity to environmental exposures or lifestyle differences vary from individual to individual because of genetic individuality. Among the factors of interest here, one may include dietary fat, energy intake, level of habitual physical activity, smoking and alcohol intake. Moreover, even though data are lacking on the topic, it is obvious that gene–gene interaction effects need to be considered. However, little research bearing directly on this topic has been reported so far.

From the research currently available (e.g. Table 1), a good number of genes seem to have the capacity to cause obesity or increase the likelihood of becoming obese. The investigation of the molecular markers of obesity has barely begun. Many additional genes will surely be identified in the future such that the panel of the human obesity genes, based on association, linkage or animal models, will grow and become relatively large. This may be a reflection of how most human obesity cases come about. In other words, the susceptibility genotypes may result from allelic variations at a number of genes.

With the advent of a comprehensive human genetic linkage map, linkage studies with a large number of markers covering most of the chromosomal length of the human genome are likely to be helpful in the identification of putative obesity genes or chromosomal regions. Recent progress in animal genetics, transfection systems, transgenic animal models, recombinant DNA technologies applied to positional cloning and methods to identify QTL have given a new impetus to this field. The stage is now set for major advances to occur in the understanding of the genetic and molecular basis of complex diseases such as human obesity.

Acknowledgement

C. B. is supported by the Medical Research Council of Canada (PG-11811, MA-10499).

References

Bouchard C 1994 Genetics of obesity: overview and research directions. In: Bouchard C (ed) The genetics of obesity. CRC Press, Boca Raton, FL, p 223–233

Bouchard C 1995a Genetics of obesity: an update on molecular markers. Int J Obes 19:10S–13S

Bouchard C 1995b The genetics of obesity: from genetic epidemiology to molecular markers. Mol Med Today 1:45–50

Bouchard C, Pérusse L 1996 Current status of the human obesity gene map. Obes Res 4:81–90

Bouchard C, Tremblay A, Després J-P et al 1990 The response to long-term overfeeding in identical twins. New Engl J Med 322:1477–1482

Bouchard C, Tremblay A, Després J-P et al 1994 The response to exercise with constant energy intake in identical twins. Obes Res 2:400–410

Davenport CB 1923 Body build and its inheritance. Carnegie Institution of Washington, Publication No. 329

Greenberg DA 1993 Linkage analysis of "necessary" disease loci versus "susceptibility" loci. Am J Hum Genet 52:135–143

Pérusse L, Bouchard C 1996 Identification of genes contributing to excess body fat and fat distribution. In: Angel A (ed) Progress in obesity research. John Libbey, London, p 281–289

Price RA 1994 The case for single gene effects on human obesity. In: Bouchard C (ed) The Genetics of Obesity. CRC Press, Boca Raton, FL, p 93–107

DISCUSSION

Swinburn: You talked about genes explaining a third of the variance in BMI but is that independent of the variation in the test environment? In other words, would a more heterogeneous environment diminish the measured variance attributable to genetic make-up?

Bouchard: In the overfeeding experiment, we isolated the twins for four months under standardized conditions, i.e. there was no significant environmental heterogeneity (Bouchard et al 1990).

Swinburn: Presumably there would be an environmental effect in your adoption studies.

Bouchard: Possibly, but there is no way we can assess it because we did not perform any intervention studies with adoptees.

James: Theoretically, a varied environment would tend to diminish the apparent significance of the variance ascribable to obesity.

Bray: You mentioned susceptibility genes, but is there any evidence for protective genes?

Bouchard: Yes, I believe that there are such protective or resistance genes. For instance, some genes have been reported to be determinants of leanness or muscle mass in animal models (e.g. the ski gene). Indeed, the ski oncogene has been shown to induce myogenic differentiation and cause selective growth of skeletal muscle in transgenic mice (Sutrave et al 1990). We have begun to study these genes but we do not yet know their significance in human body composition.

Ravussin: It is important that you have been able to follow the subjects for five years after overfeeding because in other overfeeding studies there has not been a follow-up of the subjects. The weight gain during overfeeding was related to metabolic factors (which are likely to be genetically determined), but to what extent is the variability in weight gain over the five-year period (0.7 kg/year on average) related to these same metabolic factors? In other words, do these metabolic factors play a role when overfeeding is not clamped?

Bouchard: We have not assessed that specifically. However, correlations between weight gain during the overfeeding period and the weight gain over the subsequent five years were weak.

Ravussin: Does this mean that the effect of the environment is much stronger than the genetic component identified by clamping the environment?

Bouchard: In my opinion it means that we were able to identify some types of genetic effect during the standardized overfeeding protocol but that different systems, probably related to individual differences in lifestyle, were operating during the post-overfeeding recovery. Even though there was a twin resemblance in the post-overfeeding weight changes, the effect was generally less strong than during the response to the overfeeding protocol.

Hitman: I have a comment on the power to detect associations and/or linkage between polymorphic markers and obesity. Some groups are doing sib pair analyses and looking for determinants of obesity in only 50–100 families. With this small number, one might conclude that a particular locus is not linked with disease. However, this is likely to be a false negative unless the candidate gene under study accounts for the majority of the variance to the disease.

The search for a locus for visceral fat deposition or obesity is likely to require the analysis of large numbers of families. For example, I am part of a collaborative group in the UK funded by the British Diabetic Association for collecting sib pairs with the aim of identifying genes involved in the susceptibility to type 2 diabetes. We have calculated that 600–1000 sib pairs are required to enable the identification of a locus that doubles the risk of diabetes. If you're dealing with a common trait, then you have got to have the power to find it.

Allison: I agree. From the point of view of designing future studies, the ability and necessity of pooling the sib pair data sets will become greater and greater. Take Lander & Kruglyak's recent paper in Nature Genetics, for example, which highlights the necessity to set appropriate P values (Lander & Kruglyak 1995). The problem is that it is not just one marker that is being tested. The entire length of the genome is being tested, which results in a vastly increased α value. They pointed out that before something can be declared as being significant at the 0.05 level (genome wide), a P value of 2.2×10^{-5} is required. That P value can then be put in a power analysis and it takes the 600–1000 pairs Graham Hitman mentioned multiplied by a factor of about four.

Roberts: The P values of the human linked obesity genes are marginal in all the papers that I have seen.

Hitman: This is extremely important, but what has amazed me is that, in contrast to traditional statistics, $P < 0.05$ or $P < 0.01$ in linkage studies of sib pairs is not significant. $P < 0.001$ is only barely significant for linkage analysis, and some groups would suggest a P value of less than $P < 0.0001$ should be adopted. In the literature there has been some noticeable false positives. For example, many years ago, a group claimed to have identified a gene for manic depression in a large family with a LOD score of $+3$, which represents $P = 0.001$. However, subsequently within the family just two cases changed categories from normal to manic depression and the significance was lost.

Stunkard: Could you comment on the strategy of looking for single obesity genes versus genes for what you have called intermediate phenotypes, i.e. the metabolic precursors of obesity?

Bouchard: It is essentially the same approach. For instance, we have tried to define sub-phenotypes of obesity—such as those pertaining to energy expenditure, nutrient intake or nutrient partitioning—so that we could get clearer signals, with less noise, for linkage or association studies. However, the main point is that it is much more demanding in terms of amount of laboratory work, although the pay-off is potentially much greater.

Ferro-Luzzi: Is anything known about the way in which these genes operate in terms of energy, for example? Also, in your twin study was there any difference in weight gain between the twins?

Bouchard: We have been studying about 35 candidate genes that may be associated with energy metabolism and nutrient partitioning characteristics. So far, the results have been disappointing, probably because we are limited by our understanding of the biology and the physiopathology of obesity in our attempts to select these candidate genes. Therefore, we have had to resort to a genome-wide search. This approach involves the typing of markers that are selected to cover the whole genome at regular space intervals. This approach may provide us with linkage results with chromosomal areas that potentially contain genes impacting on energy metabolism and other relevant phenotypes.

In response to your second question, there was a heterogeneity in weight gain between the twins: the range was 4–13 kg weight gain. On the average, 63% of the energy surplus was recovered as body substance gains (Dériaz et al 1993). We have calculated that the mean body weight gain reached after the 100 day overfeeding treatment represented about 55% of the expected maximal weight gain if the overfeeding conditions had prevailed indefinitely (Dériaz et al 1993).

References

Bouchard C, Tremblay A, Després JP et al 1990 The response to long-term overfeeding in identical twins. New Engl J Med 322:1477–1482

Dériaz O, Tremblay A, Bouchard C 1993 Non-linear weight gain with long term overfeeding in man. Obesity Res 1:179–185

Lander E, Kruglyak L 1995 Genetic dissection of complex traits: guidelines for interpreting and reporting linkage results. Nat Genet 11:241–247

Sutrave P, Kelly AM, Hughes SH 1990 ski can cause selective growth of skeletal muscle in transgenic mice. Genes Dev 4:1462–1472

Nutritional influences in early life upon obesity and body proportions

Alan A. Jackson, S. C. Langley-Evans and H. D. McCarthy

Department of Human Nutrition, University of Southampton, Biomedical Sciences Building, Bassett Crescent East, Southampton SO16 7PX, UK

Abstract. Close relationships exist between patterns of intra-uterine growth and the risk of ischaemic heart disease, hypertension, diabetes, insulin-resistance syndrome, obesity and some cancers later in life. Earlier studies placed emphasis on low birth weight and reduced growth, but it is now clear that disproportions in early growth are of great importance. Disproportion may be identified as disproportions of fetal and placental growth (and the risk of high blood pressure), or in head circumference, length and weight. It is hypothesized that the availability of nutrients at different times during gestation, by interacting with the maternal and fetal hormonal profile, predisposes to different patterns of growth. The same interaction programmes critical metabolic functions and determines the metabolic capacity at all later ages. People who were exposed to severe undernutrition during the Dutch hunger winter showed increased adiposity if the exposure was during early pregnancy, but decreased adiposity if the exposure was during late pregnancy. In men born in the UK, those with evidence of retarded fetal growth had significantly greater waist/hip circumference ratios for any given body mass index (the ratio fell with increasing weight at one year of age). In Mexican-Americans and non-Hispanic Caucasian Americans, people in the lowest third of birth weight had more truncal fat than those in the highest third. Offspring of rats exposed to marginally reduced protein intakes during pregnancy manifest a similar pattern of growth and metabolic change to that seen in humans, with perturbations of appetite and body fat patterning. Studies in rats suggest that programming of the hypothalamus, especially the hypothalamic-pituitary-adrenal axis might be the mechanism through which these changes are brought about.

1996 The origins and consequences of obesity. Wiley, Chichester (Ciba Foundation symposium 201) p 118–137

Growth represents a net increase in the energy content of the body (Jackson & Wootton 1990). Obesity may be characterized as the net accumulation of energy, in excess of that which can usefully be deposited as functional lean tissue, as excessive adipose tissue. Growth is a sequential process that is ordered in time, target seeking and fundamentally driven by a demand encoded in the genome. The partitioning of nutrients between linear growth, lean tissue deposition and adipose tissue formation patterns the shape, size and composition of the body. The patterning is differentially

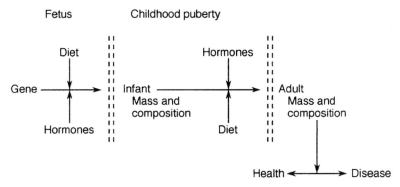

FIG. 1.   The maintenance of health or the risk of disease in an adult is determined by the interplay of their genetic potential and their nutritional and hormonal factors with their size and body composition. At each stage of development these factors interact, although the magnitude of the relative effect of the different factors varies with maturity and the stage of development.

sensitive with age to the interaction of a balance of forces that may vary with different stages of maturation. Amongst these forces, the major influences are the achieved size and body composition, the hormonal milieu and the amount and pattern of available nutrients (Fig. 1) (Wootton & Jackson 1996).

Karlberg has introduced a model of postnatal growth in which the dominant controlling influences are seen to act during three discrete, but related, periods: fetal/infant; childhood; and pubertal phases. It is thus called the ICP model of growth (Karlberg et al 1994). Within this model, fetal and infant growth are primarily limited by the availability of water, oxygen or nutrients either to the mother, the placenta or the fetus/infant. Childhood growth is driven by the growth hormone–insulin-like growth factor axis, but it may be constrained by nutrient availability. The dominant influence during puberty is the effect of sex steroids on metabolism. The extent to which the effect of an adverse influence upon growth can be reversed may be dependent upon the timing, severity and duration of the influence, with the times of maximum change being particularly sensitive to irreversible damage. However, the points of intersection of the different phases of growth also represent critical times when the system is unusually sensitive to stress or perturbations (Waterlow 1994).

The proposal by Barker and colleagues that early growth may be associated with long-term effects on metabolic and physiological function which increase the risk of disease in later life was initially identified with constraints of growth represented by small size at birth (Barker 1994). As the hypothesis has been progressively refined, it has become clear that, rather than simply size, disproportions in growth are important markers for risk and are likely to be a reflection of the process of programming (Barker 1992, 1994). Disproportions are a result of a difference in the partitioning of nutrients, which may be between the mother and the products of conception, the placenta and the fetus, or within the fetus amongst different tissues as precedence is given to the growth

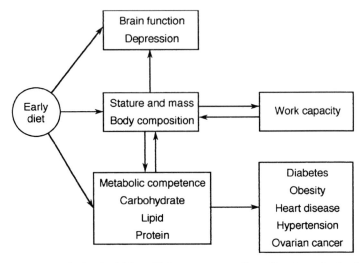

FIG. 2. Nutrition during fetal life and infancy may contribute directly to the development of brain function, the size, shape and composition of the body, and to the metabolic competence to handle macronutrients. The interaction of these factors determines physical function and work capacity, and has also been directly associated with the risk of developing chronic disease during adult life.

of the brain, if necessary at the expense of the growth of visceral or somatic tissues (Jackson & Wootton 1990).

Lucas has suggested that the term programming be used to identify a process whereby a stimulus or insult, at a critical period of development, has long-lasting or lifelong significance (Lucas 1991). This builds on the concept of sensitive periods in development, and others have used terms such as entraining to carry a similar connotation (McCance & Widdowson 1974, Dietz 1994). Barker has reviewed the cumulative evidence that the shape and size of the newborn may be related to increased risk of developing cardiovascular disease, diabetes mellitus, obstructive airways disease, depression or ovarian cancer (Barker 1994). Mechanistically, the implication is that at critical stages during early life an upper limit is set for fundamental aspects of metabolic competence. At all times thereafter the upper limit defines the maximum capacity available to cope with a metabolic stress and therefore function is constrained within this upper limit of metabolic competence. The upper limit may simply be determined by impaired growth and therefore reduced size or more subtle effects upon function because an upper limit has been set for the expression of genes for key metabolic pathways or processes (Jackson & Wootton 1990, Jackson 1992). The interaction of impaired metabolic competence with an environment that challenges the upper limit of the limited physiological capacity increases the risk of pathology developing (Fig. 2). In this sense the development of obesity may represent a special case of a general phenomenon in which differential partitioning of nutrients leads to disproportionate growth of adipose tissue and the clinically recognizable syndrome of obesity.

The purpose of this presentation is to review human evidence that relates programming to the development of adiposity or obesity; to consider the extent to which the process might be usefully modelled within animal experiments; and to consider the extent to which the animal models might provide clues to common mechanisms for the experimental and human situations.

Human evidence

The most widely quoted study that relates nutritional exposure during early life to a changed risk of obesity at later ages is that reported by Ravelli et al (1976) on the Dutch hunger winter of 1944–1945. The frequency of obesity (weight for height in excess of 120% of the median) was determined in 307 700 military inductees at 19 years of age. The men were grouped according to the period when they were born, whether they were born in the famine or control areas, and the time of the famine in relation to the period of gestation. Those individuals whose mothers had been exposed to famine during pregnancy showed the most obvious effects, with an important difference between those exposed during early pregnancy compared with those exposed during late pregnancy (Fig. 3). Young men exposed during late pregnancy had a significantly lower rate of obesity, interpreted as a constraint on the development of the number of adipocytes, and hence fat tissue mass, during the period of maximum growth in the third trimester. These observations fit in with the general concept of nutritional deprivation during the third trimester, and the increased risk of being underweight or wasted at birth, with high morbidity and mortality. The general observation that subsequent growth, body shape and size appeared to track with age (i.e. the tendency for thin individuals to remain thin, or fat individuals to remain fat) conforms with evidence from other studies (Dietz 1994).

The effect of exposure during the third trimester contrasted sharply with the remarkable observations on those who were exposed during the first two trimesters. For those in whom exposure to famine was during early pregnancy there was a twofold increased frequency of obesity compared with the control. For this group weight at birth was no different to normal, but as adults they tended to become fat. Subsequent studies have suggested evidence of a more generalized disturbance of metabolic function, for both men and women in this group, of which a tendency to obesity was but one manifestation. The effect of exposure to famine early in pregnancy was attributed by the authors to an influence being exerted upon differentiation of the hypothalamic centres that regulate food intake and growth. There are important points to note about this study. The level of food deprivation that was associated with an effect was severe: a reduction in energy intake from an average of 1400 to only 700 kcal/d. Further, care is required with the interpretation because this degree of nutritional deprivation carries with it wider metabolic consequences, amenorrhea, increased maternal morbidity and mortality, and increased fetal, neonatal and infant

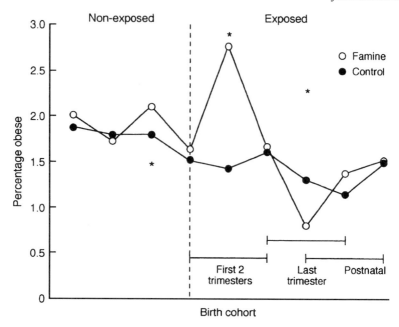

FIG. 3.   The frequency of obesity (weight-for-height greater than 120% of the median) in
307 700 military inductees aged at least 19 years, who had been conceived around the time of
the Dutch hunger winter in 1944–1946. There was a twofold increase in the frequency of
obesity in those who were exposed during early pregnancy compared with controls. In
contrast, in those exposed during late pregnancy the frequency of obesity was significantly
reduced (data from Ravelli et al 1976). *$P < 0.05$.

loss. Therefore, the population that survives is highly selected and cannot necessarily
be considered to be representative.

   The classical approach to differentiating the effect of intra-uterine environment from
genetic factors has been to carry out twin studies. This approach has been used in
attempting to identify whether birth weight tracks into adulthood independently of
genetic factors. Allison et al (1995) compared birth weight with self-reported adult
height and weight in an analysis of about 13 000 twin pairs. Differences in birth
weight correlated with adult height and adult weight, but not adult body mass index
(BMI), leading to the conclusion that the intra-uterine environment had an enduring
impact on adult height independent of weight, but not weight independent of height.
Dietz (1994) has reviewed the evidence for critical periods in childhood for the
development of obesity. He identifies three periods of increased risk: the prenatal
period; the period in childhood of adiposity rebound; and adolescence. He characterizes the 'entrainment' of a predisposition to fatness and the sexual dimorphism of fat
patterning, which might become most evident during adolescence. In his review he
does not refer directly to the ICP model of growth, nor the potential summative

consequence of effects acting during each different period, but his comments imply an effect of nutritional state on the development of fat mass and the influence of fat mass itself on metabolic function. The review adds to the impression that within a multifactorial condition there is the need to create a synthesis for the effects of metabolic demand, activity, appetite, hormonal profile and body composition.

Central fat deposition

Although BMI or measures of total adiposity show important relations with measures of risk, there are much stronger relations with the abdominal or visceral partitioning of adipose tissue (Lean et al 1995). However, there are few human data which might be used to explore the possibility that fat patterning is programmed.

Law et al (1992) have explored the possibility that abdominal fatness, rather than simply increased weight, is associated with retarded growth in fetal life and infancy. They followed a population of 845 men born between 1920 and 1930 in whom the weight at birth and weight at one year had been recorded by the health visitor, and 239 men born between 1935 and 1943 in whom the size at birth had been measured in detail. The waist/hip circumference ratio (WHR) was measured as an index of abdominal fatness. They found that the WHR rose with increasing obesity (measured by BMI). However, a higher WHR was associated with decreased growth during early life and infancy. Further, for any level of obesity there was more abdominal fat in men who weighed less at birth. These data conform with the general idea that during postnatal life weight and adiposity is entrained, but also show a separate effect of early growth on fat patterning. Thus, the relation between early growth and WHR, corrected for current BMI, suggests that abdominal fatness is programmed and inversely related to early growth. This interpretation would fit well with the observations from the Dutch hunger winter (Ravelli et al 1976).

Further support for this proposal may be derived from the San Antonio Heart Study in which the prevalence of the insulin resistance syndrome was determined in 562 subjects aged 30 years on average, who were either Mexican-American or non-Hispanic Caucasian Americans (Valdez et al 1994). For both groups there was a close relationship between birth tertile and the presence of insulin-resistance syndrome, which was much greater in the Mexican-Americans for any particular birth tertile. Moreover, there was an important interaction between birth tertile and current BMI with the prevalence of insulin-resistance syndrome for the population as a whole. The response was graded. Thus, there was no insulin-resistance syndrome for those in the highest third of birth who were in the lowest third for BMI as adults, compared with a prevalence of 25% for those in the lowest third for birth weight but the highest third for BMI as adults. When adjusted for age, gender and ethnicity, birth weight tertile was closely associated with current truncal adiposity, measured as the ratio of subscapular to triceps skinfold ratio, but only weakly to BMI and WHR.

Attempts to measure intra-abdominal fat mass with greater precision have included determinations with magnetic resonance imaging, which has been found to correlate closely with waist circumference. In 46 women aged 32 years, current body weight related to birth weight (Han et al 1996). However, in a multiple regression analysis there was a statistically significant negative relationship between birth weight and waist circumference once appropriate correction had been made for current weight.

From these data it is possible to conclude that early growth is related to later shape and size. There is probably entraining of weight related to an adverse environment and poor growth during the third trimester. When reduced growth during fetal life and infancy is associated with increased BMI in later life, obesity is especially associated with an increased risk of abdominal fat patterning. Fat mass and visceral mass relate to birth weight, but there is a need for much more detailed information on the relationships between body composition and fat patterning during early life, and the interactions of growth and body composition during childhood and later adolescence with the risk of obesity and central adiposity during adulthood. Although the most dramatic changes have been identified with severe nutritional deprivation, they can also be seen within a normal range of birth weights in people who have otherwise been considered to be normal.

Animal models

In modelling the process of programming of obesity, there is the need to identify evidence for the effect of early nutritional manipulations that have modified subsequent appetite, growth, body composition and fat patterning. The literature contains a number of examples in which extreme dietary manipulations have exerted marked effects upon physiological and metabolic function. The studies of McCance & Widdowson (1974) clearly established the general principle that diet during early life influences the rate of growth and development of form and function at later stages, and they identified the susceptibility of hypothalamic function during critical periods in early pregnancy. The idea that any particular tissue would be most sensitive to an insult (with an irreversible effect) if the insult were to act during the period of most rapid cell division has dominated thinking in this area (Winick & Noble 1966). Whilst establishing basic principles, each of these models has used extremes of dietary manipulations. Thus, it can be shown that specific appetite for macro-nutrients in the offspring can be markedly influenced by the macronutrient intake of the mother during pregnancy and lactation (Leprohon & Anderson 1980). Sexual dimorphism in growth, body composition, fat patterning and thyroid hormonal profiles were seen in the offspring from pregnancies where the total food intake was reduced to 50% during the first two thirds of pregnancy. The female offspring became relatively obese, whereas the males had evidence of preferential deposition of adipose tissue in intra-abdominal sites (Anguita et al 1993).

A model for fetal origins of adult disease

The most remarkable aspect of the epidemiological work carried out by Barker and colleagues (Barker 1994) is that the important observations have related to variations in function which lead to subsequent pathology. This pathology occurs within ranges of maternal food intakes, birth weights and growths during infancy that have in the past been considered to encompass a normal range function (Barker 1994). Therefore, we have been interested in developing an animal model with which to explore the possibility that relatively modest changes in maternal intake during pregnancy might exert an influence upon metabolic function in the offspring. The level of protein in the maternal diet has been shown to influence the development and function of the endocrine pancreas (Dahri et al 1995). We have varied the protein intake during pregnancy in a range from adequate (about 20% protein), through marginally adequate, to frankly inadequate (about 6% protein), and we have demonstrated a graded response to the programming of a wide range of metabolic functions. We gave dams different levels of protein in the diet before and during pregnancy. At birth, they received normal laboratory chow and the offspring were weaned to chow diets. Therefore, the only exposure to nutritional constraint was prenatal. With this model there is disproportionate growth of the fetus and placenta. The altered body proportions in the pups are indicative of selective protection of brain growth at the expense of viscera and somatic tissues (Levy & Jackson 1993, Langley-Evans et al 1996a). Postnatal growth is near normal except at the extremes of maternal dietary protein (6%) (Langley & Jackson 1994). When offspring are allowed macronutrient self-selection up to 100 days of age, the animals exposed to 9% protein *in utero* are significantly heavier than those exposed to 18% protein (McCarthy et al 1994). The pattern of macronutrients selected is modified in the 9% protein group, with the males and females showing different responses. Females exposed to 9% protein have statistically significantly increased adipose tissue in all regions, with increases of around 100% for intra-abdominal sites. Males have highly significant increases in omental and mesenteric sites (McCarthy et al 1994). Prenatal exposure to low protein diets alters glucose tolerance (Pickard et al 1996, Dahri et al 1995). There is a graded increase in blood pressure as the maternal dietary protein is decreased, which is identifiable from four weeks of age and persists for life (Langley & Jackson 1994). There are alterations in antioxidant capability, inflammatory responses and immune function (Langley et al 1994). Hepatic function is modulated with the appearance of direct effects upon the development of hepatic zonation (Desai et al 1995). Thus, the maternal protein intake exerts wide-ranging effects, which are specific and are not generalized, and they represent fundamental changes in aspects of metabolic competence of which changes in growth and body composition are one manifestation.

Programming of the hypothalamic-pituitary-adrenal axis

McCance & Widdowson (1974) have suggested that the critical influence exerted by nutrition during fetal life is on hypothalamic function. Edwards and colleagues have suggested that blood pressure might be critically determined through the maternal glucocorticoid axis (Edwards et al 1993). In dams given low protein diets, the activity of placental 11βOH-steroid dehydrogenase is reduced by about one-third,

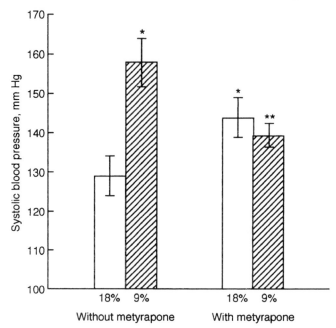

FIG. 4.   Pregnant rats were given casein diets that provided either 9% or 18% protein, and half of each group received either metyrapone (10 mg/kg body weight per day) or vehicle. At delivery the dams were placed on laboratory chow and the pups were weaned to laboratory chow. The blood pressure of pups from each group ($n = 8$–19) were measured by the tailcuff method. Data are means, S.E.M., *$P < 0.05$ vs 18% control, **$P < 0.05$ vs 9% control.

which increases the likelihood of fetal over-exposure to maternal glucocorticoids (Langley-Evans et al 1996d). The extent to which maternal glucocorticoids might directly contribute to programming fetal metabolism has been explored. Maternal administration of metyrapone abolishes the effect of maternal low protein diets upon the blood pressure of offspring (Fig. 4) (Langley-Evans et al 1996b). This provides direct evidence that part of the effect of maternal diet upon fetal programming might be attributed to changes in the hypothalamic-pituitary-adrenal axis in the mother and/ or the fetus. Further support comes from the observations that maternal low protein diets induce modulation of glucocorticoid-sensitive enzymes in the fetal brain and liver (Langley-Evans et al 1996c). There is differential regulation of glucocorticoid receptors in the brain, liver and aorta, and offspring of dams given 9% protein during pregnancy do not show a diurnal pattern of adrenocorticotrophic hormone in blood, although diurnal changes in cortisol concentrations are maintained (Langley-Evans et al 1996c).

Conclusions

The nutritional determinants of the function of a mother and her fetus have to allow for at least four different levels of interaction:

(1) maternal shape and size, which are a reflection of her genetic endowment, but may also represent the effect of intergenerational influences during her own early growth and development;
(2) maternal body composition, which relates to her chronic food intake and patterns of activity;
(3) maternal plane of nutrition, which will determine the nature of her metabolic adaptation; and
(4) current maternal food intake, which will determine the set of her homeostatic mechanisms at any particular point in time.

Within these interactions it may be difficult to differentiate genetic from intergenerational effects. For example, when the genetic model of rodent hypertension, the spontaneously hypertensive rat, is cross-fostered during lactation, the pups have a lifelong blood pressure that is in the normal range. The composition of the maternal milk appears to exert a major effect upon the development of 'genetically predisposed' increased blood pressure (McCarty & Fields-Okotcha 1994). Thus, the early life origins of adult disease are set in train through an interaction amongst maternal body composition, prenatal diet and postnatal diet (Figs 1 & 2). These directly determine the shape, size and body composition of the individual, and they interact with the hormonal profile and nutrient intake of the individual. There is clear evidence for hypothalamic programming playing a part in the process, with evidence for a contribution from glucocorticoids, growth hormone, thyroid hormone, sex steroids and the autonomic nervous system (Barker 1994).

Early growth determines later shape and size, which is probably a reflection of the adjustments required to protect brain growth and function over visceral function or somatic growth. Shape and size is related to metabolic function, and entraining of weight can be related to a severe insult during the third trimester. We can infer that at least two important processes take place during early life which will later interact with the lifestyle of the adult. During pregnancy the growth trajectory of the fetus is set at an early stage, based upon the interaction of the genetic profile with the maternal hormonal milieu and the local availability of oxygen and nutrients. This sets or programmes the 'fetal metabolic demand', probably at the level of the hypothalamus. During late gestation and infancy the achieved growth is a balance between the programmed fetal demand and the hormonal milieu (maternal and fetal) and the availability of energy and nutrients to the fetus. This interaction sets or programmes 'fetal or infant metabolic competence'. The metabolic competence determines the extent to which an individual might withstand an adverse lifestyle. A constrained metabolic competence increases the risk of metabolic dysfunction, and hence either increased total fat or central fat deposition.

Acknowledgements

We thank the Biotechnology and Biological Science Research Council, the Medical Research Council, the Wellcome Trust and the British Heart Foundation.

References

Allison DB, Paultre F, Heymsfield SB, Pi-Sunyer FX 1995 Is the intra-uterine period *really* a critical period for the development of adiposity? Int J Obes 19:397–402

Anguita RM, Sigulem DM, Sawaya AL 1993 Intrauterine food restriction is associated with obesity in young rats. J Nutr 123:1421–1428

Barker D JP 1992 Fetal and infant origins of adult disease. British Medical Association, London

Barker D JP 1994 Mothers, babies and disease in later life. British Medical Association, London

Dahri S, Reusens B, Remacle C, Hoet J J 1995 Nutritional influences on pancreatic development and potential links with non-insulin-dependent diabetes. Proc Nutr Soc 54:345–356

Desai M, Crowther NJ, Ozanne SE, Lucas A, Hales CN 1995 Adult glucose and lipid metabolism may be programmed during fetal life. Biochem Soc Trans 23:331–335

Dietz WH 1994 Critical periods in childhood for the development of obesity. Am J Clin Nutr 59:955–959

Edwards CRW, Benediktsson R, Lindsay RS, Seckl JR 1993 Dysfunction of placental glucocorticoid barrier: link between fetal environment and adult hypertension. Lancet 341:355–357

Han TS, McNeill G, Baras P, Foster MA 1996 Waist circumference predicts intra-abdominal fat mass better than waist-hip ratio in women. Proc Nutr Soc 55:85 (abstr)

Jackson AA, Wootton SA 1990 The energy requirements of growth and catch-up growth. In Schurch B, Scrimshaw NS (eds) Activity, energy expenditure and energy requirements of infants and children. International Dietary Energy Consultative Group, Lausanne, Switzerland, p 185–214

Jackson AA 1992 How can early diet influence later disease? British Nutrition Foundation. Nutrition Bulletin 17:23–30

Karlberg J, Jalil F, Lam B, Low L, Yeung CY 1994 Linear growth retardation in relation to the three phases of growth. Eur J Clin Nutr 48:25S–44S

Langley SC, Jackson AA 1994 Increased systolic blood pressure in adult rats caused by fetal exposure to maternal low protein diets. Clin Sci 86:217–222

Langley SC, Seakins M, Grimble RF, Jackson AA 1994 The acute phase response of adult rats is altered by *in utero* exposure to maternal low protein diets. J Nutr 124:1588–1596

Langley-Evans SC, Gardner DS, Jackson AA 1996a Association of disproportionate growth of fetal rats in late gestation with raised systolic blood pressure in later life. J Reprod Fertil 106:307–312

Langley-Evans SC, Phillips G J, Gardner DS, Jackson AA 1996b Role of glucocorticoids in programming of maternal diet-induced hypertension in the rat. J Nutr 126:1578–1585

Langley-Evans SC, Gardner DS, Jackson AA 1996c Role of glucocorticoids in programming of maternal diet-induced hypertension in the rat. J Nutr Biochem 7:173–178

Langley-Evans SC, Phillips G J, Benediktsson R et al 1996d Protein intake in pregnancy, placental glucocorticoid metabolism and the programming of hypertension in the rat. Placenta 17:169–172

Law CM, Barker D JP, Osmond C, Fall CHD, Simmonds S J 1992 Early growth and abdominal fatness in adult life. J Epidemiol Community Health 46:184–186

Lean ME J, Han TS, Morrison CE 1995 Waist circumference as a measure for indicating need for weight management. Br Med J 311:158–161

Leprohon CE, Anderson GH 1980 Maternal diet affects feeding behaviour of self-selecting weanling rats. Physiol Behav 24:553–559

Levy L, Jackson AA 1993 Modest restriction of dietary protein during pregnancy in the rat: fetal and placental growth. J Dev Physiol 19:113–118

Lucas A 1991 Programming by early nutrition in man. In: The childhood environment. Wiley, Chichester (Ciba Found Symp 156) p 38–55

McCance RA, Widdowson EM 1974 The determinants of growth and form. Proc Roy Soc Biol 185:1–17

McCarthy HD, Pickard CL, Speed J, Jackson AA 1994 Sexual dimorphism of macronutrient selection and regional adipose tissue accumulation following *in utero* exposure to maternal low-protein diet. Proc Nutr Soc 53:172A

McCarty R, Fields-Okotcha C 1994 Timing of preweanling maternal effects on development of hypertension in SHR rats. Physiol & Behav 55:839–844

Pickard CL, McCarthy HD, Browne RF, Jackson AA 1996 Altered insulin response to a glucose load in rats following exposure to a low protein diet in *utero*. Proc Nutr Soc 55:44 (abstr)

Ravelli G, Stein Z, Susser MW 1976 Obesity in young men after famine exposure *in utero* and early infancy. N Engl J Med 295:349–353

Valdez R, Athens MA, Thompson GH, Bradshaw BS, Stern MP 1994 Birthweight and adult health outcomes in a biethnic population in the USA. Diabetologia 37:624–631

Waterlow JC 1994 Summary of causes and mechanisms of linear growth retardation. Eur J Clin Nutr (suppl 1) 48:2105

Winick M, Noble A 1966 Cellular response in rats during malnutrition. J Nutr 89:300–306

Wootton SA, Jackson AA 1996 Influence of under-nutrition in early life on growth, body composition and metabolic competence. In: Ulijaszek SJ, Henry CJK (eds) Long term consequences of early environments. Cambridge University Press, Cambridge, p 107–121

DISCUSSION

Björntorp: The imprinting of androgens is a well-studied phenomenon. There may also be glucocorticoid imprinting of the hypothalamic-pituitary-adrenal (HPA) axis during intra-uterine life. What is your opinion of the suggestion that offspring exposed to glucocorticoids *in utero* develop a hypersensitive HPA axis later in life?

Jackson: I have suggested that the exposure of the fetus to maternal glucocorticoids may programme the sensitivity of the HPA axis. This clearly opens up the possibility of intergenerational effects in imprinting, which some may like to interpret as genetic effects or familial effects. There are ways of communicating through generations other than via genes. There is evidence that the insulin-like growth factor axis is similarly programmed, and this may also be true for the thyroid axis and the autonomic nervous system. Therefore, this may be a more general effect.

Björntorp: Is it possible to explain the hyperandrogenicity of women with visceral obesity by imprinting?

Jackson: One could develop theoretical scenarios that enable this to be included in the model, but we need more experimental evidence before we can determine if it is appropriate to include it in the model.

Björntorp: Could you elaborate on the glucocorticoid receptor data?

Jackson: Changes in glucocorticoid receptors have been measured in the hypothalamus, hippocampus and thoracic aorta, and liver. Increased specific binding is seen for type II receptors in the hippocampus and thoracic aorta in animals exposed to 9% casein diets *in utero* (Langley-Evans et al 1996a).

Forrester: Is it possible to distinguish between non-genetic intergenerational effects and genetic heritabilities?

Bouchard: There are methods that separate genetic and non-genetic heritabilities, the latter of which are sometimes referred to as cultural heritabilities. However, these methods are relatively insensitive. For example, the degree of genetic heritability can be separated from total heritability values using, for instance, adoption data. Other mechanisms may also be operating; for instance, genetic imprinting, which can be identified at the DNA level, may result in an altered pattern of expression that will not be detectable in conventional genetic epidemiology studies.

Hitman: The St. Petersburg Study was set up to investigate the thrifty phenotype hypothesis by examining people exposed to extreme famine in World War II. John Yudkin's group presented preliminary data at the British Diabetic Association Meeting suggesting no relationship between birth weight and factors associated with insulin resistance. This, however, does not necessarily disprove an association between birth weight and insulin resistance, which may only be present under certain environmental conditions or in ethnic groups with a genetic predisposition. The birth weight data can also be interpreted as evidence for the thrifty genotype hypothesis, i.e. in the face of maternal intra-uterine nutritional deficiency it is only those fetuses who carry the insulin-resistance gene who survive in adverse environmental conditions. The truth probably lies in-between the thrifty phenotype and genotype hypothesis. There is the need to design definitive experiments to tease out the answer. I personally favour a gene-to-environment interaction to explain the association between low birth weight and the insulin-resistance syndrome.

Allison: I would like to expand on the issue of whether genetic methods allow genetic and intra-uterine effects to be teased apart. Twin studies may be helpful in trying to resolve this because both dizygotic and monozygotic twins share the same intra-uterine environment. Also, many of the similarities between birth weight and adult characteristics, such as body mass index (BMI), may be due to genetic tracking. We published a paper in which we described the difference in birth weight among monozygotic twins (Allison et al 1995). If the intra-uterine environmental factors that influence birth weight have an enduring impact on adult BMI, then a correlation between the intrapair difference in birth weight and the intrapair difference in adult BMI should be observed. We did not observe such a correlation, suggesting that the tracking from birth weight to BMI was due to a genetic effect.

Bray: Birth weights of monozygotic and dizygotic twins have the same correlations ($r^2 = 0.6$), but during the first five years the concordance increases for monozygotic twins to $r^2 = 0.9$, whereas the dizygotic twins diverge further. Therefore, it may be possible to tease these things out, but it would be a challenge.

Allison: But there may still be differences in birth weights because twins do not really share the intra-uterine environment, rather they compete for it.

McKeigue: We have some relevant results from a study in Uppsala in which we tested the Barker hypothesis (Leon et al 1996, Lithell et al 1996). We studied a cohort of 1300 Swedish men with measurements at birth and follow-up to 87 years. The conclusions we reached about the role of genetics and the environment were that: (1) the relationship between birth weight and blood pressure is almost certainly not genetic; and (2) the relationship between the ponderal index and insulin resistance could be genetic. These results can be easily explained. We saw a relationship between birth weight and blood pressure, as in Barker's data. However, that relationship becomes much stronger when you look only at those who are above the median for adult height. We know from studies of the Dutch famine that the reduction in birth weight of those exposed to the famine did not affect their adult height (Stein et al 1975). Effectively, if you look at small babies who become tall adults, you are looking at a group who are deprived for nutritional reasons as opposed to people who are genetically small. In this subgroup, the relationship between birth weight and blood pressure becomes stronger than any of the relationships published by Barker's group (Law et al 1993). We have found that there is a strong relationship between the ponderal index and post-load insulin levels. However, there are examples of both animals and humans with genetic defects in insulin action, who are small at birth and insulin resistant as adults. Therefore, we cannot exclude a genetic explanation for this.

Bouchard: But, you cannot include it either.

McKeigue: It's highly unlikely that a genetic explanation would fit the relationship between birth weight and blood pressure given the interaction with adult height.

James: Do you mean that your concepts are based on adult height being an indicator of postnatal rather than fetal conditions?

McKeigue: People who are small at birth and tall as adults are likely to have been nutritionally deprived *in utero*. Those who are small at birth and short as adults are likely to have a mixture of genetic smallness and poor fetal growth.

Bennett: Do you have any information on the type of protein that is likely to produce these effects?

Jackson: During pregnancy the animals have a diet based on casein supplemented with methionine. It is likely that the exact composition of the diet produces important differences but at present I am not able to characterize the nature of those differences in any detail.

James: So why do you believe diet is important?

Jackson: We have some evidence that different levels of methionine supplementation might produce different responses (Levy et al 1993, Langley-Evans et al 1996b). The casein-based diet is 10% fat and we have evidence that the nature of the fat exerts an independent effect. This effect appears to be secondary to the effect of proteins. It is seen on the 9% protein diet, but not on the 18% diet (Langley-Evans 1996).

Björntorp: Does maternal smoking or alcohol intake play a role?

Jackson: Maternal smoking and drinking affect fetal growth, but there is no reason to believe that these are sufficient to explain the observations.

James: In the Barker studies the mothers did not smoke and usually did not drink (Barker 1992, 1994).

Jackson: And there are other studies in which they clearly don't smoke or drink (Yajnik et al 1995).

James: Is maternal protein intake in humans in any way related to the differing susceptibilities of adults in different parts of the world to adult chronic disease?

Jackson: In the rat studies the protein intake varied from 6 to 18% of dietary intake. There is a twofold difference in the availability of protein per head of population between many developing countries (around 45 g protein/caput per day) and the USA (100 g protein/caput per day). The difference in the availability of non-meat protein between the two countries is only about 5–10%, but the availability of meat protein varies by 10-fold. Thus, virtually all the difference in protein availability can be accounted for by differences in the availability in meat protein. We know that metabolic adaptations to enhance the nitrogen economy of the body are operating on a protein intake of 45 g/day (Jackson & Margetts 1993). Therefore, it is likely that the habitual protein available to many women in developing countries is equivalent to the levels of protein at which we see important changes in our experimental rat model.

James: I was intrigued by the idea that Indian rice-based diets lead to the subsequent vulnerability of the Indians to abdominal adiposity hyperinsulinaemia and diabetes (James 1995).

Stunkard: What is your opinion of the recent report by Rolland-Cachera that an elevated fat content of the diet of children is not responsible for adiposity, adiposity rebound and possibly also adult obesity, but that elevated protein content is responsible (Rolland-Cachera et al 1995)?

Jackson: I'm not familiar with that report, but the concept is not difficult to explain. Studies on macronutrient disposal show that during rapid catch-up growth in severely malnourished children, there are constraints on the deposition of lean tissue (Jackson & Wootton 1990). The need to replete lost tissue generates a profound hunger drive, but the diet does not provide the appropriate mix of nutrients to enable repletion of muscle, and there is preferential adipose deposition. It has been difficult to achieve a diet that enables both growth and good quality of growth.

Stunkard: A low protein diet might lead to obesity because people would be overeating in order to get adequate amino acids.

Jackson: There's reasonable evidence that a low protein diet, in the same way as a marginal intake of any other nutrient, makes one energetically inefficient. Therefore, it is possible that a high protein intake makes one energetically more efficient, so that one retains more energy rather than expending it.

Shaper: I have a point relating to the types of diets on which one becomes fat. The internal biochemical environment in an individual might be influenced by the dietary patterns of the specific society. For example, a mother with a BMI of 21 kg/m^2 in Jamaica may have a different internal biochemical environment from a mother of the same BMI in Chicago.

Jackson: I agree. In my opinion, a large part of nutrition relates to the control of the internal environment nourishing the tissues. Food is one component that contributes to this internal environment, but there are other equally important contributors. I have simply suggested that the shape, size and body composition of the mother have important effects on her ability to carry a fetus, and that the developmental form of the fetus plays an important role in its own metabolic competence, and the way in which it will grow and relate to its own environment, including its diet. Therefore, current food intake is a large contributor to the overall variability that is seen in populations, but unless you recognize the potential for other confounding factors, such as early life programming, you are in danger of drawing inappropriate conclusions. I am happy to accept that there are important differences between populations, but these differences have not been adequately characterized.

Shetty: Bill Dietz published a report last year that described the phenomenon of adiposity rebound seen during growth in childhood and adolescence (Dietz 1994). He proposed that the early development of adiposity rebound may provide a longer period of fat deposition and therefore result in the development of obesity. Because we are so preoccupied with Barker's most exciting hypothesis, are we ignoring the environmental influences of early childhood and adolescence? This period is also a critical period that may influence the development of late obesity.

Jackson: I don't disagree with you. Childhood is a long and complicated process, but in a limited period of time one has to be selective about what one is going to discuss. Studies of the transitions from one growth phase to another are desperately needed, and it is extremely difficult to do decent studies during adolescence, but this doesn't mean to say that they're not important.

Björntorp: I heard recently that the Dutch famine study was followed up in more detail. Do you have any information on this?

Jackson: Professor Clive Osmond is conducting those studies with support from the Medical Research Council. I do not think that the data have been analysed as yet.

Garrow: I would like to take this opportunity to point out that there is an important confounding effect in the Dutch famine study (Stein et al 1975). During the famine, 50% of the women of child-bearing age become amenorrhoeic. Therefore, those women who became pregnant during the famine were a selected set of women. The observation that these women had a higher proportion of obese children does not necessarily imply that this was caused by the famine.

Prentice: The effects of programming on BMI and waist/hip circumference ratio (WHR) are relatively modest compared to the effects on other outcomes, such as blood pressure and syndrome X. Therefore, one should not underestimate the power of programming by looking specifically for effects on BMI and WHR. The effect of programming on the modulation of the effect of obesity on disease outcome may be more important.

Jackson: This is a legitimate and important point. The fact that we are able to measure changes in outcomes such as blood pressure or blood glucose control in some individuals does not mean that these are the only processes which have been programmed in these individuals. We have a problem of identifying which are the underlying factors and which are the secondary manifestations. However, the observation that there are no measurable changes in WHR doesn't necessarily mean that a propensity for change is not present.

McKeigue: We have also found in our Swedish studies that being thin at birth changes the slope of the relationship between BMI and blood pressure, or between BMI and post-load insulin levels (Leon et al 1996, Lithell et al 1996).

Blundell: It seems to have been implied that the causal mechanism induces a neonatal shift in metabolism which then expresses itself in adulthood. It's also possible that there is an indirect route, i.e. that what happens in the fetus changes some behavioural lifestyle factor, which could have implications in adulthood. Is there any way of distinguishing between direct (metabolic) and indirect (behavioural) mediation of the effects of early experiences on adult states?

Jackson: You have made a big jump from early life to adulthood for a process that is continuous throughout life. I have suggested that the experience of the fetus changes the metabolic competence of that fetus. However, because of metabolic redundancy or reserve metabolic capacity the limit of metabolic competence may not become exposed as a constraint on function or illness until adulthood. Studies during childhood, either in Salisbury in the UK or Pune in India, show that by four years of age there are differences in metabolic function, or the metabolic set, which will predispose to later disease (Law et al 1991, Yajnik et al 1995). There are metabolic differences which are present from birth, and there may also be behavioural differences. For example, growth during the first year of life might be related to mood, depression and risk of suicide in adulthood (Barker et al 1995).

Prentice: Do you have any information on muscle function as a possible mediator of obesity, both in terms of behaviour, i.e. propensity towards physical activity, and metabolic fuel selection?

Jackson: The evidence we've collected so far supports this. I've drawn the two extremes — the epidemiological and the intervention studies in rats — to justify that there is something happening. Clearly, it is necessary to determine how these general mechanisms operate in individuals. Wootton et al (1994) have looked at glucose and by implication lipid handling in muscle, and there are indications that these relate to birth size. However, the extent to which this is simply related to the mass of the muscle, or some other quality of muscle, is for future exploration.

Forrester: There have been limited comparative studies of anthropometry and metabolic functioning. The literature has described protein turnover and urea salvage as adaptive mechanisms to ensure that nitrogen requirements are met throughout pregnancy. Alan Jackson's data and David Barker's data in the UK are tantalizing, but they are also incomplete (Langley-Evans & Jackson 1994). In Jamaican women there is a rapid rate of protein turnover in early pregnancy. Efforts to adapt for what we infer is a mismatch between amino acid demand and supply is indicated by an increased rate of urea nitrogen salvage. The high rate of protein turnover and the pressure to match the demand and supply decreases as pregnancy proceeds. This is the opposite of what has been observed in women from the UK. We measured the differences in height, weight and BMI of mothers from Jamaica and the UK, and we found that most Jamaican mothers had a BMI of 21–24 kg/m², whereas most mothers from the UK had a BMI of at least 25 kg/m². Therefore, mothers who are too thin may be unable to match amino acid supply with demand at the beginning of pregnancy, and this may contribute to whether fetuses grow proportionately or not. We are now designing strategies to follow, at various stages of pregnancy, both fetal growth with ultrasound, and maternal anthropopometry, body composition and metabolic processes.

James: Is it possible to modify the fetal outcome of Jamaican women by changing their diet?

Forrester: We don't know this yet.

Prentice: In The Gambia there is a pronounced seasonality in energy balance, so the population is the same except for the time that they conceive. Within this population there are variations in birth weight and weight gain during pregnancy. We have recently found that the weight of adult females, corrected for season, differs by about 3 kg, according to their month of birth. This is only a small change, but one could imagine that given an environment in which obesity was more likely to develop this could develop into a major change.

Ravussin: I would like to make the comment that in Pima Indians, despite the usual J-shaped curve between birth weight and the incidence of diabetes, most cases of diabetes occurred in subjects with intermediate birth weights or high birth weights (McCance et al 1994). I believe that a similar situation is occurring for obesity in westernized societies, i.e. that those with a low birth weight account for a minor proportion of the total number of cases of obesity.

McKeigue: Although the relationship between low birth weight and diabetes is weak, when there is a more refined measure of fetal growth, such as the ponderal index, the relationship becomes stronger. We've shown that the relationship also becomes stronger when you restrict the analysis to term births, so that low birth weights which are the result of prematurity are excluded. Therefore, some of the weakness of these relationships may be attributable to the limitations of birth weight alone as a measure of restricted fetal growth.

Prentice: The effects that David Barker has shown are apparent in spite of the fact that no correction was made for maternal size. But Paul McKeigue is saying that when corrections are made the effects are stronger.

Jackson: One has to establish whether or not one is using shape and size as a proxy for metabolic function. For metabolism the rate of delivery of nutrients is important; and shape and size, or the plane of nutrition, may be an expression of the set of the control points for rate-limiting function in terms of the delivery of nutrients to the fetus. It is proposed, therefore, that if the fetus itself is on a low growth trajectory during critical periods early in pregnancy, it is relatively protected at later points in time because the setting of the control point has a low expectation. Those fetuses that start off on a high growth trajectory with a high set point are at much greater risk if at a later stage they have to slow down because of a limitation in the provision of critical nutrients. Postnatally, the period during catch-up to the early growth trajectory appears to carry a significant risk in perturbing metabolic control. Therefore, there is a complicated series of relationships in a process which is constantly changing in time.

Campfield: I have a comment on the issue of imprinting (in the sense of altered function) and searching for imprinting in both muscle fibre types and fat cells. The brain is a site of imprinting, and changes in critical neural networks in the brain of these individuals would be sufficient to make them more energetically and metabolically efficient. The areas of the brain that are involved with energy balance and metabolic efficiencies are black-box areas. I hope that further genetic research will allow us to identify those areas and study them in these critical growth periods. We shouldn't restrict our analysis to muscle fibres and fat cells. A different brain that arises as a result of a different fetal environment may be a sufficient explanation.

Jackson: We're not at the stage where we can afford to exclude any of the areas. One of the more important aspects of nutrition is that it is an integrated system, so that a perturbation of one component will have a consequence elsewhere. One of the traps that we've fallen into too frequently is to simply explore an isolated component without then putting it back into the whole context. I would like to believe that the way in which muscle functions and develops is related to the body's ability to satisfy the functioning of the brain.

Campfield: That's exactly my point. I want to bring back integrated studies. This field often looks at fragments of the organism that are ultimately matched in terms of energy intake and expenditure. The brain is one of the great matchers of these two terms of the energy balance equation. A major research goal is the identification of the decision rules and the algorithms used by the CNS to perform this matching. I like the term 'metabolic competence'. It suggests that either something is too ambiguous to understand or that it is the result of an integrative process. I favour the latter.

References

Allison DB, Paultre F, Heymsfield SB, Pi-Sunyer FX 1995 Is the intra-uterine period really a critical period for the development of adiposity? Int J Obesity 19:397–402

Barker D JP 1992 Fetal and infant origins of adult disease. British Medical Association, London

Barker D JP 1994 Mothers, babies and disease in later life. British Medical Association, London

Barker D JP, Osmond C, Rodin I, Fall CHD, Winter PD 1995 Low weight gain in infancy and suicide in adult life. Br Med J 311:1203

Dietz WH 1994 Critical periods in childhood for the development of obesity. Am J Clin Nutr 59:955–959

Jackson AA, Margetts BM 1993 Protein intakes in the adult population of the UK. Int J Food Sci Nutr 44:95–104

Jackson AA, Wootton SA 1990 The energy requirements for growth and catch-up growth. In: Schurch B, Scrimshaw NS (eds) Activity, energy expenditure and energy requirements of infants and children. International Dietary Energy Consultative Group, Switzerland, p 185–214

James WPT 1995 Coronary heart disease in Indians. Possible role of nutritional factors. Bull Nutr Found India 16:1–4

Langley-Evans SC 1996 Intrauterine programming of hypertension in the rat: nutrient interactions. Comp Biochem Physiol 114:327A–333A

Langley-Evans SC, Jackson AA 1994 Increased systolic blood pressure in adult rats induced by fetal exposure to material low protein diet. Clin Sci 86:217–222

Langley-Evans SC, Gardner DS, Jackson AA 1996a Evidence of programming of the hypotha-lamic-pituitary-adrenal axis by maternal protein restriction during pregnancy. J Nutr 126:1578–1585

Langley-Evans SC, Gardner DS, Jackson AA 1996b Association of disproportionate growth of fetal rats in late gestation with raised systolic blood pressure in later life. J Reproduc Fertility 106:307–312

Law CM, Barker DJP, Bull AR, Osmond C 1991 Maternal and fetal influences on blood pressure. Arch Dis Child 66:1291–1295

Law CM, de Swiet M, Osmond C et al 1993 Initiation of hypertension *in utero* and its amplification throughout life. Br Med J 306:24–27

Leon DA, Koupilova I, Lithell HO et al 1996 Failure to realize growth potential *in utero* and adult obesity in relation to blood pressure in 50-year old Swedish men. Br Med J 312:401–406

Levy L, Jackson AA 1993 Modest restriction of dietary protein during pregnancy in the rat: fetal and placental growth. J Dev Physiol 19:113–118

Lithell HO, McKeigue PM, Berglund L, Mohsen R, Lithell U-B, Leon DS 1996 Relationship of size at birth to non-insulin-dependent diabetes and insulin concentrations in men aged 50–60 years. Br Med J 312:406–410

McCance DR, Pettitt DJ, Hanson RL, Jacobsson LTH, Knowler WC, Bennett PH 1994 Birth weight and non-insulin dependent diabetes: thrifty genotype, thrifty phenotype, or surviving small baby genotype? Br Med J 308:942–945

Rolland-Cachera ML, Detfeeger M, Akront M, Bellisle F 1995 Influence of macronutrients on adiposity development: a follow-up study of nutritional growth from 10 months to eight years of age. Int J Obes 19:573–578

Stein Z, Susser M, Saenger G, Marolla F 1975 Famine and human development. In: The Dutch hunger winter of 1944–1945. Oxford University Press, New York, p 119–148

Yajnik CS, Fall CHD, Vaidya U et al 1995 Fetal growth and glucose and insulin metabolism in four-year-old Indian children. Diabetic Med 12:330–336

Wootton SA, Murphy JL, Wilson F, Phillips D 1994 Energy expenditure and substrate metabolism after carbohydrate ingestion in relation to fetal growth in women born in Preston. Proc Nutr Soc 53:174 (abstr)

Overconsumption as a cause of weight gain: behavioural–physiological interactions in the control of food intake (appetite)

John E. Blundell and Neil A. King

BioPsychology Group, Department of Psychology, University of Leeds, Leeds LS2 9JT, UK

Abstract. There is an asymmetry in the operation of physiological processes that maintain body weight. The body exerts a strong defence against undernutrition and weight loss, but applies a much weaker resistance to overconsumption and weight gain. These principles influence how appetite control operates and this constitutes one form of vulnerability to weight gain. The expression of appetite is reflected in an episodic pattern of eating behaviour, the selection of dietary commodities and an associated profile of conscious sensations such as hunger, preferences, aversions and fullness. The onset and termination of eating episodes are subject to facilitatory and inhibitory physiological processes, and are held in place by strong environmental contingencies and habitual routines. Energy intake resulting from physiological and environmental control of behaviour is generally in balance with energy expenditure, although changes in energy expenditure do not inevitably trigger changes in food intake. Excess energy intake over expenditure may be due to aberrant positive drive to seek energy or a permissive response to strong external stimuli. The former could arise from a defect in a lipostatic regulatory system, and the latter from the weakness of inhibitory signals or from strong facilitatory responses to superpotent physical features of food. Taste and textural qualities of food give rise to hedonic responses via opioidergic and aminergic systems. Inhibitory responses to macronutrients include adjustment of gastric volume, rate of gastric emptying, release of cholecystokinin and enterostatin, and changes in plasma levels of products of digestion. These peripheral responses lead to a series of changes in brain neurotransmitter networks. Proteins, fats and carbohydrates generate different sets of physiological responses that produce different effects on the intensity and duration of satiety. The nutrient composition of food and the overall energy density influence control of meal size and post-ingestive inhibition. Particular sensory and nutrient combinations in foods can facilitate passive overconsumption. Overriding physiological satiety signals can lead to a positive energy balance and weight gain.

1996 The origins and consequences of obesity. Wiley, Chichester (Ciba Foundation Symposium 201) p 138–158

Vulnerability to weight gain

What factors give rise to the positive energy balance leading to increments in body weight that may eventually lead to obesity? What role is played by an appetite system (which controls food intake) in the development of a positive energy balance? Initially, the relationship between food intake and body weight regulation can be approached by asking the simple question: is overeating (too much food intake) a cause of obesity (too much body fat)?

Is the current prevalence of obesity a legacy of the evolutionary development of our physiological system coupled with an aggressive environment? Two scenarios can be envisaged: one in which energy expenditure is high and food is scarce (or periodically scarce), and the other in which energy expenditure is low and food is abundant. It can be argued that the first situation prevailed during most of the course of human evolution, the latter situation occurring only in the last 50–60 years. Consequently, biological processes concerning food intake and energy conservation are well adapted to the first situation and very poorly adapted to the second (the present) situation.

Therefore, the current epidemic of weight gain in many cultures is an understandable function of a changed relationship between biology and the environment. The mechanisms controlling food intake have beneficial consequences (weight regulation, prevention of death by starvation) under one relationship but disadvantageous consequences (weight increase, obesity) under another. The prevalence of obesity in humans does not require the postulation of a specific obesity-inducing mechanism such as those occurring in certain rodent mutations. Is this a reasonable deduction? The argument is, of course, similar to the proposals of Neel (1962) concerning the thrifty genotype, which suggests that an intrinsically adaptive capacity has become maladaptive due to changes in environmental circumstances.

A symmetrical control of appetite

A consideration of anthropological, epidemiological and experimental evidence suggests that it is easier for humans to gain weight than to reduce weight. This implies that the control of appetite (by the psychobiological system) is asymmetrical. Figure 1 shows how this arises. The extension of Claude Bernard's principle of homeostasis to include behaviour has been referred to as the behavioural regulation of internal states (Richter 1943). Logic demands that behaviour (eating) is controlled in accordance with biological states of need. This constitutes a form of biological regulation. However, the expression of behaviour is also subject to environmental demands, and behaviour is adapted in the face of particular circumstances. In the case of human appetite, consideration should be given to the conscious and deliberate control over eating behaviour. Humans can decide to alter their own behaviour to meet particular objectives; for example, a display of moral conviction (political hunger strike) or a demonstration of aesthetic achievement (e.g. dieting). In both of these examples eating is curtailed thereby interrupting the nutrition supply.

Regulatory mechanisms will tend to oppose this undersupply and generate a drive to eat. In many parts of the world environmental adaptation also means adjusting to a food supply characterized by an abundance of palatable, energy-dense (mainly high fat) foods or by a large proportion of fatty items. Exposure to such diets usually gives rise to an

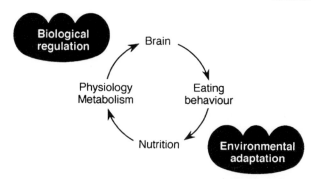

FIG. 1. Schema indicating the way in which eating behaviour contributes to biological regulation and environmental adaptation. Eating is influenced by both biological and environmental forces.

overconsumption of energy. Since this does not appear to be biologically driven (by a need state) or consciously intended, this phenomenon has been referred to as passive overconsumption (Blundell et al 1993a). This, in turn, interacts with genetic vulnerability leading to an increase in fat deposition (Bouchard 1985). A good example of this is the changes in dietary habits and levels of obesity occurring in the Pacific Islands of Polynesia and Micronesia (Zimmet 1992). This appears to be due to the high energy density of foods and since fat is the most dense nutrient, fat contributes most to the energy density and therefore most to the phenomenon of passive over-consumption. But it should be remembered that a number of nutrient and sensory features of foods may contribute in differing degrees to the stimulation of hyperphagia.

However, this passive overconsumption leading to the accumulation of body fat does not appear to generate any biological drive to undereat. Indeed it is now well accepted that energy intake of obese individuals is, on average, greater than that of lean subjects in order to attain balance with the higher rate of energy expenditure (Prentice et al 1989). Obese people do not get any help from their adipose tissue to reduce their appetites (although eventually the increase in fat deposits will increase fat oxidation and ultimately restore fat and energy balance). Hence, the operation of the regulatory system is not symmetrical. Two principles may be deduced. Firstly, that biological processes exert a strong defence against undereating which serves to protect the body from an energy (nutritional) deficit. Therefore, undereating must normally be an active and deliberate process. Secondly, in general biological defences against overconsumption are weak or inadequate. This means that overeating may occur despite the best efforts of people to prevent it.

Eating behaviour bridges the gap between environment and physiology

It is worth keeping in mind that food intake (the expression of appetite) is a form of behaviour usually regarded as being under voluntary control. This behaviour can be described by terms such as amount of energy ingested, structure of dietary pattern or macronutrient profile. However, all of these terms are the consequences of behaviour (food being seized by the hands and transported to the mouth). Therefore, a study of food intake should concentrate on the way in which environmental, cognitive or biological events can be translated into effects upon the act of behaviour. It is also worth mentioning that not eating (one aspect of which is satiety) is also a form of behaviour. Therefore, events which prevent eating are also important. Of course, to declare that food intake is a form of voluntary behaviour does not necessarily mean that it can be easily changed by a conscious decision. Behaviour can resist change if it is firmly locked into place by environmental contingencies and cognitions.

At a fundamental level, body weight regulation can be said to reflect the outcome of an interaction between biology and the environment. It is worth considering the critical role played by behaviour in such interactions. It is behaviour which allows biological processes to exert effective action upon the environment, and it is also behaviour which mediates (in part) the impact of the environment upon biology. When the environment is represented by the nutritional characteristics of the food supply, and biology is represented by those processes involved in energy balance and adipose tissue metabolism, the importance of eating behaviour can be readily appreciated. Eating behaviour bridges the gap between the nutritional environment and the physiological/biochemical mechanisms of weight control.

Food habits and positive energy balance

The conceptualization of behaviour as a bridge draws attention to the way in which the nutritional environment (food supply) can influence the form of eating and energy consumed. We can refer to this behaviour as food habits. Is it the nature of these food habits (food selection, pattern of eating, nutrient composition) which causes energy intake to exceed energy expenditure?

This issue can be turned into questions concerning the extent of the influence of physiology over eating behaviour (food habits). Why is it that a low energy expenditure does not exert a restraining effect over food intake? Why does a positive energy balance fail to generate a negative signal to suppress food intake? Does the body contain a mechanism capable of detecting a positive energy balance (or positive nutrient balances)?

When energy intake continuously exceeds energy expenditure, is this due to: (1) the presence or potency of mechanisms which stimulate or facilitate intake; or (2) to the weakness or failure of mechanisms which could prevent or inhibit intake. In other words, are the facilitatory influences too strong or the inhibitory influences too weak? In the event of a positive energy (or nutrient) balance, why do the inhibitory signals not become stronger in order to suppress intake and restore balance? What is the evidence concerning the operation of these signals, and is it possible for food habits to overcome inhibitory physiological signals?

Satiety signals

Some physiological responses that follow food consumption are identified as signals which terminate eating and/or maintain inhibition over further intake. These responses are usually referred to as satiety signals. What are the features of foods which are believed to be monitored and which give rise to satiety signals? What is the status of the putative satiety signals?

It has been assumed or claimed that volume, weight, energy content, macronutrient proportion and energy density may all be monitored and constitute the source of specific satiety signals. These may be divided into general factors (e.g. weight, volume) which apply to all foods, and specific factors (nutrient content) which depend on the particular food consumed. Why should weight and volume appear as important features in some studies? (A litre of water would have weight and volume but would provide no energy or nutrients.) All physiological satiety signals, (e.g. rate of gastric emptying and release of cholecystokinin) have functions in addition to their role in a negative feedback system. A satiety signal is a function assumed by some underlying physiological property. Given a history of food seeking and consumption it is inevitable that weight and volume of food will have become associated with (conditioned to) the important biological components of food, namely energy value and nutrient composition. The system has learned how to operate in a real environment, and the objective of the system is to produce a veridical response. Brunswick's theory of perception provides a model for understanding this issue (Brunswick 1950). Weight and volume are learned cues with high functional validity (proximal cues which correlate well with more distal cues such as hormone release, contact with gastro-intestinal receptors etc.). This is why weight and volume often appear to be important monitored variables (rather than energy or nutrient content) when nutritional composition of food has been covertly manipulated. The system is operating sensibly according to its previous experience; but it does not mean that weight is fundamentally more important than energy content. However, it does mean that humans (and animals) have learned during the course of their lives (and long-term exposure to food) that weight is very often a good predictor of energy value or nutrient content

Satiety cascade: satiation and satiety

How can the issue of satiety signals be incorporated into a model for thinking about the relationship between the nutritional environment, eating behaviour and physiology? One way is to consider how eating behaviour is held in place by the interaction between the characteristics of food and the biological responses to ingestion. These biological responses are often thought of as satiety signals.

The biological drive to eat can be linked with the satiating power or efficiency of food — the capacity of any consumed food to suppress hunger and to inhibit the onset of a further period of eating. Food brings about this effect by mediating certain processes

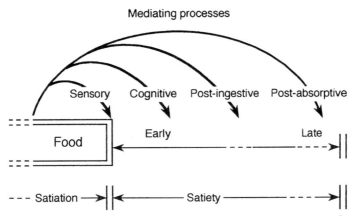

FIG. 2. The 'satiety cascade' indicating the distinction between satiation and satiety, and illustrating major processes which contribute to post-ingestive satiety.

that can be roughly classified as sensory, cognitive, post-ingestive and post-absorptive. The operation of these processes results from the effects of food on physiological and biochemical mechanisms. Collectively these processes (Fig. 2) have been referred to as the satiety cascade. The way that food is sensed and processed by the biological system generates neural and humoral signals that control appetite. It follows that any self-imposed or externally applied reduction in the food supply, creating a calorie deficit, will weaken the satiating power of food. One consequence of this will be the failure of food to suppress hunger (the biological drive) adequately. The satiety cascade appears to operate as efficiently in obese people as in lean individuals. Therefore, a normal appetite response to reduced calorie intake is evident in obese subjects.

Technically, satiety can be defined as the inhibition of hunger and eating that arises as a consequence of food consumption. It can be distinguished from satiation, which is the process that brings a period of eating to a halt. Consequently, satiation and satiety act conjointly to determine the pattern of eating behaviour and the accompanying profile of motivation. Together, these two processes control events operating within meals or between meals. The conscious sensation of hunger is one index of motivation and reflects the strength of satiation and satiety. Hunger as a biologically useful sensation is a nagging, irritating feeling that prompts thoughts of food and reminds us that the body needs energy; it can therefore be used as one index of the drive for food and as a consequence of the appetite control system.

Satiating efficiency of foods: effects of macronutrients

The satiety cascade implies that foods of varying nutritional composition will engage differently with the mediating processes and will therefore exert differing effects upon satiation and satiety. A procedure widely used to assess the action of food on satiety is the preload strategy. Provided that no contaminating stimuli are introduced between the preload and the test meal (Blundell & Rogers 1991, 1994), this procedure can be used to assess the satiating power of a wide variety of foods varying in macronutrient composition. Even before food touches the mouth, physiological signals are generated by the sight and smell of it. These events constitute the cephalic phase of appetite (Powley 1977). Cephalic phase responses are generated in many parts of the gastro-intestinal tract; their function is to prepare for the ingestion of food.

During and immediately after eating, afferent information provides the major control over appetite. It has been noted that 'afferent information from ingested food acting in the mouth provides primarily positive feedback for eating; that from the stomach and small intestine primarily negative feedback' (Smith et al 1990). This draws attention to the relative potency of oral and post-ingestive stimulation in controlling the amount of food that is eaten.

Initially, the brain is informed about the amount of food ingested and its nutrient content via afferent input. This afferent information constitutes one class of 'satiety signals' and forms part of the post-ingestive control of appetite. It is usual to identify a postabsorptive phase that arises when nutrients have undergone digestion and have crossed the intestinal wall and entered the circulation. These products, which accurately reflect the food consumed, may be metabolized in peripheral tissues or organs or may enter the brain directly via the circulation. In either case, these products constitute a further class of satiety signals. There is evidence that the degree of oxidative metabolism of glucose and free fatty acids in the liver constitutes a significant source of metabolic information which influences the expression of appetite (Friedman et al 1986).

It is clear that the balance between oro-sensory effects, post-ingestive (but preabsorptive) and postabsorptive events will contribute markedly to the action of different types of foods on the control of appetite. In what way do the macronutrients influence this control?

It is generally accepted that dietary protein exerts a potent effect on satiety (De Castro 1987) and provides the strongest inhibition over appetite. This is in keeping with the maintenance of protein intake at 11–14% of daily energy, suggesting that the intake of protein is tightly controlled.

Carbohydrates may influence a number of mechanisms involved in satiety. These include glucoreceptors within the gastro-intestinal tract (Mei 1985) that send afferent information via the vagus and splanchnic nerves to the nucleus tractus solitarius and hypothalamic regions of the brain and cells in the liver that respond to glucose which monitor postabsorptive effects of glucose (Oomura 1988). These mechanisms form the basis of the so-called energostatic control of feeding (Booth 1972). Although sweet carbohydrates induce some positive feedback for eating through oral afferent stimulation, this may be countered by the potent inhibitory action via post-ingestive (preabsorptive) and postabsorptive mechanisms.

One clear finding from these studies is that carbohydrates are efficient appetite suppressants; that is, they contribute markedly to the satiating efficiency of food and exert a potent effect on satiety (Rogers et al 1988, Blundell et al 1994). This evidence is precisely complemented by studies showing that an analogue of glucose, 2-deoxy-D-glucose (which blocks the utilization of glucose by cells), actually increases hunger when given to human subjects (Thompson & Campbell 1977). On the basis of studies on rats, it was argued some years ago that 'if the cumulative inhibitory effects of carbohydrate on feeding are indeed energostatic . . . then any substance which can readily be used by the animal to provide energy should produce an appropriate food intake compensation over a period of several hours after loading' (Booth 1972). Studies have shown a similar situation in humans. A variety of carbohydrates, including glucose, fructose, sucrose and maltodextrins, have rather similar effects when given in a preload: they suppress later intake by an amount roughly equivalent to their calorie value, although the time course of the suppressive action may vary according to the rate at which the carbohydrate loads are metabolized (Van Amelsvoort & Weststrate 1992).

Nutrients and overconsumption

Perhaps the most controversial area of research on macronutrients involves comparisons of fat and carbohydrate. The outcome of experiments is critically dependent on the methodology employed. There are signs that general agreement is beginning to emerge. For some time, it has been known that subjects exposed to high fat foods tend to overconsume energy (e.g. Lissner et al 1987). This effect depends in large part on the high energy density of the high fat foods, and the overeating effect has been referred to as 'passive overconsumption' (Blundell & Burley 1991). It should be noted that the stimulatory effect of fatty foods on energy intake is not only due to the high energy density but also to the likely facilitatory action of fat in the mouth (Tordoff & Reed 1991, Smith & Greenberg 1992). For many years it has been known that offering subjects high fat or high carbohydrate foods which have been manipulated to be equally energy dense, eliminates the high fat overeating phenomenon (Van Stratum et al 1977). This effect has recently been confirmed (Stubbs et al 1993).

The 'passive overconsumption' effect of fat on energy intake occurs due to an action during consumption (it is an intra-meal effect). This can be investigated through techniques referred to by Kissileff (1984) as concurrent evaluation. Interestingly, this procedure of evaluating the action of foods on appetite control has been virtually neglected by researchers in favour of the procedure of measuring satiating efficiency (preload design). This term refers to the capacity of a food to suppress appetite following ingestion of the food. The experimental evidence on the relative effectiveness of isocaloric loads of high carbohydrate or high fat foods to influence post-ingestive satiety is equivocal. Some studies have reported equivalent satiety of fat and carbohydrate (Rolls et al 1994, Foltin et al 1990), whilst others have indicated a weaker satiating effect of fat (on a joule for joule basis) (Blundell et al 1993b, Rolls et al 1994, Cotton et al 1994).

The fat paradox

The apparently ambivalent effects of fat have generated a phenomenon referred to as the fat paradox. On the one hand, a fat such as corn oil, infused into the jejunum has been shown to slow gastric emptying, increase feelings of fullness and reduce food intake in a test meal (Welch et al 1985). Infusions into the ileum bring about similar effects and also reduce feelings of hunger (Welch et al 1988). However, similar infusions made intravenously exerted no effect on gastric emptying or measures of appetite. Similar experiments have been carried out in rats where intra-duodenal infusions inhibited food intake whilst intravenous infusions did not (Greenberg et al 1989). These findings imply that, after the ingestion of fat, potent fat-induced satiety signals are generated which are mediated primarily by preabsorptive rather than postabsorptive physiological responses. In addition, this effect is blocked by the cholecystokinin type A antagonist lorglumide, thus pointing to the mediation of cholecystokinin in the inhibitory effect of fat on appetite (Greenberg et al 1989). In human subjects the inhibitory effect of infused fat on appetite is also attenuated by lorglumide (Lieverse et al 1994).

However, a number of studies (of short- and medium-term duration) have demonstrated the existence of very high intakes of energy with high fat foods. These studies have demonstrated that high fat foods constitute a sufficient, but not a necessary, condition for passive overconsumption (also referred to as high fat hyperphagia). This form of hyperphagia should not be possible if fat generates potent satiety signals which impede further eating. How can these two features be reconciled?

There are now some data to indicate that fat-induced satiety signals are not incompatible with the phenomenon of high fat hyperphagia. In certain studies in which subjects have been exposed to ranges of high fat and high carbohydrate foods, the fat foods give rise to a markedly higher consumption of energy associated with a lower weight of food eaten (e.g. Green et al 1994). The function of a satiety signal should be to reduce the amount of food that people put into their mouths. This appears to occur with high fat foods (in normal weight subjects) indicating the operation of an inhibitory influence over eating. However, in the face of the high energy density and possible oral facilitation of fatty foods, this inhibition is either too weak or too slow acting to prevent the intake of a significant amount of energy. This interpretation means that in considering the action of dietary fat on appetite control it is necessary to distinguish between fat *per se* and fat as a contributor to the high energy density of foods. These deductions also suggest behavioural, nutritional and pharmacological strategies for reducing fat (energy) intake (Blundell et al 1995).

Overconsumption and carbohydrate

While considering the issue of overeating and weight gain, it is worth mentioning that fat is not the only nutrient which can form the basis for overconsumption. There is evidence that high carbohydrate diets can also generate a high energy intake, as for example in the Guru Walla phenomenon, which leads to weight gain (Pasquet et al 1992). It should of course be noted that the Guru Walla syndrome is not a form of passive overconsumption but represents a voluntary and determined attempt to gain weight by young Cameroon men. The forceful striving to ingest the red sorghum and cows' milk diet (70.1% carbohydrate energy) sometimes leads to reflux and vomiting. It would be expected that high fat diets would be more efficient at inducing weight gain, but the phenomenon of weight gain with high carbohydrate diets must be explained. Does this mean that the metabolism of carbohydrate does not generate a potent physiological response which serves as an inhibitory signal for the control of appetite?

In a recent study subjects were fed isoenergetic amounts (50% above requirements) of fat and carbohydrate for 14 days each (Horton et al 1995). A whole-room calorimeter was used to measure energy expenditure and nutrient oxidation on four separate days during the overfeeding period. This obligatory fat overfeeding had minimal effects on fat oxidation and total energy expenditure with the consequence that 90–95% of the excess fat energy was stored. The obligatory carbohydrate overfeeding gave rise to progressive increases in carbohydrate oxidation and total energy expenditure resulting in 75–85% of excess energy being stored. On Day 14 of the overfeeding period the proportion of total energy that was stored as body fat did not differ significantly between the two diets. However, when the total 14 day overfeeding period was considered substantially more total energy and total fat was stored when the dietary excess was fat rather than carbohydrate.

It is often widely believed that weight gain is not possible on a high carbohydrate diet because of the low rate of *de novo* lipogenesis in humans (Acheson et al 1989). In the study by Horton et al (1995) referred to above the calorimetry data indicated that net lipogenesis from carbohydrate did not occur. However, with the carbohydrate feeding, fat storage (positive fat balance) occurred due to the suppression of fat oxidation accompanying the increase in carbohydrate oxidation.

What are the implications of this phenomenon for the control of food intake? First, it should be recognized that the study by Horton et al (1995), like the Guru Walla syndrome, involved mandatory overfeeding (experimenter imposed rather than self-imposed). In practice, it is much more difficult to freely overconsume carbohydrate than fat due to the usually lower energy density of carbohydrate-rich foods. In addition, as noted previously, carbohydrate is widely regarded as being more satiating than fat. Therefore 'passive overconsumption' of carbohydrates is unlikely to be a frequently occurring phenomenon.

There is also one other interesting consequence of these studies which has implications for the relationship between that pattern of food intake and weight gain. It has been argued that small but sustained overeating over a long period of time would give rise to weight gain but the nutrient composition of the excess would be rather unimportant (Horton et al 1995). However, in the case of a positive energy balance arising from multiple periods of overeating over a single day or over a few days, the difference in fat storage would be greater with fat than with carbohydrate. This second scenario has been identified as a pathological form of eating behaviour arising from the passive overconsumption of high fat foods (Lawton et al 1993). Consequently, obesity could arise from quite different patterns of eating involving different nutrient profiles.

Hedonics: food and pleasure

In considering the capacity for energy intake to rise above energy expenditure the weakness of inhibitory factors has to be set against the potency of facilitatory processes. The palatability of food is clearly one feature that could exert a positive influence over behaviour. The independent index of palatability is usually considered to be the subjective appreciation of pleasantness. This subjective sensation is quantified by expressing it on an objective scale according to standard psychophysical procedures. This sensation is often taken to reflect the hedonic dimension of food. The nature of the relationship between palatability and food consumption has never been systematically determined, although palatability does influence the cumulative intake curve and palatability has been invoked as a mediating principle to account for the prolongation of ingestion from a variety of foods due to sensory specific satiety (e.g. Rolls et al 1988).

It may be hypothesized that palatability would exert a powerful effect on intra-meal satiety (whilst food was being consumed), and there is evidence for an enduring legacy which influences post-ingestive satiety. For example, it has been demonstrated that high palatability can maintain the level of post-ingestive hunger (Hill et al 1984). Palatability also influences the rate of eating and the experience of hunger during a meal. There are compelling logical reasons why energy intake should be strongly influenced by palatability; a phenomenon readily appreciated by the food manufacturing industry in which much food technology is devoted to developing foods with increasingly potent and pleasurable mouth sensations.

Pleasure and reward

One mechanism frequently overlooked appears to be the capacity of the pleasurable sensations of food to act as a reward. Such reward or reinforcement would condition those behavioural acts instrumental in generating the reward — in other words, the behaviour of eating. In addition stimuli which set the scene for the eating would acquire particular salience or discriminative properties.

Consequently it should not be overlooked that eating is an important source of pleasure and that the sensations arising from eating constitutes the basis for a reward. In a recent analysis (Berridge 1996) it has been argued that reward has two separable components which may be termed 'liking' and 'wanting'. In terms of psychological functions these can be defined as 'palatability' and 'incentive'. It follows that the greater the positive sensations arising from foods then the greater should be the satisfaction of those responses causing the eating, and the greater the willingness to maintain or re-initiate those responses. This view again draws attention to the interrelationships between hedonics and hunger (Blundell & Rogers 1991).

In simple terms, the essence of this analysis is that the ever-increasing intensity and quality of sensory experiences derived from food (pleasure) constitute a factor favouring overconsumption.

Sweetness

Sweetness is one of the most powerful and easily recognized taste sensations. Sweetness is clearly a potent psychobiological phenomenon. Foods are made sweet in order to increase their attractiveness (raise palatability) and, in turn, to increase consumption (by the eater and purchaser). The most economical account of sweetness is that, like the more general attribute of palatability, it facilitates food intake. This should apply independent of the energy or macronutrient profile associated with the sweetness. However, the effects of the associated energy and nutrients should be considered when assessing the overall action of sweetness in foods (Blundell & Green 1996).

Some attempts have been made to uncouple sweetness and energy experimentally so as to evaluate the relative contribution of each factor to the control of appetite (Blundell et al 1988). According to the foregoing argument it may be supposed that sweetness would facilitate whilst energy would inhibit. After some lively debate, it now seems to be agreed that the consumption of sugars (sweetness plus energy) does lead to energy compensation (a subsequent suppression of intake by an amount roughly equivalent to the amount provided by the sugars). This conclusion is supported by a recent interpretation of the experimental literature (Anderson 1995). It was concluded that 'the ingestion of > 50g sugar within 20–60 min of a meal results in a reduced meal time food intake, which suggests that appetite regulatory centres respond to sugar's energy content' (Anderson 1995). It follows that if sugars are replaced in foods by a non-caloric sweetener then the regulatory centres will have no energy to which they can respond. However, different sugars (mono- or disaccharides) may exert somewhat different effects. Since industrial manufacturers are largely agreed that it is the addition of sweetness to foods which is believed to enhance consumption (a stimulatory effect), it is difficult to argue that it is the sweetness *per se* which causes the compensation. From this it follows that high intensity sweeteners and sucrose should produce different effects on food intake by virtue of their distinctive physiological effects. The suppressive effect of sugar is presumably due to carbohydrate metabolism (see earlier discussion). However, sucrose-like high intensity sweeteners will also confer a facilitatory action on appetite via sweetness *per se*. This means that the effects of sweetness will be manifest when present in combination with other nutrients. For example, what would be the effect of high fat foods whose palatability has been raised further by the addition of sweetness? Would the effect be detected on satiation or satiety? For some years it has been claimed that sweet/fat mixtures in foods would form a potent stimulatory complex and this would be particularly important for women who report a preference for sweet fat foods (Drewnowski et al 1992). Recently, it has been demonstrated that passive overconsumption was markedly enhanced by foods characterized by the sweet/fat combination (Green & Blundell 1995) in comparison with salty/fatty foods. It is likely that investigations of the interaction between the sensory and nutritional dimensions of food will lead to further revelations about the capacity of particular foods to influence food intake and weight control.

One implication of this issue concerns the interpretation of recent analyses of the relationship between obesity, and sugar and fat consumption. Using a large database, it has been shown that the consumption of fat is positively related to body mass index while an inverse relationship is seen for sucrose (Bolton-Smith & Woodward 1994). Initially, these data suggest that sucrose intake is quite unrelated to obesity. Indeed, it could be argued that consuming sucrose either prevents obesity or is the cure for obesity. One deduction that could be made from these data is that a reduction in sugar intake (by substituting a low calorie sweetener) could lead to a reciprocal augmentation of fat intake. This would conform to the idea of the sugar/fat see-saw. This phenomenon is actually apparent in some of the early landmark studies on the substitution of sugar by aspartame (Porikos et al 1982). In addition, it has recently been reported in an intervention study that 'the substitution of artificial sweeteners for sugar caused an increase of 11% in total fat intake' (Naismith & Rhodes 1995). However, at the present time the analysis does not indicate how the overall profile of nutrient intake relates to the selection of particular food groups or to actual eating behaviour. Indeed, it is quite possible for the food supply to reflect a positive relationship between sugar and fat content (Macdiarmid et al 1995). In other words, eaten foods can contain significant quantities of both sugar and fat. Several scenarios could be envisaged. One of these would involve a subgroup of people who are overweight, or gaining weight, and whose sugar intake is low but the sugar is consumed along with fat. Other sweetening agents may also be involved. Some proposals concerning the effects of sweet and fat foods have been made (e.g. Heaton & Emmett 1994). This issue is part of a larger problem involving sensory and nutrient interactions in foods and their capacity to stimulate or inhibit food intake (Greenough et al 1994). For the moment, it should be recognized that some foods with particular sensory–nutrient combinations are likely to be particularly potent in generating overconsumption.

Overconsumption and the origins of obesity

The evidence discussed here has provided a formulation for thinking about appetite control in relation to obesity. The biological system involved in the expression of appetite clearly permits overconsumption to occur leading to a positive energy balance. This phenomenon is related to asymmetrical control of body weight by which any loss of body weight is more strongly resisted than any increase.

Although sedentariness clearly contributes to a positive energy balance, it is argued here that overconsumption is an independent risk factor in obesity. The overconsumption has been termed passive since it does not appear to entail any volitional intent on the part of the consumer. However the term passive does not mean that the overconsumption does not have causes. Indeed the causes can be identified. High energy density of foods in the food supply is one factor; many of these are fat-containing foods which can overcome fat-induced satiety signals. Such foods are highly palatable and the fatty texture can arouse oro-sensory facilitation of eating. Once consumed fat appears to exert a relative weak effect on post-ingestive satiety kilojoule for kilojoule in comparison with the other macronutrients. However, it is clear that a high fat diet is not a necessary condition for overconsumption; under particular circumstances it is possible for high carbohydrate diets to generate a positive energy balance.

The tendency of energy-dense (high fat) foods to lead to overconsumption can be intensified by the sensory qualities of the food consumed. Particular features which raise palatability (hedonic value) of foods can lead to sensory–nutrient combinations which generate high levels of consumption-overriding satiety signals. Moreover, particular food habits (based on personal food choices or environmental circumstances) will favour overconsumption. Of course these food habits will involve foods with those sensory–nutrient combinations (e.g. sweet/fat) previously identified as able to overcome satiety signals and weaken satiation. It follows that certain food habits (selection of low density, high carbohydrate, low fat foods) will protect against overconsumption and will tend to prevent a positive energy balance and weight gain.

These arguments draw attention to the relationship between environmental and biological features in the control of energy intake. In a number of cases it appears that physiological mechanisms can be overridden by nutritional or behavioural characteristics. For example, the quality of foods (sensory–nutrient combination) can overcome quick-acting preabsorptive satiety signals (physiological responses not strong enough to inhibit eating). In addition, substantial metabolic fluctuations in fuel balances (postabsorptive physiology) appear to have a negligible effect on the pattern of eating. Taken together, these findings suggest that the pattern of eating is expressed to a significant degree independent of many physiological processes. This issue has been addressed earlier in questioning whether obesity is a biogenetic or biobehavioural problem (Schlundt et al 1990).

In the light of the above discussion, it can be deduced that the problem of overconsumption has its origins in behaviour (food habits) and the environment (hedonic–nutrient combinations in the food supply) in the face of a permissive physiological system. Consequently, overconsumption can be tackled most obviously at the level of behaviour and the food supply. However, physiological procedures are also important in order to develop techniques to enable the biological system to resist more strongly the behavioural and environmental factors. The overall picture suggests clear strategies — behavioural, nutritional and pharmacological — to protect against overconsumption and to prevent weight gain.

Acknowledgements

The authors are grateful to the Biotechnology and Biological Sciences Research Council for their support, to L. Gill for help with the preparation of the manuscript, and to C. Lawton and S. Green for scientific collaboration.

References

Acheson K J, Schutz Y, Bessard T, Anantharaman K, Flatt JP, Sequier E 1989 Glycogen storage capacity and *de novo* lipogenesis during massive carbohydrate overfeeding in man. Am J Clin Nutr 50:307–314

Anderson GH 1995 Sugars, sweetness, and food intake. Am J Clin Nutr 62:195S–202S

Berridge KC 1996 Food reward: brain substrates of wanting and liking. Neurosci Biobehav Rev 20:1–25

Blundell JE, Burley VJ 1991 Evaluation of satiating power of dietary fat in man. In: Oomura Y, Baba S, Shimazu T (eds) Progress in obesity research 1990. Libbey, London, p 453–457

Blundell JE, Green SM 1996 Effect of sucrose and sweeteners on appetite and energy intake. Int J Obes 20:12S–17S

Blundell JE, Rogers PJ 1991 Hunger, hedonics and the control of satiation and satiety. In: Friedman M, Kare M (eds) Chemical senses, vol 4: Appetite and nutrition. Marcel Dekker, New York, p 127–148

Blundell JE, Rogers PJ 1994 Sweet carbohydrate substitutes (intense sweeteners) and the control of appetite: scientific issues. In: Fernstrom JD, Miller GD (eds) Appetite and body weight regulation: sugar, fat and macronutrient substrates. CRC Press, Boca Raton, FL, p 113–124

Blundell JE, Rogers PJ, Hill AJ 1988 Uncoupling sweetness and calories: methodological aspects of laboratory studies on appetite control. Appetite 11:54–61

Blundell JE, Lawton CL, Hill AJ 1993a Mechanisms of appetite control and their abnormality in obese patients. Hormone Res 39:72–76

Blundell JE, Burley VJ, Cotton JR, Lawton CL 1993b Dietary fat and the control of energy intake: evaluating the effects of fat on meal size and post-meal satiety. Am J Clin Nutr 557:772S–778S

Blundell JE, Green S, Burley V 1994 Carbohydrates and human appetite. Am J Clin Nutr (suppl) 59:728S–734S

Blundell JE, Cotton JR, De Largy H et al 1995 The fat paradox: fat-induced satiety signals versus high-fat overconsumption. Int J Obes 19:832–835

Bolton-Smith C, Woodward M 1994 Dietary composition and fat to sugar ratios in relation to obesity. Int J Obes 18:820–828

Booth DA 1972 Postabsorptively induced suppression of appetite and the energostatic control of feeding. Physiol Behav 9:199–202

Bouchard C 1985 Inheritance of fat distribution and adipose tissue metabolism. In: Vague J, Björntorp P, Guy-Grand B, Rebuffe-Scrive M, Vague P (eds) Metabolic complications of human obesities. Excerpta Medica, Amsterdam, p 87–96

Brunswick E 1950 The conceptual framework of psychology. University of Chicago Press, Chicago, IL, p 102

Cotton JR, Burley VJ, Weststrate JA, Blundell JE 1994 Dietary fat and appetite: similarities and differences in the satiating effect of meals supplemented with either fat and/or carbohydrate. J Hum Nutr Diet 7:11–24

De Castro JM 1987 Macronutrient relationships with meal patterns and mood in the spontaneous feeding behavior of humans. Physiol Behav 39:561–569

Drewnowski A, Kurth C, Holden-Wiltse J, Saari J 1992 Food preferences in human obesity: carbohydrates versus fats. Appetite 18:207–221

Foltin RW, Fischman MW, Moran TH, Rolls BJ, Kelly TH 1990 Caloric compensation for lunches varying in fat and carbohydrate content by humans in a residential laboratory. Am J Clin Nutr 52:969–980

Friedman MI, Tordoff MG, Ramirez I 1986 Integrated metabolic control of food intake. Brain Res Bull 17:855–859

Green S, Blundell JE 1995 Comparison of the perceived fillingness and actual food intake of snack foods. Int J Obes (suppl 2) 19:28

Green S, Burley VJ, Blundell JE 1994 Effect of fat-containing and sucrose-containing foods on the size of eating episodes and energy intake in lean males: potential for causing overconsumption. Eur J Clin Nutr 48:547–555

Greenberg D, Torres NI, Smith GP, Gibbs J 1989 The satiating effect of fats is attenuated by the cholecystokinin antagonist lorglumide. Ann N Y Acad Sci 575:517–520

Greenough A, Lawton CL, Delargy HJ, Blundell JE 1994 Uncoupling the effect of sensory and nutrient combinations (sweetness and fat) on the pattern of meals. Int J Obes (suppl 2) 18:29

Heaton KW, Emmett PM 1994 Extrinsic sugars and the consumption of fat. Am J Clin Nutr (suppl) 59:774S

Hill AJ, Magson LD, Blundell JE 1984 Hunger and palatability: tracking ratings of subjective experience before, during and after the consumption of preferred and less preferred food. Appetite 5:361–371

Horton TJ, Drougas H, Brachey A, Reed GW, Peter JC, Hill JO 1995 Fat and carbohydrate overfeeding in humans: different effects on energy storage. Am J Clin Nutr 62:19–29

Kissileff HR 1984 Satiating efficiency and a strategy for conducting food loading experiments. Neurosci Biobehav Rev 8:129–135

Lawton CL, Burley VJ, Wales JK, Blundell JE 1993 Dietary fat and appetite control in obese subjects: weak effects on satiation and satiety. Int J Obes 17:409–416

Lieverse RJ, Jansen JMBJ, Masclee AAM, Lamers CBHW 1994 Role of cholecystokinin in the regulation of satiation and satiety in humans. Ann N Y Acad Sci 713:268–272

Lissner L, Levitsky DA, Strupp BJ, Kalkwarf HJ, Roe DA 1987 Dietary fat and the regulation of energy intake in human subjects. Am J Clin Nutr 46:886–892

Macdiarmid JI, Cade JE, Blundell JE 1995 Extrinsic sugar as vehicle for dietary fat. Lancet 346:696–697

Mei N 1985 Intestinal chemosensitivity. Physiol Rev 65:211–237

Naismith DJ, Rhodes C 1995 Adjustment in energy intake following the covert removal of sugar from the diet. J Hum Nutr Diet 8:167–175

Neel JV 1962 Diabetes mellitus: a thrifty genotype rendered detrimental by 'progress'? Am J Hum Genet 14:353–362

Oomura Y 1988 Chemical and neuronal control of feeding motivation. Physiol Behav 44:555–560

Pasquet P, Brigant L, Froment A et al 1992 Massive overfeeding and energy balance in men: the Guru Walla model. Am J Clin Nutr 56:483–490

Porikos KP, Hesser MF, Van Itallie TB 1982 Caloric regulation in normal-weight men maintained on a palatable diet of conventional foods. Physiol Behav 29:293–300

Powley J 1977 The ventromedial hypothalamic syndrome, satiety and a cephalic phase hypothesis. Physiol Rev 84:89–126

Prentice AM, Black AE, Murgatroyd PR, Goldberg GR, Coward WA 1989 Metabolism or appetite: questions of energy balance with particular reference to obesity. J Hum Nutr Diet 2: 95–103

Richter CP 1943 Total self-regulatory functions in animals and human beings. Harvey Lect 38:63–103

Rogers PJ, Carlyle J-A, Hill AJ, Blundell JE 1988 Uncoupling sweet taste and calories: comparison of the effects of glucose and three intense sweeteners on hunger and food intake. Physiol Behav 43:547–552

Rolls BJ, Hetherington M, Burley VJ 1988 The specificity of satiety: the influence of foods of different macronutrient content on the development of satiety. Physiol Behav 43:145–153

Rolls BJ, Kim-Harris S, Fischman MW, Foltin RW, Moran TH, Stoner SA 1994 Satiety after preloads with different amounts of fat and carbohydrate: implications for obesity. Am J Clin Nutr 60:476–487

Schlundt DG, Hill JO, Sbrocco T, Pope-Cordle J, Kasser T 1990 Obesity: a biogenetic or biobehavioral problem. Int J Obes 14:815–828

Smith GP, Greenberg D 1992 The investigation of orosensory stimuli in the intake and preference of oils in the rat. In: Mela DJ (ed) Dietary fats: determinants of preference, selection and consumption. Elsevier, London, p 167–178

Smith GP, Greenberg D, Corp E, Gibbs J 1990 Afferent information in the control of eating. In: Bray GA (ed) Obesity: towards a molecular approach. Alan R Liss, New York, p 63–79

Stubbs RJ, Murgatroyd PR, Goldberg GR, Prentice AM 1993 Carbohydrate balance and the regulation of day-to-day food intake in humans. Am J Clin Nutr 57:897–903

Thompson DA, Campbell RG 1977 Hunger in humans induced by 2-deoxy-D-glucose: glucoprivic control of taste preference and food intake. Science 198:1065–1068

Tordoff MG, Reed DR 1991 Sham-feeding sucrose or corn oil stimulates food intake in rats. Appetite 17:97–103

Van Ameslvoort JMM, Weststrate JA 1992 Amylose–amylopectin ratio in a meal affects postprandial variables in male volunteers. Am J Clin Nutr 55:712–718

Van Stratum P, Lussenburg RN, Van Wenzel LA, Vergroesen AJ, Cremer HD 1977 The effect of dietary carbohydrate : fat ratio on energy intake by adult women. Am J Clin Nutr 31:206–212

Welch I, Saunders K, Read NW 1985 Effect of ileal and intravenous infusions of fat emulsions on feeding and satiety in human volunteers. Gastroenterology 89:1297

Welch IML, Sepple CP, Read NW 1988 Comparisons of the effects on satiety and eating behaviour of infusions of lipid into the different regions of the small intestine. Gut 29:306–311

Zimmet PZ 1992 Kelly West Lecture 1991. Challenges in diabetes epidemiology: from West to the rest. Diabetes Care 15:232–252

DISCUSSION

Garrow: You pointed out that inhibition of hunger is maximal soon after the meal and, therefore, preabsorptive stimuli are involved. I used to be convinced by David Booth's contention that satiety was a conditioned reflex and that it was experienced on the basis of the events following the previous meal (Booth 1977). Were you using protocols for which that wasn't a possible explanation?

Blundell: The protocols don't allow us to assess that but I would agree that the inhibition of hunger following a meal is in part a result of a conditioning process. Indeed, whenever subjects take part in an appetite study they bring with them a lifetime of eating experiences, not just an experience of the previous meal. The biological system has therefore been exposed to a multitude of meals varying in weight, volume, energy density and macronutrient composition. The system will have learnt (been conditioned) that certain immediate sensations predict later nutritional satisfaction and the response (hunger) will be based, in part, on these early sensations. It is therefore inevitable that whenever meal characteristics are manipulated in an experiment, the response to that meal will be based partly on unconditioned responses to the food consumed and partly on conditioned responses established over the years.

James: But David Booth has suggested that an individual's behaviour is conditioned over a relatively short period of time, even when it is based on physiological signals of which the subject is totally unaware.

Blundell: Conditioning can take place over a short period of time but the effects can endure for much longer. This type of classical conditioning is usually called cue-consequence learning. It means that the sensory experiences of food in the mouth become closely linked to the subsequent metabolic effects of that food. Accordingly, the mouth sensations serve as a predictor of the nutritional value of food and this has been regarded as one way in which the 'wisdom of the body' is built up and used for the control of food intake. The problem is that with a rapidly changing food supply there is the potential for a similar taste sensation to be linked to a variety of metabolic responses and vice versa. Consequently, this form of wisdom is undermined.

James: An individual's weight gain amounts to an average of 0.7 kg per year, which occurs with a turnover of hundreds of thousands of calories. We are concerned with the average weight gain of populations as they go through industrialization, so we are talking about a variety of processes that presumably involve everything you've been talking about. Are you saying that out of all these control systems, there are only one or two principal components, and that these relate to dietary fat or to the energy density of the diet when these interact with a sedentary lifestyle?

Blundell: It is true that the average weight gain across populations seems quite small but this does not mean that all individuals gain weight at such a low rate. Moreover, weight gain does not necessarily depend upon a tiny excess of energy being consumed uniformly on a day-to-day basis. When we consider the weight gain of populations as they are exposed to a changing environment of industrialization it should be recognized that a complex system can be influenced in a variety of ways. Indeed, there are likely to be many pathways to obesity. The control systems operating on the ingestion and utilization of nutrients can become impaired in many ways (see Blundell 1991). However, if we consider the most potent and obvious pathway the evidence suggests that people with a low energy expenditure (sedentary lifestyle) exposed to very palatable, high density (probably fat rich) foods will be induced most easily into a positive energy balance and consequent weight gain. The problem does seem to be passive overconsumption with a permissive biological system.

Campfield: We have been studying the transient changes in blood glucose that occur before meals in rats, and we've demonstrated that this signal initiates feeding behaviour in rats (Campfield & Smith 1990a,b). It was first identified by Louis-Sylvestre & Le Magnen (1980). We've now done the same studies in humans, and we have found that people who have a transient 10% decrease in blood glucose increase their hunger ratings and request meals (Campfield et al 1996). Therefore, in the case of blood glucose, a pattern of change imposed upon the steady-state level has important signal information that makes people request food. In the case of insulin and its patterns of change, there are three or four peaks of insulin during the preabsorptive to postabsorptive phase. Therefore, the pattern of insulin, and the context of that pattern when it gets to the CNS, is important. The levels of leptin do not change with meals, but there appears to be a 90 min rhythm around a steady-state concentration of leptin (Considine et al 1996). The same investigators have also shown that there is a major increase in the levels of leptin when subjects are sleeping. Therefore, we have a gene product coming from fat cells that is elevated in obese people, suggesting that they are insensitive or resistant to that signal. However, this protein also has 90 min rhythm around a stable mean value, it is elevated in the sleeping state and there is a 90% decrease in its levels with 24 h of fasting. It is a complicated situation, suggesting that leptin is not just involved in energy balance.

Bray: Why do you think a high level of leptin in obese people reflects insensitivity? Does it affect food intake?

Campfield: It affects food intake and metabolism. If obese people have an elevated level, yet they continue to have increased body fat stores, one has to argue that they are insensitive to leptin.

Bray: But leptin may not be involved with food intake.

Campfield: An increase in adipose tissue mass leads to increased levels of leptin. This results in a decreased food intake, an increase in both activity and metabolic rate, and ultimately a decrease in fat storage. This suggests that it is impossible to have dietary-induced obesity in animals, unless AKR/J and SWR mice have low and high levels of leptin, respectively. Dietary-induced obesity in humans is intermediate between *ob/ob*, the mouse that has no leptin (and there seems to be no human counterparts for that), and *db/db*, the mouse that doesn't respond. We showed that a fivefold increase in the levels of leptin was necessary to reduce food intake and cause weight loss, which suggests a degree of insensitivity.

Swinburn: As people gain weight they become insulin resistant. Their metabolic rate increases and they burn more fat. All of these changes serve to counter that weight gain. Leptin may respond in a similar fashion by increased expression in response to increased fat mass and therefore acting as another measure that slows down weight gain.

Campfield: Peripheral administration of leptin in mice results in reductions in food intake, body weight and fat mass, and an increased metabolic activity (Campfield et al 1995, Halaas et al 1995, Pelleymounter et al 1995). We injected it into the lateral ventricles of the brain, and showed that this has a striking effect on food intake and other processes that are centrally mediated (Campfield et al 1995). Further work has to be carried out to find out what else it is doing. It clearly has a metabolic action, and it acts over a long period of time: a single injection has effects on food intake and other parameters that last for 24 h.

James: George Bray, why don't you think it's important?

Bray: I didn't say leptin wasn't important. I wanted to know the evidence that high levels of leptin in obesity reflects insensitivity. David York and I have performed adrenalectomies, which produce the same effects, but we don't say that the animals are steroid resistant. There is the issue of whether the food intake system is what you go after when you want to interpret the effect of leptin. When the gene was first cloned there were three hypotheses: (1) that obese people have an mRNA deficiency; (2) that a partially active protein is circulating in obese people; and (3) that obese people have normal levels of protein but that the protein is faulty and does not adjust food intake and fat mass to the expected level. The more we learn about its biology, the more we may move our attention away from food intake and focus on other functions. We have some preliminary data using animal models which suggest that leptin has some interesting effects on metabolic processes unrelated to food intake.

James: Do different patterns of food intake, such as a high level of fat intake, affect the levels of leptin?

York: The level of protein has not been studied, but the mRNA level increases rapidly if a rat is put on a high fat diet (Lin et al 1995).

Garrow: I was interested in the comment that people only change weight by 0.7 kg per year, which suggests that the system is not under close control (Gordon & Kannel 1973). The Framingham Study suggests that the average weight of individuals over a period of a decade or so fluctuates by about 10 kg. Therefore, it may be misleading to focus on short-term control, such as in the response to a single meal. These fluctuations don't continue indefinitely, which suggests that a long-term control mechanism is operating. This may be related to an individual's ability, or inability, to gain and lose weight rapidly. I believe there is a cognitive control mechanism.

Blundell: If we accept the argument that a daily small positive energy balance will eventually build up into a sizeable gain in weight, then I believe that it is appropriate to focus on single eating episodes, such as a meal. The inability of physiological satiety signals to inhibit eating sufficiently strongly represents one short-term control mechanism, whose inefficiency could account for long-term weight changes. Cognitions are important, and we know from the research on dietary restraint that many individuals in weight-conscious societies are attempting to substitute cognitive control for biological control. This often serves to make matters worse by disregulating the control over appetite (Blundell 1990).

Allison: The observation that some peoples' weights fluctuate widely, but that the mean stays roughly constant, is consistent with the idea that a control system is operating, whether it's cognitive or otherwise. However, it's also consistent with just random fluctuation, i.e. the roughly constant tendency for each person to eat a particular amount and expend a particular amount of energy, combined with a particular random perturbation (with a normal distribution or otherwise) on any given day.

Prentice: There is an argument in favour of a more robust protection against a low body weight, and that most decreases in weight — such as in the Framingham population — are as a result of a former gain of weight. A system that is always trying to regulate against loss of body weight will be much better designed. The control will be maximal when there is a high level of physical activity and a low fat diet.

Roberts: I agree. If young people are overfed they typically lose that weight and return back to normal. However, if they are underfed they subsequently overeat so that they become heavier than their original weight. Also, in the majority of overfeeding and unfeeding studies there are larger decreases in energy expenditure in response to underfeeding than increases in energy expenditure as a result of overfeeding (Saltzman & Roberts 1995).

Swinburn: Energy intake is intermittent and highly variable. Energy expenditure is also highly variable but continuous. An individual's weight does not fluctuate to the extent that one might expect given the wide variations between energy input and output. This suggests that there are mechanisms to even out changes in weight and restore the equilibrium. Leptin may be involved in this restoration, rather than being involved in a resistance pathway.

Blundell: I support the view that there is a much greater defence against undernutrition than against overnutrition. Moreover, in considering overconsumption we should probably make a distinction between obligatory overfeeding (mandatory experimental protocol) and volitional overeating. Biological compensatory mechanisms are more likely to be invoked in response to obligatory energy overloading than with overeating achieved without coercion. In a number of experimental studies with forced overfeeding, a reasonable degree of compensation often follows the cessation of the regime so that body weight is returned to near initial value. This does not appear to occur under natural circumstances in which overeating (positive energy balance) and weight gain occurs in response to incidental vagaries of physiology or the environment.

References

Booth DA 1977 Satiety and appetite are conditioned reactions. Psychosom Med 39:76–81

Blundell JE 1990 How culture undermines the biopsychological system of appetite control. Appetite 14:113–115

Blundell JE 1991 Pharmacological approaches to appetite suppression. Trends Pharmacol Sci 12:147–157

Campfield LA, Smith FJ 1990a Systemic factors in the control of food intake: evidence for patterns as signals. In: Sricker EM (ed) Handbook of behavioral neurobiology, vol 10: Neurobiology of food and fluid intake. Plenum, New York, p 183–206

Campfield LA, Smith FJ 1990b Transient declines in blood glucose signal meal initiation. Int J Obes 14:15–33

Campfield LA, Smith FJ, Guisez Y, Devos R, Burn P 1995 Recombinant mouse OB protein: evidence for a peripheral signal linking adiposity and central neural networks. Science 269:546–549

Campfield LA, Smith FJ, Rosenbaum M, Hirsch J 1996 Human eating: evidence for a physiological basis using a modified paradigm. Neurosci Biobehav Rev 20:133–137

Gordon T, Kannel WB 1973 The effects of overweight on cardiovascular disease. Geriatrics 28:80–88

Halaas JL, Gajiwala KS, Maffei M et al 1995 Weight-reducing effects of the plasma protein encoded by the obese gene. Science 269:543–546

Lin X, York DA, Harris RBS, Bray GA, Bruch RC 1995 The effect of high fat diets on expression of *Ob* mRNA in a model of diet-induced obesity. Obesity Res 3:389(abstr)

Louis-Sylvestre J, Le Magnen J 1980 A fall in blood glucose level precedes meal onset in free-feeding rats. Neurosci Biobehav Rev 4:13–15

Pelleymounter M, Cullen M, Baker M et al 1995 Effects of the obese gene product on body weight regulation in *ob/ob* mice. Science 269:540–543

Saltzman E, Roberts SB 1995 The role of energy expenditure in energy regulation: finding from a decade of research. Nutr Rev 53:209–220

Obesity and metabolic efficiency

Arne Astrup

The Research Department of Human Nutrition & Centre of Food Research, The Royal Veterinary & Agricultural University, Rolighedsvej 30, DK-1958 Frederiksberg C, Copenhagen, Denmark

Abstract. Obesity has a strong genetic component, which should be viewed as a predisposition only if certain environmental factors are present. Impaired regulation of both sides of the energy balance equation plays a role in the propensity to gain weight and develop obesity. Overeating may be induced in susceptible individuals by high dietary fat content, large portion sizes and low meal frequency. Increased metabolic efficiency in the form of a low resting metabolic rate has been identified in pre- and post-obese subjects, and the impact on total energy expenditure may be amplified by a low level of physical activity. A low thermic effect of food has been shown not to be a risk factor for weight gain, and post-obese subjects have a normal thermic effect of food. A genetically determined enhanced metabolic efficiency during overfeeding has been reported to contribute to fat gain. The heterogeneous nature of obesity indicates that different mechanisms, such as changes in the partitioning of fat (due to lipoprotein lipase activity, fat oxidative muscle enzymes) and carbohydrate, and an altered responsiveness of the sympathoadrenal system and thyroid hormones to a positive energy balance, seem to be involved.

1996 The origins and consequences of obesity. Wiley, Chichester (Ciba Foundation Symposium 201) p 159–173

Much attention has been given to factors likely to influence the efficiency of a given metabolic process and its relationship to the propensity to leanness or obesity. It is irrelevant to assess the energy output of the body without taking the other side of the energy equation, energy intake, into consideration. The energy content of an individual represents only a minute fraction of the total energy consumed during their life span; therefore, the variables influencing energy intake and expenditure are not nearly as critical for body weight maintenance and obesity as are the mechanisms responsible for the adjustment of energy intake to expenditure, regardless of the overall rate of energy turnover (Astrup & Flatt 1996). Although energy intake is normally regulated to equal expenditure, the adjustments of appetite to maintain constant body carbohydrate and fat stores are less precise when energy expenditure is low. Consequently, an increased metabolic efficiency may be seen when energy expenditure is lower than predicted, and a changed nutrient partitioning of macronutrients with consequences for appetite control and energy intake may also take place. Studies of twins and adoptees have provided evidence of an important genetic basis for the development of obesity (Poehlman et al 1986) but, because body fat gain and obesity are usually triggered by environmental factors, it is of particular interest to address the question as to how the typical modern, high fat, low carbohydrate diet interacts with the genetic make-up of individuals.

Increased energetic efficiency as a predisposing factor of obesity

Low energy expenditure as a risk factor for weight gain

A low energy expenditure for a given body size and composition (relative energy expenditure) is one of the genetically determined factors that may contribute to weight gain (Bogardus et al 1986, Ravussin et al 1988). In a cross-sectional study of Pima Indians, Bogardus et al (1986) reported that 83% of the variance of resting energy expenditure could be accounted for by fat-free mass, age and sex. Moreover, they reported that family membership accounted for an additional 11%, so that 94% of the total variability of resting energy expenditure could be explained. Together with support from twin studies these results suggest that the relative resting energy expenditure is at least partly genetically determined. In a subsequent prospective study in Pima Indians, Ravussin et al (1988) demonstrated that both a low relative resting energy expenditure and a low relative 24 h energy expenditure were risk factors for body weight gain. Follow-up four years later showed that the risk of gaining 10 kg was approximately seven times greater in those subjects with the lowest relative resting energy expenditure (lower tertile) than in those with the highest resting energy expenditure (higher tertile). The rate of relative 24 h energy expenditure was estimated to be responsible for up to 40% of the weight change. Other studies are, however, less unequivocal (Roberts 1995). Moreover, Seidell et al (1992) found no link between resting energy expenditure and weight gain over 10 years in 775 lean and obese men. In a long-term study of post-obese and non-obese women, Weisnier et al (1995) were unable to find any relationship between resting energy expenditure and subsequent weight gain.

Why do some families have a lower resting energy expenditure than others? Resting energy expenditure for a given body composition, as assessed by family studies in the Pima Indians, is a family trait. There is also a clear familial aggregation of both 24 h energy expenditure and resting energy expenditure, as indicated by the highly significant intraclass correlation coefficients of 0.44 and 0.58, respectively, in Caucasian siblings. Similar figures have been reported from twin studies. However, in Caucasian siblings the familial effect on energy expenditure can be explained entirely by a familial resemblance of fat-free mass and fat mass; even though plasma concentrations of free T_3 (triiodothyronine) and noradrenaline (indices of sympathetic activity) explain, independent of body composition, an additional proportion of the interindividual variation in energy expenditure (Toubro et al 1996). This pattern of findings suggests that non-additive genetic factors are operating (perhaps major genes which are particularly prevalent among Pima Indians). It remains to be determined whether low absolute and relative energy expenditures are risk factors for weight gain in Caucasians and longitudinal studies in Caucasians are therefore warranted.

Low energy expenditure in post-obese subjects

The investigation of possible causal abnormalities of energy expenditure and metabolic efficiency in obese subjects may be misleading because increased body size and changed body composition influences energy expenditure, substrate utilization, hormones and substrates. It is important to note that, due to the increased fat-free mass accompanying the obese state, both resting metabolic rate and 24 h energy expenditure are higher in obese individuals than in normal weight controls (Fig. 1). This is a classic shortcoming of the cross-sectional and case-control design, and this is certainly a pitfall in obesity research. Longitudinal studies overcome these obstacles to a certain degree, but they are time consuming and require large resources. The results obtained from studies comparing normal weight, either predisposed (pre-obese) or formerly obese individuals (post-obese), with matched controls without a weight problem history, are much easier to interpret, despite the difficulties involved in identifying predisposed subjects and producing weight-stable post-obese subjects.

The contention that post-obese individuals display a subnormal resting energy expenditure for a given body composition is questioned by eight out of 11 studies comparing post-obese with matched controls (Table 1). Although the significantly lower resting energy expenditure reported in three studies could be spurious, a pooled analysis of the 11 studies provides a larger sample size, and the 4–5% difference in resting energy expenditure now becomes significant (Astrup et al 1996). We have recently tested a group of 28 post-obese women, matched with respect to age, gender, fat-free mass and fat mass to a control group, and found that the mean relative resting energy expenditure was 8% lower in the post-obese group ($P < 0.02$). One should also take into consideration that a low relative resting energy expenditure is unlikely to be a pathophysiological factor involved in all obesities, and a mean difference of 4–5% cannot be detected consistently by the low statistical power provided by groups of six to 10 subjects. Unfortunately, the reported studies have not been composed of a sufficient number of post-obese subjects to allow another analysis, namely to test if a higher proportion of post-obese subjects have a relative energy expenditure lower than a given percentile of the never obese population.

Thermic effect of food

Meal-induced thermogenesis, or the thermic effect of food (TEF), has been found to be subnormal in obesity (Astrup et al 1987), and it has been suggested that the facultative component mediated by the sympathoadrenal system is reduced in obese subjects, and that it could play a causal role in the development and maintenance of obesity. The

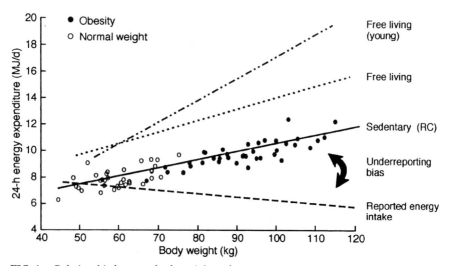

FIG. 1.   Relationship between body weight and energy requirements assessed by measurement of energy expenditure and reported energy intake in normal weight and overweight/obese (body mass index > 25 kg/m²) subjects. Sedentary 24 h energy expenditure is measured in a respiration chamber (RC) on a fixed physical activity programme, whereas the data on free-living energy expenditure are from measurements of double-labelled water. Modified from Astrup & Raben 1996.

importance of the role of the sympathetic system has been further supported by the finding that TEF remained decreased after a major weight loss, and that the sympathetic response to carbohydrate also remained smaller than seen in a non-obese control group (Astrup et al 1990). However, in a more carefully controlled study post-obese subjects were entirely weight normalized and weight stable before examination, and TEF did not differ between post-obese and controls under these conditions (Raben et al 1994). Furthermore, in a prospective study a low TEF was not found to be associated with subsequent weight gain (Tataranni et al 1995). There is therefore no evidence to support a causal role in obesity for a low TEF.

Enhanced metabolic efficiency in fat partitioning

Energy-related considerations cannot be expected to provide realistic answers to body weight regulation and obesity issues because 'energy' is an abstract concept, which does not have an equivalent in a biological system (Astrup & Flatt 1996). Weight maintenance is only possible when the fuel mixture oxidized matches the macronutrient mixture consumed, in amount and in composition. Substrate oxidation is determined by the need to regenerate ATP (which is primarily a function of body size and physical activity) and by the availability of intracellular metabolites that reflect circulating substrate levels. The mobilization of fuel reserves is controlled

TABLE 1   Resting energy expenditure (EE) of 114 post-obese subjects (PO) and 109 matched controls (C)[a]

Reference	Group size (PO/C)	Adjusted resting EE[b] (ΔPO versus C)	Significance of difference
Lean & James 1988	7/6	↓10%	$P < 0.01$
Goldberg et al 1991	9/9	↓4%	ns
McNeill et al 1990	6/6	↓8%	ns
Bukkens et al 1991	6/6	↓5%	ns
Nelson et al 1992	24/24	↓3%	ns
de Peuter et al 1992	6/6	↓4%	ns
Buemann et al 1992	8/8	↓5%	$P = 0.04$
Amatruda et al 1993	18/14	↓6%	ns
Astrup et al 1994	9/9	↓1%	ns
Toubro et al 1994	9/9	↓13%	$P < 0.05$
Raben et al 1994	12/12	↓3%	ns
Weighted average difference	114/109	↓5%	

[a]Studies are included only if the body weight of PO is within the normal range (body mass index $\leqslant 25$ kg/m²). Studies providing an antecedent low fat, high carbohydrate diet are excluded.
[b]Resting energy expenditure, or preferably basal metabolic rate and sleeping energy expenditure, are used after division by fat-free mass or by proper adjustment.

by endocrine regulatory signals and by the degree of replenishment of the body's fuel reserves. If the fuel mix oxidized does not match the macronutrient mixture consumed then the oxidative autoregulation adjusts the respiratory quotient (RQ), but in susceptible individuals nutrient partitioning causes changes in body composition. This continues until a body weight and size is reached where body composition complements endocrine and substrate level regulation in such a way that the fuel mix oxidized matches the macronutrient mixture consumed. Recent investigations have therefore increasingly focused on factors likely to effect and regulate substrate balances.

Carbohydrate and protein balances are achieved without obvious or readily measurable changes in the body's glycogen stores and protein pools. Adjustment of fat oxidation to intake is far less accurate, and the differences and changes in the body's stores that contribute to weight maintenance are greater. The degree of fatness at which weight gain tends to plateau to a steady-state of weight maintenance may be an elemental clue to the understanding of how the interactions between genetic, acquired and lifestyle factors influence the adjustment of fat oxidation and fat intake.

It is now clear that factors influencing food intake play a much greater role for weight maintenance than changes in energy expenditure, as the former can reverse, whereas the latter can only attenuate the effect of previous differences between energy intake and expenditure. Our great tolerance for substantial daily variations in energy expenditure and food intake makes it difficult to establish which of the many known regulatory effects are likely to play dominant roles.

Macronutrient partitioning in humans

During a 100-day 4.2 MJ/d overfeeding experiment with 12 pairs of monozygotic twins, weight gain varied from 4.3 to 13.3 kg, but within each pair fat gain was very similar (Bouchard et al 1990). The difference in weight gain between pairs could only partly be explained by differences in gain of fat and fat-free mass, and in the pair who gained the least weight about 60% of the extra energy must have been dissipated. In this study energy intake was fixed, but under *ad libitum* conditions the partitioning between fat storage and oxidation may have feedback implications for appetite and energy intake. It has been suggested that an increased proportion of fat in the diet of obesity-prone individuals may exceed the immediate capacity of the autoregulation to raise fat oxidation, i.e. cause the nutrient partitioning of fat to favour storage over oxidation. The increased fat deposition may, in turn, be responsible for adaptive mechanisms, such as increased levels of fat substrates and insulin resistance, which increase fat oxidation. According to this hypothesis, the accompanying negative carbohydrate balance, and inappropriate replenishment of the glycogen stores and subsequent metabolism of fuels in the liver, plays a crucial role by stimulating appetite to increase intake, resulting in amplification of the positive energy and fat balances (Friedman 1995).

This concept has been challenged by some studies in humans where *ad libitum* intake was found to be unaffected subsequent to dietary manipulation of the glycogen status. This suggests that appropriate glycogen stores are not maintained by subsequent increases or decreases in carbohydrate intake, rather by adjustments of RQ (Stubbs 1995). Interestingly, the same researchers have also shown that a positive carbohydrate balance at the end of one day is related to a negative energy balance at the end of the subsequent day, whereas there is a positive relationship between one day's fat balance and the following day's energy balance (Stubbs et al 1995). This study demonstrates that protein and carbohydrate, but not fat, may suppress subsequent energy intake. In obesity-prone individuals a disturbed nutrient partitioning may further amplify these macronutrient-specific effects on appetite. Indeed, some studies show that obesity-prone subjects respond differently to normal controls when exposed to a fat-rich diet. Heitmann et al (1995) found that weight gain after a six-year follow-up was only weakly associated with dietary fat at baseline. The association between dietary fat energy and weight gain, however, was sevenfold stronger in overweight and obese subjects, and the relationship was 15-fold stronger in those at familial risk. Moreover, covert manipulation of different isoenergetic amounts of fat and carbohydrate in preload tests showed that, in obese and non-obese restrained subjects, high fat preloads suppress subsequent intake to a lesser extent than do high carbohydrate preloads. In contrast, in normal weight subjects, who are unconcerned about body weight and eating (unrestrained), an accurate

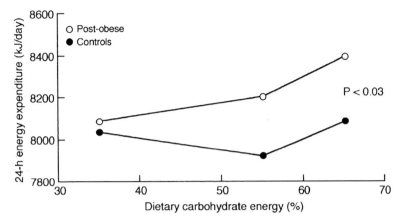

FIG. 2. The effect of controlled isocaloric changes in dietary carbohydrate content on 24 h energy expenditure in post-obese women and matched never-obese controls. 24 h energy expenditure was not influenced by dietary carbohydrate among the controls, but in the post-obese group 24 h energy expenditure was increased by increased carbohydrate content. Modified from Astrup et al 1994.

compensation for energy differences in the preloads occurs independent of macronutrient composition (Rolls et al 1994). These results suggest that high fat foods cause an inappropriate appetite response in susceptible individuals. A metabolic background for this response has been demonstrated by Verboeket-van de Venne et al (1994), who found that restrained eating subjects showed a lower fat oxidation in response to a high fat diet than unrestrained subjects. Prospective studies also support the theory that nutrient partitioning of fat, favouring storage over oxidation, is involved in the aetiology of obesity. However, the concept that fat oxidation may be impaired in predisposed subjects is supported by studies in post-obese subjects. One study using 24 h calorimetry examined the ability of post-obese women to adjust macronutrient oxidation in response to three different isocaloric diets providing 20%, 30% or 50% fat as energy (Astrup et al 1992). No differences were found between post-obese and controls on the two lower fat diets. On the high fat diet, however, the post-obese women failed to increase the ratio of fat to carbohydrate oxidation appropriately, which caused a positive fat balance. In another study increased carbohydrate oxidation and decreased fat oxidation were reported in post-obese women challenged with a high fat meal (Raben et al 1994). There is some evidence to support the finding that the accompanying negative carbohydrate balance causes decreased satiety and increased hunger in the post-obese, but this crucial link from glycogen stores to appetite remains to be proven. It is quite possible that the glycogen levels (in the liver, CNS or elsewhere) is not the signal which is directly linked to hunger. As proposed by Friedman (1995), the oxidative metabolism is a more likely candidate to provide a relation between fuel metabolism and appetite.

Energetic efficiency and diet composition

The twin overfeeding study by Bouchard et al (1990) mentioned above provided evidence of an energy-dissipating mechanism under strong genetic influence. The variability in fat gain may be partly related to different abilities to increase sympathetic activity and T_3 concentration, and hence increase adaptive thermogenesis. Even during isocaloric circumstances, a carbohydrate-rich diet increases both sympathetic activity and plasma T_3 levels as compared with a low carbohydrate diet, but parallel changes in 24 h energy expenditure can only be detected in subjects with the propensity to obesity (Fig. 2) (Astrup et al 1994). Overeating results in a variable increase in 24 h energy expenditure (Larson et al 1995), and the energetic efficiency is clearly less during carbohydrate overfeeding than during fat overfeeding (Horton et al 1995). Therefore, diet composition, or more particularly the carbohydrate/fat ratio, plays a role not only in appetite and energy intake, but also in energetic efficiency and fat deposition (Astrup & Raben 1995).

Acknowledgements

These studies were supported by the Danish Medical Research Council and the Danish Research and Development Programme for Food Technology.

References

Amatruda JM, Statt MC, Welle SL 1993 Total and resting energy expenditure in obese women reduced to ideal body weight. J Clin Invest 92:1236–1242

Astrup A, Flatt JP 1996 Metabolic determinants of body weight regulation. In: Bouchard C, Bray GA (eds) Regulation of body weight. Biological and behavioral mechanisms. Life Sciences Research Report 57. John Wiley & Sons, Chichester, p 193–210

Astrup A, Raben A 1995 Carbohydrates and obesity. Int J Obes (suppl 5) 19:27–37

Astrup A, Raben A 1996 Mono- and disaccharides: nutritional aspects. In: Eliasson A-C (ed) Carbohydrates in food. Marcel Dekker, New York, p 159–189

Astrup A, Andersen T, Henriksen O et al 1987 Impaired glucose-induced thermogenesis in skeletal muscle in obesity. The role of the sympathoadrenal system. Int J Obes 11:51–66

Astrup A, Andersen T, Christensen NJ et al 1990 Impaired glucose-induced thermogenesis and arterial norepinephrine response persist after weight reduction in obese humans. Am J Clin Nutr 51:331–337

Astrup A, Buemann B, Christensen NJ, Madsen J 1992 24 h energy expenditure and sympathetic activity in postobese women consuming a high-carbohydrate diet. Am J Physiol 262: 282E–288E

Astrup A, Buemann B, Christensen NJ, Toubro S 1994 Failure to increase lipid oxidation in response to increasing dietary fat content in formerly obese women. Am J Physiol 266:592E–599E

Astrup A, Buemann B, Toubro S, Ranneries C, Raben A 1996 Low resting metabolic rate in subjects predisposed to obesity: a role for thyroid status. Am J Clin Nutr 63:879–883

Bogardus C, Lillioja S, Ravussin E et al 1986 Familial dependence of the resting metabolic rate. N Engl J Med 315:96–100

Bouchard C, Tremblay A, Després J-P et al 1990 The response to long-term overfeeding in identical twins. New Engl J Med 322:1477–1482

Buemann B, Astrup A, Christensen NJ, Madsen J 1992 Effect of moderate cold exposure on 24-hour energy expenditure. Similar response in post-obese and non-obese women. Am J Physiol 263:1040E–1045E

Bukkens SGF, McNeill G, Smith JS, Morrison DC 1991 Postprandial thermogenesis in post-obese women and weight-matched controls. Int J Obes 15:147–154

de Peuter R, Withers RL, Brinkman M, Tomas FM, Clark DG 1992 No differences in rates of energy expenditure between post-obese women. Int J Obes 16:801–808

Friedman MI 1995 Control of energy intake by energy metabolism. Am J Clin Nutr (Suppl) 62:1096S–1100S

Goldberg GR, Black AE, Prentice AM, Coward WA 1991 No evidence of lower energy expenditure in post-obese women. Proc Nutr Soc 50:109A

Heitmann BL, Lissner L, Sørensen TIA, Bengtsson C 1995 Dietary fat intake and weight gain in women genetically predisposed for obesity. Am J Clin Nutr 61:1213–1217

Horton TJ, Drougas H, Brachey A, Reed GW, Peters JC, Hill JO 1995 Fat and carbohydrate overfeeding in humans: different effects on energy storage. Am J Clin Nutr 62:19–29

Larson DE, Tataranni PA, Ferraro RT, Ravussin E 1995 *Ad libitum* food intake on a 'cafeteria diet' in Native American women: relations with body composition and 24h energy expenditure. Am J Clin Nutr 62:911–917

Lean MEJ, James WPT 1988 Metabolic effects of isoenergetic nutrient exchange over 24 hours in relation to obesity in women. Int J Obes 12:15–27

McNeill G, Bukkens SGF, Morrison DC, Smith JS 1990 Energy intake and energy expenditure in post-obese women and weight-matched controls. Proc Nutr Soc 49:14A

Nelson KM, Weinsier RL, James LD, Darnell B, Hunter G, Long CL 1992 Effect of weight reduction on resting energy expenditure, substrate utilization and the thermic effect of food in moderately obese women. Am J Clin Nutr 55:924–933

Poehlman ET, Tremblay A, Després JP et al 1986 Genotype-controlled changes in body composition and fat morphology following overfeeding in twins. Am J Clin Nutr 43:723–731

Raben A, Andersen HB, Christensen NJ, Madsen J, Holst JJ, Astrup A 1994 Evidence for an abnormal postprandial response to a high-fat meal in women predisposed to obesity. Am J Physiol 30:549E–559E

Ravussin E, Lillioja S, Knowler WC et al 1988 Reduced rate of energy expenditure as a risk factor for body-weight gain. N Engl J Med 318:467–472

Roberts SB 1995 Abnormalities of energy expenditure and the development of obesity. Obesity Res (suppl 2) 3:155S–163S

Rolls BJ, Kim-Harris S, Fischman MW, Foltin RW, Moran TH, Stoner SA 1994 Satiety after preloads with different amounts of fat and carbohydrate: implications for obesity. Am J Clin Nutr 60:476–487

Seidell JC, Muller DC, Sorkin JD, Andres R 1992 Fasting respiratory exchange ratio and resting metabolic rate as predictors of weight gain: the Baltimore Longitudinal Study on ageing. Int J Obes 16:667–674

Stubbs RJ 1995 Macronutrient effects on appetite. Int J Obes (suppl 5) 19:11–19

Stubbs RJ, Harbron CG, Murgatroyd PR, Prentice AM 1995 Covert manipulation of dietary fat and energy density: effect on substrate flux and food intake in men eating *ad libitum*. Am J Clin Nutr 62:316–329

Tataranni PA, Larson DE, Snitker S, Ravussin E 1995 Thermal effect of food in humans: methods and results from use of a respiratory chamber. Am J Clin Nutr 61:1013–1019

Toubro S, Sørensen TIA, Rønn B, Christensen NJ, Astrup A 1996 24-h energy expenditure: the role of body composition, thyroid status, sympathetic activity and family membership. J Clin Endocrinol Metab 81:2670–2674

Verboeket-van de Venne WPHG, Westerterp KR, ten Hoor F 1994 Substrate utilization in man: effects of dietary fat and carbohydrate. Metabolism 43:152–156

Weinsier RL, Nelson KM, Hensrud DD, Darnell BE, Hunter GR, Schutz Y 1995 Metabolic
    predictors of obesity: contribution of resting energy expenditure, thermal effect of food, and
    fuel utilization to 4-year weight gain of post-obese and never-obese women. J Clin Invest
    95:980–985

DISCUSSION

Bray: How can you be sure that two different diets with different fat contents are
isocaloric?

Astrup: It's difficult to achieve isocaloric conditions. However, it is possible to do
this by using respiration chambers, in which an approximate energy balance can be
obtained by estimating the energy requirements by prediction equations using fat-free
mass, fat mass, age and gender. We also analysed the chemical components of the diets.

Bray: What was the exact procedure of making diet adjustments?

Astrup: The subjects were fed different diets about three or four days prior to being
measured in the respiration chamber. We already had initial baseline information about
the energy requirement during a chamber stay, so we knew exactly how much energy
they required during the 24 h period in the chamber. On the low fat, high carbohydrate
diet 24 h energy expenditure was 4–5% higher than on the high fat diet, so those on the
high carbohydrate diet were slightly underfed because they had a high energy
expenditure.

Swinburn: Did you measure the relationship between respiratory quotient (RQ) and
food quotient in the obese people before they lost weight?

Astrup: It's rather difficult to compare obese and post-obese in terms of RQ because
obese subjects tend to consume a diet with a higher fat content. Therefore, obese
subjects will tend to have a lower RQ than normal subjects. Post-obese subjects had
stable weights and their diets were controlled for three to four days before we measured
them in the chambers. We did a subsequent study where we kept them for five days in
the chambers. On the first day they were given a low fat diet and they were in energy
and macronutrient balance. On the second day they were given a high fat diet, and we
observed the dynamics of how they increased their fat oxidation. It was clear that post-
obese subjects had a pronounced suppression of post-prandial fat oxidation that could
be switched off by changing the diet composition. They expressed the suppression of
post-prandial fat oxidation only when they were challenged with a high fat diet. It
disappears if they are given a medium or a low fat diet. To address whether this is
causal, we would have to do longitudinal studies similar to those that the Phoenix
group have done (Zurlo et al 1990). We are performing longitudinal studies to
determine whether a low fat oxidation (high RQ) is a risk factor for weight gain in
Caucasians.

Ferro-Luzzi: You showed that even normal subjects responded to carbohydrate diet
with a higher energy expenditure, but your study period was only two weeks. Do you
believe that this is a short-lived response, or would the increase in energy expenditure

persist if the subjects were maintained on this diet? I am thinking of the real world, where developing country populations obtain a higher proportion of their calories from carbohydrates, while not having an energy expenditure which is higher than that of Europeans.

Astrup: It's impossible to answer this question at the moment, because other cultural and ethnic differences may confound the relationship. There are some indications that vegetarians have a higher resting metabolic rate. But we don't know whether this is caused by carbohydrate or other nutrients, or even behavioural differences. We are participating in a European multicentre trial that is just about to start. It is a six-month dietary intervention trial that will compare high and low fat diets, and look at different carbohydrate sources. The 24 h energy expenditure will also be one of the measurements. Therefore, this study may tell us if these changes in energy expenditure are permanent or only short-term.

Prentice: We performed some whole-body calorimeter experiments in the Gambia (Minghelli et al 1990). We matched Gambian and Swiss men in terms of body composition, and put them in the chamber on an RQ of around 0.93, which represents a high carbohydrate diet. We found that the energy expenditure is lower in the Gambian men. This may not be a carbohydrate effect, but rather may be caused by other confounding effects of a long-term chronic energy insufficiency.

York: Arne Astrup emphasized the importance of diet composition affecting metabolism, but there's now evidence from animal studies that the metabolic profile of an animal may determine diet selection. Examples of this include our model of dietary obesity in OM and S5B rats that George Bray and I have been looking at (Bray et al 1990). Also, in David West's mouse model (West et al 1994) the mice that get fat are the mice that, given a choice, selected a high fat diet before they became fat (Smith et al 1995). In addition, if carbohydrate metabolism is blocked there is selective stimulation of macronutrient intake. These experiments suggest that the activities of metabolic pathways themselves determine the selection of macronutrients. These systems may be interactive or may be controlled by the same signals.

Heymsfield: I would like to make two comments. The first is a general comment about post-obesity. I've studied a few post-obese patients over the past few years but they're not easy to find, so the sample size is small. However, I have found that all of these subjects are not particularly healthy. In women osteoporosis, amenorrhoea and menstrual abnormalities seem to be very common. Therefore, post-obese subjects may be a biased group or they may have some abnormalities that are peculiar to that population.

My second point is that we assume that fat-free mass is the metabolically active compartment, and we adjust energy expenditure against that. We have consistently found that post-obese subjects (i.e. those that lose 30–40 kg over five years or so) tend to be overhydrated. Their extracellular fluid compartment, compared to their fat-free mass, is relatively large, so body composition may be an important difference between post-obese and never-obese subjects of similar body weight.

Astrup: Our post-obese subjects are not recruited from the general population, they are post-obese as a result of our own intervention studies. Therefore, the females are normal and healthy. If they had any of the disturbances that you mentioned, they would be excluded from the study.

In relation to your second point about fluid retention, this possibility can probably be ruled out. We have been unable to find any differences in body composition between post-obese and controls using dual energy X-ray absorptiometry scanning and magnetic resonance imaging (MRI).

Heymsfield: We also did computed tomography (CT) and MRI, and did not find any differences, but these imaging techniques examine organs and tissues. If you look instead at fluid compartments you will see that there are differences between post-obese and never-obese subjects in extracellular fluid volume.

Prentice: The work of John Blundell and Arne Astrup, and our studies, suggest that carbohydrate is protective in terms of weight gain (e.g. Hill & Prentice 1995, Prentice 1995). Is there any evidence that obesity is occurring in any of the Afro-Caribbean groups that have a high carbohydrate diet? Or can we ascribe the high prevalence of obesity by the transition to a high fat diet?

Jackson: What is your definition of a high carbohydrate diet?

Prentice: I'm more used to thinking about carbohydrate diets in terms of the per cent of fat, so I would say about 30% energy from fat or less. I'm unconvinced that we would find people who were becoming obese on a diet from which they obtained less than 30% energy from fat.

Astrup: It may be possible if they have a very low level of physical activity.

Bouchard: Exactly, most people think that chronic overfeeding with fat or carbohydrate is the main cause of obesity. However, this may be incorrect. The level of macronutrient intake or of total energy intake may be reasonable or may have remained at the same level in these countries, but the level of energy expenditure may have decreased considerably.

Prentice: John Blundell's data suggest that a low fat diet is protective even in typical sedentary populations.

Bouchard: Yes, but the levels of fat intake in these studies were below or above current values. A number of studies have shown that, with a fat intake of about 35–38% of calories from fat, sedentary people tend to be in positive energy balance.

Shuper: The kind of data that Andrew Prentice is asking for have to come from studies of individuals, because in populations there will be some people who become fat even when only 15% of their calorie intake is obtained from fat.

Forrester: We don't have any data for individuals, but the food balance data from Jamaica indicate that at least 30–40% of calories are obtained from fat.

Jackson: If fat is providing 30% of calorie intake then this is close to the level identified by Andrew Prentice as a high carbohydrate diet, on which he said people were unlikely to become obese.

James: Patrick Francois has suggested that the break point is about 20%, which would fit the Chinese data with minimal obesity rates on an average dietary fat content of 14% (Francois & James 1994).

Bray: Berit Heitmann was a co-author of a review on dietary fat and obesity (Lissner & Heitmann 1995). After reading her review, I was not convinced that dietary fat played a major role in human obesity, in contrast to the animal studies, which show that obesity readily results from a high fat diet. Berit, would you like to comment on that?

Heitmann: The picture from cross-sectional studies is clear-cut, i.e. there is a significant association between fat intake and obesity (Lissner & Heitmann 1995), but the picture from prospective studies is not clear-cut. On the other hand, although none of the intervention studies had the primary aim of looking at fat intake in relation to weight change, the intervention studies reducing fat intake in relation to breast cancer, for instance, show that people who reduce their fat intake do lose weight.

Stunkard: Also, vegetarians have a very low fat intake, and Havala & Dwyer (1993) have shown that there are virtually no obese vegetarians.

Roberts: When we talk about low fat diets, they are usually low fat, low energy-dense, high fibre and less palatable diets. We need to separate these factors out. We've recently completed some studies in which we've separated fat from palatability and energy density and fibre content (Roberts 1995). In lean people, at least, we find that there is only a small effect of fat intake on caloric intake when we control for these other factors. They switch from carbohydrate to fat oxidation very easily.

Blundell: In considering the relationship between dietary fat and obesity, we can probably say that a low fat diet protects against the development of obesity. Analysis of the National Diet and Nutrition Survey of British Adults data has revealed that in the low fat consumers (<35% energy from fat) there was only one case of obesity (Macdiarmid et al 1996). In the Leeds High Fat Study we have found that certain cases of obesity among current low fat consumers have recently changed from a high fat to a low fat diet. Consequently, in cross-sectional studies the relationship between dietary fat and obesity may be artificially weakened by the presence of people who have recently reduced their fat intake in response to health messages. When we consider whether obesity is brought about by overconsumption or underactivity, we can identify high fat foods as one cause of overconsumption (but not necessarily the only cause). It is worth recognizing that it is possible to consume double the average daily fat intake in one single meal. However, we should resist the temptation to apply these general formulas universally. It is not necessary to claim that obesity is due exclusively to underactivity or to overconsumption; there will be particular cases where each of these formulas (and others) can be applied.

Astrup: It's meaningless to discuss whether a low physical activity, a high fat diet or genetic factors are causing obesity. All three factors interact, so some people who have a low level of physical activity and consume a low fat diet may have normal body weights.

Bouchard: I disagree. If an individual is sedentary and has a fat intake that is too low, then there is a risk that the low level of fat intake will not be sustained. Food or fat intake may therefore increase because these levels of intake were not 'comfortable' for the individual. This is probably a scenario that occurs often in our highly sedentary mode of life.

Garrow: In my opinion, metabolic efficiency is not an important factor in obesity for two reasons. Firstly, Ravussin et al (1988a) have shown that among Pima Indians, those who have a lower metabolic rate than one would expect considering their body composition have a higher propensity to gain weight. However, having gained weight they then have a higher than expected metabolic rate. Secondly, if having a low energy expenditure was really a powerful predictor of obesity, all short people should be fat. However, there is no relationship between stature and the prevalence of obesity.

Ravussin: I agree. Metabolic efficiency alone cannot explain obesity. Pima Indians, a population with a very high prevalence of obesity, have a 'normal' resting metabolic rate when compared to Caucasians. However, as John Garrow has mentioned, within the Pima population, those with a low metabolic rate for a given body weight and body composition gain more weight than those with a high metabolic rate (Ravussin et al 1988b). Despite this observation, we could only explain approximately one-third of the weight gain by differences in metabolic rate. Furthermore, a weight gain of about 3 kg would easily offset the 50–70 kcal/day deficit observed in those who had gained weight. This is also true for other metabolic predictors of weight gain, such as a high RQ, low spontaneous physical activity or insulin sensitivity (Ravussin & Swinburn 1993). Taken together, these results indicate that other factors—such as food intake and physical inactivity—play important roles in the aetiology of obesity in Pima Indians; for example, Arne Astrup's group has shown that a blunted plasma norepinephrine response is associated with higher food intake in Caucasians (Raben et al 1996). In addition, Leibel et al (1995) have shown that most of the metabolic adaptation in response to body weight gain or body weight loss is attributable to the energy cost of physical activity. When these same subjects were measured in our respiratory chamber, only marginal differences in 'metabolic efficiencies' were found.

References

Bray GA, York DA, Fisler JS 1990 Experimental obesity: a homeostatic failure due to defective nutrient stimulation of the sympathetic nervous system. Vitam Horm 45:1–25

Francois PJ, James WPT 1994 An assessment of nutritional factors affecting the BMI of a population. Eur J Clin Nutr 48:110S–114S

Havala S, Dwyer J 1993 Position of the American Dietetic Association: vegetarian diets. J Am Diet Assoc 93:1317–1319

Hill JO, Prentice AM 1995 Sugar and body weight regulation. Am J Clin Nutr 62:264S–274S

Leibel RL, Rosenbaum M, Hirsch J 1995 Changes in energy expenditure resulting from altered body weight. N Engl J Med 332:621–628

Lissner L, Heitmann BL 1995 Dietary fat and obesity: evidence from epidemiology. Eur J Clin Nutr 49:79–90

Macdiarmid JI, Cade JE, Blundell JE 1996 High and low fat consumers, their macronutrient intake and body mass index: further analysis of the National Diet and Nutrition Survey of British Adults. Eur J Clin Nutr, in press

Minghelli G, Schutz Y, Charbonnier A, Whitehead RG, Jéquier E 1990 Twenty-four-hour energy expenditure and basal metabolic rate measured in a whole-body indirect calorimeter in Gambian men. Am J Clin Nutr 51:563–570

Prentice AM 1995 Are all calories equal? In: Cottrell R (ed) Weight control. The current perspective. Chapman & Hall, London, p 8–33

Raben A, Holst JJ, Christensen NJ, Astrup A 1996 Determinants of postprandial appetite sensations: macronutrient intake and glucose metabolism. Int J Obes 20:161–169

Ravussin E, Lillioja S, Knowler WC et al 1988a Reduced rate of energy expenditure at a risk factor for body-weight gain. N Engl J Med 318:467–462

Ravussin E, Lillioja S, Knowler WC et al 1988b Reduced rate of energy expenditure as a risk factor for body-weight gain. N Engl J Med 318:467–472

Ravussin E, Swinburn BA 1993 Metabolic predictors of obesity: cross-sectional versus longitudinal data. Int J Obes (suppl 3) 17:28S–31S

Roberts SB 1995 Abnormalities of energy expenditure and the development of obesity. Obesity Res (suppl 2) 3:155S–163S

Smith BK, West DB, York DA 1995 Carbohydrate vs. fat preference: evidence for differing patterns of macronutrient selection in two inbred mouse strains. Obesity Res 3:411 (abstr)

Stunkard AJ, Messick S 1985 The three-factor eating questionnaire to measure dietary restraint, disinhibition and hunger. J Psychosom Res 29:71–83

West DB, Goudey-Lefevre J, York B, Truett GE 1994 Dietary obesity linked to genetic loci on chromosome 9 and 15 in a polygenic mouse model. J Clin Invest 94:1410–1416

Zurlo F, Lillioja S, Esposita-Del Pueule A et al 1990 Low ratio of fat to carbohydrate oxidation as a predictor of weight gain: study of 24 h RQ. Am J Physiol 259:650E–657E

Socioeconomic status and obesity

Albert J. Stunkard

Department of Psychiatry, University of Pennsylvania, 3600 Market Street, PA 19104, USA

Abstract. Two recent developments have thrown into bold relief the importance of environmental forces in determining the prevalence of human obesity. The first is genetic studies that estimate the heritability of human obesity at no more than 33%. The second is the 33% increase in the prevalence of obesity in the USA during the past decade. The importance of the environment in influencing obesity is matched only by the extent of our ignorance of how it exerts its effects and of how we may favourably alter them. The most thoroughly studied measure of environmental influences is socioeconomic status. Among women in developed societies socioeconomic status is strongly (negatively) correlated with the prevalence of obesity: the lower the social class the more the obesity. Prospective studies have shown that this correlation reflects, in part, causation: socioeconomic status helps to determine the prevalence of obesity and thinness. Likewise, the presence of obesity helps to determine socioeconomic status. In developing societies there is also a strong relationship between socioeconomic status and obesity, but it is a positive one: the higher the socioeconomic status the more the obesity. Unfortunately, we know of few other social determinants of obesity and studies on the social determinants of this disorder are desperately needed.

1996 The origins and consequences of obesity. Wiley, Chichester (Ciba Foundation Symposium 201) p 174–187

Two recent developments have thrown into bold relief the importance of the environment in determining the prevalence of obesity in western society. The first is the striking increase in the prevalence of obesity in the USA during the past decade (Kuczmarski et al 1994). The second is quantitative genetic studies that have revealed only a modest heritability of human obesity (Vogler et al 1995), leaving a large role for the environment.

Environmental determinants

Compelling evidence for an influence of environmental factors on the prevalence of obesity lies in the results of two National Health and Nutrition Examination Surveys (NHANES) conducted in 1976–1980 and again in 1988–1991 (Kuczmarski et al 1994). In the first of these surveys the overall prevalence of obesity was estimated at about 25%; no more than 10 years later this figure had risen to 33%, or an increase of one third. Furthermore, the increase in body weight was not confined to obese persons. It included all weight classes, with an increase in the body weight of all Americans that averaged 3.6 kg. This increase over a 10-year period was hardly due to a change in the American gene pool. The primary responsibility must lie in changes in the environment.

Genetic determinants

The existence of numerous forms of genetic obesity in animals and the ease with which adiposity can be produced by the selective breeding of farm animals have long suggested that genetic factors can play an important role in human obesity. But stunning advances in our knowledge during the past decade have made it clear that genetic factors do play an important role in human obesity (Bouchard et al 1994).

The first studies, utilizing the classic twin method, estimated very high levels of heritability (the percentage of variance accounted for by genetic influences) for the body mass index (BMI), i.e. weight(kg)/height(m)^2, of the order of 80% (Stunkard et al 1986). Even the more conservative estimates derived from studies of identical twins separated at birth were as high as 66% (Stunkard et al 1990). There is now a general belief that these studies overestimated the role of heredity and that a more reasonable estimate is that derived from adoption and family studies, i.e. about 33% (Vogler et al 1995).

If the heritability of BMI is no more than 33%, then 67% of the variance must be environmental. Thus, although human obesity develops within the constraints imposed upon it by genetic factors, environmental determinants play an enormously important part in its development. These two determinants are not in conflict, but they interact, as shown in the idealized representation of genetic vulnerability and environmental challenge in Fig. 1 (Stunkard 1990).

The extent of environmental influences on human obesity is matched only by the extent of our ignorance of how these influences exert their effects and so of how we may favourably alter them. Compared to the flood of research on genetic influences on obesity, studies of environmental influences are painfully limited. Of these, the most systematic have been those of socioeconomic status.

Socioeconomic status and obesity

The first study of socioeconomic status and obesity 30 years ago established the basic relationships between these two variables (Goldblatt et al 1965). In a stratified sample of 1660 persons in Midtown Manhattan, as shown in Fig. 2, obesity was six times more prevalent among women of lower socioeconomic status than among those of upper socioeconomic status. These results were important because of the strength of the relationship between current socioeconomic status and obesity, but the study went further.

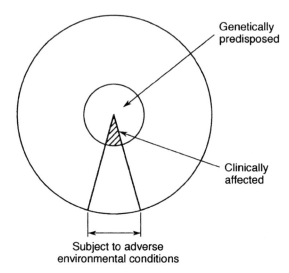

FIG. 1.   Genetics and environment. The small inner circle represents those persons who are genetically predisposed to a disorder. The wedge represents adverse environmental conditions to which these individuals may be exposed. The model indicates that only those genetically predisposed persons who are exposed to adverse environmental conditions are clinically affected, as in the case of obesity.

In addition to current socioeconomic status, the Midtown Manhattan Study measured parental socioeconomic status when the respondents were eight years old, the so-called 'socioeconomic status of origin', and assessed its relationship to the prevalence of obesity. As shown in Fig. 2, the socioeconomic status of origin was related to the prevalence of obesity almost as strongly as was the respondents' own socioeconomic status. The respondents' obesity could hardly have influenced their socioeconomic status of origin, suggesting that socioeconomic status of origin was a determinant of obesity, at least in this population. Note, however, that the prevalence of obesity in the socioeconomic status of origin was lower among persons of lower socioeconomic status and was higher among persons of upper socioeconomic status, than was the case for current socioeconomic status. These differences indicate that, in addition to socioeconomic status influencing obesity, obesity also influenced socioeconomic status.

Analysis of the social mobility of the population (the rise or fall in social class) confirmed the importance of obesity in determining social class. Thus, the prevalence of obesity was nearly twice as high (22%) among women who fell in social class as it was (12%) among those who rose in social class (Goldblatt et al 1965). The recent prospective study of Gortmaker et al (1993) helps to elucidate the mechanisms for this fall. Obesity has a deleterious influence on social functioning in women: those who had been obese in adolescence suffered significant social disability in adult life.

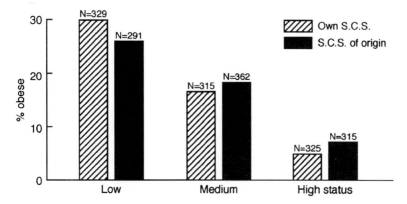

FIG. 2.   Socioeconomic status (S.C.S.) and obesity. The percentage of the population that is obese is noted on the y-axis. The shaded bars show that, among women of lower socioeconomic status, 30% were obese, compared to 16% and 5% among women of middle and lower socioeconomic status. The hatched bars show the percentage of women who were obese as a function of 'socioeconomic status of origin' or the socioeconomic status of their parents when they were eight years of age.

These findings have been confirmed in no fewer than 54 studies in developed countries, which found a strong inverse relationship between socioeconomic status and obesity among women (Sobal & Stunkard 1989). Furthermore, two prospective longitudinal studies from the UK have confirmed that socioeconomic status is a determinant of body weight (Braddon et al 1986, Power & Moynihan 1988). They have shown that both girls and boys born into a lower socioeconomic status were more overweight as adults than those born into an upper socioeconomic status.

The direction of causality

The simplest explanation for these findings is that the relation of socioeconomic status and obesity is bidirectional: socioeconomic status determines the prevalence of obesity and obesity leads to a decline in socioeconomic status. There is, however, a complication. Another factor or factors may influence both socioeconomic status and obesity (Stunkard & Sørensen 1993). An example of such a common factor is heredity. As has been noted, genetic factors influence obesity. It is less well known that genetic factors may also influence socioeconomic status. Thus, studies of Danish adoptees have revealed that the socioeconomic status of biological parents influences the socioeconomic status of their offspring, even though they have had no personal contact with them (Teasdale & Sørensen 1983).

A path analysis helps to explain this surprising finding. It shows that the influence of socioeconomic status on obesity is mediated by factors measured by the intelligence quotient (IQ). Biological parents influence the IQ of their children and IQ, in turn, influences obesity: the higher the IQ the lower the prevalence of obesity. Adoptive parents also influence the socioeconomic status of their offspring but the mechanism is different: the path goes through the years of education that they afford their children. It is noteworthy that these influences were present even when the socioeconomic status of the adoptee was controlled. The relationship between socioeconomic status and obesity is not a simple one (Stunkard & Sørensen 1993).

Discordant findings on the relationship between socioeconomic status and obesity

The exquisite relationship between socioeconomic status and obesity among women in developed societies is not found regularly among men or children. Among them, a significant percentage manifest either no relationship between socioeconomic status and obesity or a direct relationship: the higher the socioeconomic status the greater the prevalence of obesity (Sobal & Stunkard 1989).

An even more striking difference in the relationship between socioeconomic status and obesity is found in developing societies. When we turn from developed to developing societies, there is a complete reversal in the relationship between socioeconomic status and obesity. Among every developing society that has been studied, there is a direct and often very strong relationship between socioeconomic status and the prevalence of obesity (Sobal & Stunkard 1989) in men, women and children.

Mediators of the relationship between socioeconomic status and obesity

Clearly, there are powerful relationships between socioeconomic status and obesity. A first step in controlling the environment that predisposes to obesity is understanding the factors which mediate these relationships. In developed societies the most revealing of these relationships is that of the difference between men and women in terms of socioeconomic status and obesity. As we have seen, among women socioeconomic status is strongly related to obesity, and among men it is not (Sobal & Stunkard 1989). A first step is to assess the difference in social forces acting on men and women, forces which continue their action to the present time. Over a period of 20 years there has been little change in the BMI of men (Flegal et al 1988a). In contrast, the BMI of women has risen and, significantly, risen more rapidly among women of lower socioeconomic status than it has among women of upper socioeconomic status (Flegal et al 1988b). In the light of these facts, let us consider what may mediate the relationship between socioeconomic status and obesity.

At least five factors may mediate the inverse relationship between socioeconomic status and obesity among women in developed societies, particularly factors that control obesity among women of upper socioeconomic status.

The first important influence constraining the prevalence of obesity among woman of upper socioeconomic status in developed societies is dieting and dietary restraint. Women of higher socioeconomic status diet more often than do women of lower socioeconomic status, they have greater access to resources that facilitate dieting, they have greater knowledge of nutrition, and they are more committed to the view that slimness is desirable and are therefore more motivated to achieve a slim figure.

A second closely related influence is dietary preference, which differs considerably among the social classes. Among those of upper socioeconomic status, foods high in fat are avoided and low fat foods are favoured, a ranking not found among persons of lower socioeconomic status who consume a higher proportion of fatty foods. This difference in preference is dictated partially by the lower cost of high fat foods and partly by social pressure; the two are probably closely linked.

A third direct influence on the control of obesity among women of higher socioeconomic status is their greater physical activity, derived from their greater leisure time and greater opportunity for recreational exercise. Interestingly, pathologically increased physical activity characterizes the young women of upper socioeconomic status whose dieting leads to anorexia nervosa.

A fourth factor mediating the inverse relationship between socioeconomic status and obesity among women is social mobility. As we have noted in the Midtown Manhattan Study (Goldblatt et al 1965), the prevalence of obesity is nearly twice as high among women who fall in social class as it is among women who rise in it. One of the longitudinal studies in the UK confirmed and extended this finding. It showed that obesity was significantly less prevalent (5%) among women who rose in social status than among those (11%) who remained in their social class of origin (Braddon et al 1986). As is the case with socioeconomic status itself, social mobility plays a far less important part in determining the prevalence of obesity among men.

A fifth factor influencing the relationship between socioeconomic status and obesity is heredity. Parents can influence the body weight of their children through both a direct influence on body weight and an indirect influence via socioeconomic status. As we have seen, studies of Danish adoptees have revealed a significant influence of the socioeconomic status of biological parents upon the prevalence of obesity in their children, with whom they have had no personal contact (Teasdale & Sørensen 1983). This influence appears to be genetically transmitted, via the transmission of IQ.

The strong direct relationship between socioeconomic status and obesity in developing societies has a more straightforward rationale than does the inverse relationship in developed societies. The low prevalence of obesity in developing societies appears to be due to a lack of food, often coupled with a high energy expenditure. The greater prevalence of obesity among persons of higher socioeconomic status appears to be due to their social influence in obtaining larger amounts of food, coupled with cultural values favouring fat bodies. Obesity may be a sign of health and wealth in these societies, the opposite of its significance in developed societies. In such societies the biological propensity to store fat is associated with, and may even influence, cultural evolution, which selects 'fatness' as a valued trait. Among most of the 58 traditional cultures for which information is available, 'plumpness' is viewed as an ideal of feminine beauty and a symbol of prestige (Brown & Konner 1987). In circumstances of relative deprivation, members of the upper socioeconomic status may have access to sufficient food to become fat,

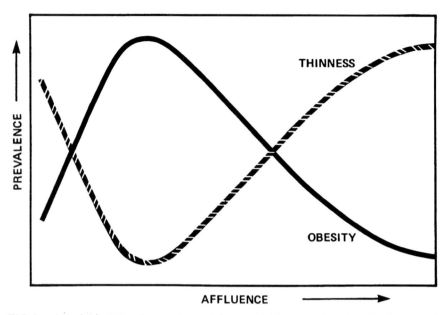

FIG. 3.   A model depicting the prevalence of obesity and thinness as a function of socioeconomic status. Obesity is rare among the poor because of the scarcity of food. As more food becomes available, the prevalences of obesity and thinness increase and decrease, respectively. With greater affluence, fashion dictates a decrease in obesity and an increase in thinness.

whereas members of lower socioeconomic status do not. A model reflecting the relationship between socioeconomic status and obesity across the spectrum from extreme poverty to extreme affluence is depicted in Fig. 3.

Other social factors and obesity

Because of the enormous importance of environmental factors in determining obesity, it is unfortunate that our information about factors influencing the prevalence of obesity is largely limited to socioeconomic status. The effort to control obesity will require a far better understanding of the social factors that promote it than is now available. There is, therefore, an urgent need to explore social factors in addition to socioeconomic status. A few recent examples illustrate the direction in which such a study may be conducted profitably.

A first approach is disaggregation of the measure of socioeconomic status. Traditionally, socioeconomic status has been defined by income, education and occupation. Studies in developing societies have found that education is far more closely related to obesity than is either occupation or income. Even within the USA such disaggregation appears fruitful. Thus, the NHANES study of secular trends also found that education was more closely related to changes in BMI and skinfold thickness than was occupation (Flegal et al 1988a,b).

Among adolescent girls in the USA, the inverse relationship between socio-economic status and obesity, which has been so firmly established among women, has been reported to be absent among North American Black adolescent girls, even though it was present in Caucasian girls (Moore 1993). Evidently these North American Black girls were not affected by the messages on body shape that play such an important part in the prevailing culture.

Analysis of the recent Hispanic Health and Nutrition Examination Survey (HANES) has revealed a similar lack of relationship between socioeconomic status and obesity among certain groups. Not only Puerto Rican women but also Mexican-Americans and Cuban-Americans of both genders showed no relationship between socioeconomic status and the prevalence of obesity (L. K. Kahn, personal communication). This study also suggests the involvement of social determinants different from those that have been the subject of most of the research to date.

Finally, acculturation to a dominant culture appears to influence the prevalence of obesity, but the method whereby it exerts this influence is still unclear. In the previously described Midtown Manhattan Study it was found that the prevalence of obesity decreased in a monotonic manner over four levels of increasing acculturation: foreign-born, second generation in the USA, one parent second generation and, finally, third and later generations (Goldblatt et al 1965). In striking contrast are the results of the Hispanic HANES study. Among Mexican-American men the prevalence of obesity increased with increasing acculturation to American society (L.K. Kahn, personal communication).

Future directions

In the future, epidemiological studies of obesity will benefit from measurement and control of genetic influences. There is already a convenient measure of genetic influence — the extent of parental obesity — and more precise measures will become available with the discovery of genetic markers.

There is an urgent need to move beyond the traditional environmental measure of socioeconomic status as a determinant of the prevalence of obesity. One useful measure has been disaggregation of the three traditional components of socioeconomic status — income, occupation and education — relating each of them individually to the prevalence of obesity. Among the three components, years of education is the easiest to measure and the one with the greatest cross-cultural relevance. It may also be the most powerful.

New measures of social influence are urgently needed. Acculturation is a promising candidate and other measures will undoubtedly present themselves to the inquisitive investigator. They should be explored with vigour and dispatch.

References

Bouchard C 1994 The genetics of obesity. CRC Press, Boca Raton, FL

Braddon FEM, Rodgers B, Wadsworth MEJ, Davies JMC 1986 Onset of obesity in a 36 year birth cohort study. Br Med J 293:299–303

Brown PJ, Konner M 1987 An anthropological perspective on obesity. Ann N Y Acad Sci 499:29–46

Flegal KM, Harlan WR, Landis JR 1988a Secular trends in body mass index and skinfold thickness with socioeconomic factors in young adult men. Am J Clin Nutr 48:544–551

Flegal KM, Harlan WR, Landis JR 1988b Secular trends in body mass index and skinfold thickness with socioeconomic factors in young adult women. Am J Clin Nutr 48:535–543

Goldblatt PB, Moore ME, Stunkard AJ 1965 Social factors in obesity. JAMA 192:1039–1044

Gortmaker SL, Must A, Perrin JM, Sobol AM, Dietz WH 1993 Social and economic consequences of overweight in adolescence and young adulthood. N Engl J Med 329:1008–1012

Kuczmarski RJ, Flegal KM, Campbell SM, Johnson CL 1994 Increasing prevalence of overweight among US adults: the national health and nutrition examination surveys, 1960 to 1991. JAMA 272:205–211

Moore DE 1993 Body image and eating behavior in adolescents. J Am Coll Nutr 12:505–510

Power C, Moynihan C 1988 Social class changes and weight-for-height between childhood and early adulthood. Int J Obes 12:445–453

Sobal J, Stunkard AJ 1989 Socioeconomic status and obesity: a review of the literature. Psychol Bull 105:260–275

Stunkard AJ 1990 Genetic contributions to human obesity. In: McHugh PR, McKusick VA (eds) Genes, brain, and behavior. Raven, New York, p 205–219

Stunkard AJ, Sørenson TIA 1993 Obesity and socioeconomic status: a complex relation. New Engl J Med 329:1036–1037

Stunkard AJ, Foch TT, Hrubec Z 1986 A twin study of human obesity. JAMA 256:51–54

Stunkard AJ, Harris JR, Pederson NL, McClearn GE 1990 The body mass index of twins who have been reared apart. New Engl J Med 322:1483–1487

Teasdale TW, Sørensen TIA 1983 Educational attainment and social class in adoptees: genetic and environmental contributions. J Biosoc Sci 15:509–518

Vogler GP, Sørensen TIA, Stunkard AJ, Srinivasan MR, Rao DC 1995 Influences of genes and shared family environment on adult body mass index assessed in an adoption study by a comprehensive path model. Int J Obes 19:40–45

DISCUSSION

Fraser: One of the issues that hasn't been mentioned so far at this symposium is pregnancy. People who have looked at pregnancy in Caucasian populations have often been surprised by the relatively small amount of weight gain. I've studied 60 overweight Barbadian women who have been treated with Isomeride™, a weight-reducing medication, and I have the clear impression that most of their weight gain occurs after they have had children. Prakesh Shetty and I have a colleague who is currently doing a large study on weight gain in pregnant women and the impression is that their weight gain is greater than that reported for Caucasian populations.

Stunkard: The amount of weight gain during pregnancy is probably also linked to social class. The best study of weight gain during pregnancy is that by Stefan Rössner in Stockholm. He has shown that a year after delivery most women weigh little more than before they became pregnant. However, 15–20% of women weigh a lot more (10 kg or so) a year later. This is almost certainly due to a genetic susceptibility that is brought out by pregnancy (Ohlin & Rössner et al 1994).

Rissanen: A prospective Finnish study looked at parity, weight gain and social class in 6200 women over six years (Rissanen et al 1991). The study revealed that the most important factors influencing weight gain were education, physical activity and parity in women of a low social class. Educated women did not retain excess weight following pregnancy.

Allison: There are two studies in the USA showing that Afro-American women have much higher postpartum weight retention than Caucasian women (Smith et al 1994, Scholl et al 1995).

Albert Stunkard mentioned that there was a general consensus that the level of heritability is about 30%. I disagree with this statement. Claude Bouchard has described how different types of studies yield different estimates, with the twin studies generally yielding higher estimates in the range of 70%. It is possible that estimates based on twin studies are wrong because of a violation of the equal environments assumption, i.e. that monozygotic twins are treated more similarly than are dizygotic twins. However, there has been at least one test within the field of obesity (DeCastro 1993), and there have been numerous tests in other fields (Loehlin 1992), which show that there is no reason to suspect that this assumption is violated. Conversely, there are many reasons to believe that the higher estimate of body mass index (BMI) heritability based on twin studies is correct. These primarily involve evidence for non-additivity of gene effects. For example, Claude Bouchard presented the results of segregation studies which showed a recessive pattern of non-additivity. His overfeeding study suggests that the response to food has a strong genetic component; and DeCastro showed that food intake has a strong genetic component. Food intake and the response to food intake is multiplicative, and it will be apparent in studies of monozygotic twins who are concordant not just for genes but for patterns of genes. Therefore, in the presence of non-additivity, studies of monozygotic twins and dizygotic twins will give correct, high heritability estimates. This has been confirmed in studies of monozygotic twins reared apart, where the same estimates of heritability are obtained even when the equal environment assumption is not made (Allison et al 1996).

Bouchard: The true size of the heritability coefficient for obesity is not a critical point at this time. Indeed, once we have identified the genes, the interest in the heritability concept will fade away. For instance, the results of twin studies cannot be validated by external criteria allowing full control over all the assumptions of the design. I personally believe that these assumptions are partly violated in the case of phenotypes such as overweight or obesity. This limitation is likely to disappear when we have the genes in hand for genetic or intervention studies.

Roberts: I disagree. Determining the importance of genetic inheritance versus environmental influences is important because it determines which approaches are taken for prevention and treatment of fatness. It is likely that environment versus genetic susceptibility to fatness will result from entirely different sets of problems.

Bouchard: There are many factors that have an effect on the value of heritability; for instance, sample size.

Allison: There's a difference between the sampling variation around something you're trying to estimate and saying there's nothing to estimate. The point is that small sample sizes may allow heritability estimates to vary from one study to another but have no effect on the actual value of heritability in a population.

Stunkard: The problems with the twin studies don't arise from violation of the equal environments assumption because in at least one study the twins were separated early in life and did not share a common (or equal) environment (Stunkard et al 1990), yet they showed a very high heritability. A more likely theory is that people create their own environments and that twins create unusually similar environments. Living in those similar environments, they are subjected to very similar environmental influences. But these influences are counted as genetic and not as environmental. In contrast, the adoption studies suggest a heritability that is only about half that of the twin studies.

Allison: This does not explain the difference between twins and adoptees because adoptees can also create their own environments. People's genotypes lead them to create environments, i.e. it's a gene–environment correlation. You're correct in saying that this will be picked up as being genetic in a twin study, but it will also be picked up as genetic in other family studies and adoption studies. Therefore, it does not explain the discrepancy.

Swinburn: I would like to make a comment on weight gain in women. Educated women do not seem to be gaining weight, but this is potentially at the cost of suffering from eating disorders due to dietary restraint. Therefore, I wonder whether these women are really the appropriate models for overweight women.

Heitmann: The only study that has examined the effect of social class in women is the Finnish study. In the three other Scandinavian countries the data have not yet been differentiated according to socioeconomic status. However, the trend in BMI for women is an overall decline (Mikkelson et al 1995).

James: In Finland do educated women watch their weight with great precision, or can this be explained by changes in physical activity or smoking?

Rissanen: From what is known (Pietinen et al 1996), overall differences in diet, physical activity or smoking habits do not generally seem to explain the observed educational or socioeconomic gradient in obesity. However, because we have witnessed an eating disorder epidemic among young women and an increased level of dietary restraint in middle-aged women, I believe that dietary restriction is the preferred method of weight control among educated women.

Ferro-Luzzi: Is there any information on whether these educated women were never obese or whether they had been obese in the past but slimmed and then had an unusually low relapse rate?

Stunkard: They are far less likely to become obese. A striking example is the finding of Flegal et al (1988) that women of an upper social class showed no secular trend towards obesity over a 10-year period, whereas women of a lower social class showed a marked increase in obesity.

Prentice: One can add to that the data from Power & Moynihon (1988) in the 1958 birth cohort. They looked at children aged seven who were overweight, and they found that those in a low social class at birth go on to become obese at age 23, but those who were in a high social class have resolved by the time they're 23.

Heitmann: Is the level of education as an indicator of socioeconomic status higher in the USA compared to Scandinavian countries?

Stunkard: I'm not sure but it would probably be lower. Epidemiologists have suggested that the number of years of schooling is the best indicator of socioeconomic status because it's easier to equate across cultures than are the other two elements of socioeconomic status (income and occupation).

Prentice: We've all been making a plea that this is an interesting alley to go down for trying to untangle the influences on obesity. I've been looking at the Health Survey of England 1993 data, and I have observed that for women there is a highly significant inverse relationship between both social class and educational level and obesity (Bennett et al 1995). There are also the usual associations with physical activity, smoking and alcohol, but unfortunately we don't have good diet data. However, we can still only explain about 10% of the variance, and if those other variables — such as physical activity, smoking and alcohol — are included, we do not eliminate the social class or educational level effects. These relationships are robust and something we don't understand. Restraint probably plays a big part in the maintenance of slimness in well-educated, high social class women.

Rissanen: In Finland we have observed this phenomenon in women for several decades, whereas in men the association between lower socioeconomic status and obesity emerged only in the 1970s. The difference in the prevalence of obesity between the social classes has been documented from several countries. There are some recent data from The Netherlands showing a four- to sixfold difference in the prevalence of obesity between those of a high and low educational standard, and an increasing gradient between the educational classes (Seidell et al 1995).

Bray: Are you saying that your data for men are as strong as the data for women.

Rissanen: Yes, the recent data are almost as strong in men, but this was not so in male data sets from 1967 to 1970.

Bray: This surprises me. I had assumed that this was a universal difference between men and women. It may or may not be true for data sets from any other countries. It's not true for the Nurses Health Surveys data—there is a weaker relationship between obesity and educational status in men than in women.

Bennett: Do the Finnish men suffer from eating disorders to the same extent as Finnish women?

Rissanen: Within the last few years we have seen a few cases of men with bulimia. Before this, there were no reported cases.

Bouchard: Let me go back to the education issue. If education is important, then it must index something that influences energy balance. For example, education may impact on the selection of food because educated people know more about nutrition. It also has an effect on the level of leisure time physical activity. Studies in the USA, Canada and Australia indicate that the proportion of those who are totally inactive and sedentary in the high educational class is smaller than those in the low educational class.

James: But that's not what Andrew Prentice has found.

Prentice: No, I have found that. But when the regression model is incorporated, it does not throw out the social class influence.

Bouchard: But you have shown that these variables are only surrogates for energy balance variables. They are not true estimates of energy expenditure or of energy intake.

James: So how do you cope with the power issue in relation to your activity analysis? A relationship may be poor but it's still there, and it may be an energetically significant component.

Prentice: One of the answers is that we need better data.

Ferro-Luzzi: The modern western woman still spends time doing household chores. It seems reasonable that higher educated women will maintain these activities, adding them to their work schedule, which will obviously add to their overall physical activity. If these women also spend their free time in more active forms of leisure than the less educated women, wouldn't that increase their daily energy expenditure to a level which would protect them from becoming obese?

James: Patrick François (unpublished observations 1995) has analysed socioeconomic time use in many countries, including Scandinavia, and Finland in particular. He found that working women had the highest rates of physical activity, and they were under tremendous pressure, because they were essentially running a household at the same time as managing their career. I gather that Finland has the highest proportion of working women.

Rissanen: Yes. Most women have paid work, so there are no major differences in the job stress levels of well-educated and less-educated women. Therefore, this does not explain the socioeconomic relationship, which remains largely unknown at the moment.

James: Do you have dietary data for this?

Rissanen: Yes. Dietary differences between the educational classes of the Finnish population have virtually disappeared in recent years (P. Pietinen, unpublished results 1995).

Heitmann: We have to realize that when we talk about socioeconomic classes there may be a different reporting pattern of diet intake in different socioeconomic groups. For instance, there is some indication that in relation to under-reporting of food intake, the more educated people are more likely to give biased diet information. This could also apply to physical activity.

James: Andrew Prentice have you got any double-labelled water data which indicate that educated women exaggerate the amount of physical activity they do?

Prentice: No, I cannot answer that question yet.

Heymsfield: We published some physical activity estimates and double-labelled water measurements (Lichtman et al 1992). We found that most women over-reported their physical activity level, but this was not associated with social class.

Hitman: Isn't this just peer group pressure? In higher socioeconomic classes most women are thinner, so the women will strive to be in that norm. However, this norm may be different in a different social class, or even in a different country. The norm may be what women are striving for, which may be thin or fat depending on the setting. Or is this too simplistic for an explanation?

Prentice: No, it not too simplistic. We have a lot of indirect evidence that this is happening; for example, the increased prevalence of both smoking and eating disorders in young girls. These are corrective behaviours, and they're very damaging corrective behaviours.

Stunkard: It also is related to an individual's idea of beauty, which varies according to social class. Fallon & Rozin (1985) presented young upper class girls with silhouettes of body shape varying from thin to fat and asked them how they viewed themselves in relation to these shapes. They identified their shapes, and said they thought that boys would want them to be thinner. However, when he asked the boys about the girls, they said that the girls were fine as they were.

Fraser: These sociocultural differences are important. I would like to see a collaborative, in-depth comparison of the attitudes of individuals to their own body image and that of their partners across a wide variety of cultures.

McKeigue: A preference for a low waist–hip circumference ratio (WHR) may be more universal than a preference for slimness. Singh (1994) has studied college students that have arrived in the USA from different parts of the world, and has found that although they vary in their preference for slimness, they all share a preference for female forms that have a low WHR.

Allison: His data are interesting. However, his manipulation of WHR in silhouettes is confounded, at least by my eye, with the total width of the silhouette. Therefore, silhouettes with smaller WHRs are thinner overall, so it's difficult to say that people are just keen on WHR independent of total mass.

References

Allison DB, Kaprio J, Korkeila`M, Koskenvuo M, Neale MC, Hayakawa K The heritability of body mass index among an international sample of monozygotic twins reared apart. Int J Obes 20:501–506

Bennett N, Dodd T, Flatley J, Freeth S, Bolling K 1995 Health Survey for England. Series HS No 3. HMSO, London

DeCastro JM 1993 Genetic influences on daily intake and meal patterns of humans. Physiol Behav 53:777–782

Fallon AE, Rozin P 1985 Sex differences in perceptions of desirable body shape. J Abn Psychol 94:102–105

Flegal KM, Harlan WR, Landis JR 1988 Secular trends in body mass index and skinfold thickness with socioeconomic factors in young adult women. Am J Clin Nutr 48:535–543

Loehlin JC 1992 Genes and environment in personality development. Sage, Newbury Park, CA

Lichtman SW, Pisarska K, Raynes Berman E et al 1992 Discrepancy between self-reported and actual caloric intake and exercise in obese subjects. New Engl J Med 327:1893–1898

Mikkelsen KL, Heitmann BL, Sørensen TIA 1995 Secular changes in mean body mass index and in the prevalence of obesity — three Danish population studies of 31 000 subjects. Int J Obes 19:30

Ohlin A, Rössner S 1994 Trends in eating patterns, physical activity and sociodemographic factors in relation to postpartum body weight development. Br J Nutr 71:457–470

Pietinen P, Vartiainen E, Männistö S 1992 Trends in body mass index and obesity among adults in Finland from 1972 to 1992. Int J Obes 20:114–120

Power C, Moynihan C 1988 Social class and changes in weight-for-height between childhood and early adulthood. Int J Obes 12:445–453

Rissanen A, Heliövaara M, Knekt P, Reunanen A, Aromaa A 1991 Determinants of weight gain and overweight in adult Finns. Eur J Clin Nutr 45:419–430

Seidell JC, Verschuren WMM, Kromhout D 1995 Prevalence and trends of obesity in The Netherlands 1987–1991. Int J Obes 19:924–927

Singh D 1994 Waist-to-hip ratio and judgement of attractiveness and healthiness of female figures by male and female physicians. Int J Obes 18:731–737

Scholl TO, Hediger ML, Schall JI, Ances IG, Smith WK 1995 Gestational weight gain, pregnancy outcome and post-partum weight retention. Obstet Gynecol 86:423–427

Smith DE, Lewis CE, Caveny JL, Perkins LL, Burke GL, Bild DE 1994 Longitudinal changes in adiposity associated with pregnancy. JAMA 271:1747–1751

Stunkard AJ, Harris JR, Pederson NL, McClearn GE 1990 The body mass index of twins who have been reared apart. New Engl J Med 322:1483–1487

General discussion II

Swinburn: Is there an association between eating disorders and social class?

Rissanen: Eating disorders used to be largely confined to women of upper social classes. However, they have now become common in all social strata.

Heitmann: I'm not sure how many adults in Denmark have eating disorders. In the Danish MONICA (MONItoring of trends and determinants in CArdiovascular diseases) cohort we asked people questions related to binge eating, bulimia and anorexia nervosa and there are certainly not many people above the age of 35 that suffer from these eating disorders. I would expect that this is true also in other countries.

Allison: The catchment area studies, which were some of the major epidemiological studies in psychiatry in the 1980s in the USA show that the prevalence of anorexia nervosa among young Caucasian women was only about 0.1%, and it was virtually 0% among young Black women (French et al 1994, Eaton et al 1984).

Stunkard: Other studies of eating disorders in the USA have estimated that they affect less than 3% of women in the 15–25 year age group. Therefore, it's not a big public health problem. In an unpublished study, Christopher Fairburn in Oxford has looked into the determinants of eating disorders. Dieting is one factor, and another is the presence of psychiatric disturbance. This suggests that dieting is only a small contributor to this problem and in terms of weight control the benefits would seem to outweigh the costs.

James: How is the socioeconomic gradient obtained in which educated middle-aged women are less obese but do not practise restraint behaviour, i.e. they do not have eating disorders?

Heitmann: They're probably dieting and have a different reporting pattern, so that they are more likely to give biased diet information. This is not the same as having restrained behaviour.

Rissanen: These women are chronic dieters. They have a high level of dietary restraint, but they seldom have the profoundly disturbed behaviours and cognitive characteristics of eating disorders. Chronic dieting can be considered to be a kind of eating disorder when it is associated with inappropriate or extreme weight control practices, excessive anxiety and feelings of guilt.

Jackson: I would like to be clear what is meant by 'restraint behaviour'. It has been clearly recommended for a number of countries that populations should alter their diets to a pattern which will enable them to remain slim. Now, I hear a suggestion that these changes might be characterized as 'restraint behaviour', which implies an eating disorder or a psychosocial abnormality.

Rissanen: Conforming to a diet that enables you to stay thin in rich environments usually means constant dietary restraint, if you have low energy expenditure. Extreme dietary restraint may have adverse consequences in predisposed persons. These could be avoided, if healthy weight was maintained by lifestyle modification including increased physical activity.

Prentice: The important point is that people are using inappropriate methods of restraint, which includes chronic dieting. As Aila Rissanen has mentioned, what is required is a change in overall lifestyle rather than these inappropriate dieting episodes which can lead onto eating disorders. Modifications such as changing the amount of fat in one's diet or taking more exercise are modifications that do not, as far as we know, lead to eating disorders.

Swinburn: Women in the upper socioeconomic classes have a lower prevalence of obesity, but we don't know what methods they have employed to achieve this and the costs in the form of eating disorders.

Jackson: Who are these people? What age are they? I am a little concerned that some explanations of population shifts and population gradients are based on anecdotal stories restricted to a small proportion of the population that are then extrapolated beyond what the evidence justifies. I am happy to accept justified evidence, but one has to be careful how appropriate the evidence is around the margins.

Rissanen: Let me try to clarify this using the US population as an example. According to a recent report by the National Institutes of Health (1993) about 40% of American women and 24% of men are currently trying to lose weight. Many of them are overweight, and have lost and regained weight repeatedly. However, about one-sixth of Americans who are not overweight also try to lose weight at any given time. These efforts may have adverse physical and psychological consequences. The level of dietary restraint is enormously high in these people.

James: What do you mean by enormously high?

Rissanen: When given questionnaires on their eating patterns, those people are very conscious of what they eat, and they make strict rules about their diet.

James: I'm going to make the assumption that when you're talking about restraint you're talking about responses to formal questionnaires, and when you're talking about a high prevalence rate you mean about 75%.

Rissanen: Yes, most chronic dieters and especially those trying to maintain weight show a high level of dietary restraint.

Blundell: In considering the roles of physical activity and food consumption in populations, in principle we should be able to measure these parameters and relate them to obesity. We should be able to identify the high sedentary ones and the high energy intakers. The problem is that the tools which we have to measure these phenotypes are rather poor. On the activity side, I'm not impressed by surrogate measures of activity, such as car ownership or hours of television viewing. I suggest that we need to see how they convert to kilojoules of energy expended per day. The instruments for measuring dietary intake are so unreliable that they are almost worthless. Certainly, the distorted reporting (particularly selective or non-selective under-reporting) makes it extremely hazardous to draw any firm conclusions about relationships between dietary intakes and other variables.

Roberts: I'm distressed by dietary methods in general, but not all dietary methods are equally as bad. We have just completed a study showing that measurements of food frequency are better predictions of total energy expenditure in individuals than seven-day food records (Sawaya et al 1996).

Blundell: I accept that some techniques are better than others but it doesn't undermine the point I made, since all the currently used procedures produce dietary data that are unreliable as indicators of habitual intake.

Prentice: One of the problems is that under-reporting is another feature of restraint. We may be able to learn more about the aetiology of overconsumption in Africa and the Caribbean, where restraint is much less prevalent and where we probably have more realistic records of food intake. Appetite studies may be more informative if they were carried out in these populations.

Astrup: I would like to ask Aila Rissanen to clarify whether, in her opinion, subjects who are trying to stick to dietary recommendations are restrained?

Rissanen: This depends on the person and the food choices available. Most people trying to adhere to the recommendations would not need to be restrained if the recommended diet is easily available. More restraint is required when rich and fatty foods abound.

Allison: As far as I know, there isn't any evidence to support that dieting leads to eating disorders. It's appropriate to say that dieting precedes eating disorders because it is rare that anyone develops these disorders without first passing through a dieting phase, but it's not necessarily causal. Dieting and the development of these disorders are both likely to be due to the social pressures to be thin combined with some other severe psychopathology.

Garrow: People who were in concentration camps were undernourished for long periods. After they were liberated they developed eating disorders (Keys et al 1950).

Allison: It's not appropriate to compare the experience of being confined to a concentration camp with choosing to go on a diet under the supposedly supported supervision of health care professionals living in an outpatient setting. Also, people have looked at whether going on diets under health care supervision in an outpatient setting results in the development of binge eating, for example. French & Jeffery (1994) have shown that there is a normalization of eating patterns. There is no evidence of bingeing or any other eating disorders.

Garrow: We have discussed the desirability of recommending a lower fat intake. I would like to clarify whether people are making this recommendation on the basis that a high fat intake is energy dense and palatable or for other metabolic reasons. I suggest that an important part of the reason why high fat diets predispose to obesity is that they have a high energy density and they are palatable. van Stratum et al (1978) studied nuns, and fed them soup that had a constant taste and energy density but was either high or low in fat, and he found that it had no effect on intake.

Blundell: It has been proposed that when people are in negative energy balance the proportion of macronutrients in the diet has little effect on body weight. When people are in energy balance then the prevalence of fat in the diet has a small effect, since fat may be more readily assimilated into adipose tissue. But when someone is in positive energy balance then the macronutrient composition of the diet can exert a large effect. I'm impressed by both the laboratory studies and field studies that draw attention to the amount of fat which can be consumed in a single eating episode without any conscious recognition of this by the subject. This is referred to as passive overconsumption since the subjects do not intend to consume so much fat (often more than 100 g in a single meal). Indeed most people are unaware of the macronutrient composition of the foods they are consuming. When overconsumption is so readily achieved I can't support the idea that obesity is due largely to underactivity.

Jackson: Activity may not necessarily be a mechanism for consuming energy but a mechanism for setting metabolic control points and making metabolic control operative.

Bouchard: We have found that there are people who, in the sedentary state, have a higher skeletal muscle oxidative potential than others (Simoneau & Bouchard 1995). When challenged by excess calories, these people have a greater tendency to remain in energy balance than those with a lower skeletal muscle oxidative potential. The most reliable way to establish whether an individual is a high or a low lipid oxidizer is to assay key enzymes from a muscle biopsy sample. We have also found that there are family lines in which parents and children are high lipid oxidizers but others who are low lipid oxidizers. The phenotype is somewhat correlated with muscle fibre type distribution but even more strongly with mitochondrial markers.

Heitmann: I agree that passive overconsumption plays an important role in weight gain but a genetic susceptibility to gain weight may also be important. For specific interactions — such as between fat intake and familial disposition to weight gain from a high fat diet — only a few per cent of the population would seem to be genetically susceptible (Heitmann et al 1995), but this is only one gene–environment interaction mechanism. Another mechanism by which interactions between genes and environment could play a role is physical activity and susceptibility to weight gain from inactivity, or different predispositions to lose weight from smoking. There are several levels by which gene–environment interactions could play a role, and if we add these, we may start seeing larger numbers than a few per cent of the population who are susceptible to gain weight from the different gene–environment interactions.

Jackson: I would like to add *in utero* programming of metabolic competence to your list of factors which may be important: either by exposing a risk in a genetically susceptible individual or by generating a risk through the modulation of appetite or other aspects of metabolic competence.

Astrup: There may be other differences between fats and carbohydrates apart from their energy densities that are important in these overfeeding experiments. The overfeeding study by Horton et al (1995) demonstrated that the metabolic efficiency is higher on a high fat diet compared with a high carbohydrate diet. Therefore, genetic and dietary determined differences in metabolic efficiency are also important for the overall energy balance.

Garrow: Is there a consensus about whether the intake side or the metabolic side is quantitatively predominant?

Astrup: In my opinion the intake side predominates. However, it is probably not possible to separate them because the oxidation of nutrients affects appetite and vice versa.

Prentice: We have performed experiments where we have given people in whole-body calorimeters identical foods and checked for palatability with feeding panels, and we have shown that they show this phenomenon of passive overconsumption (Stubbs et al 1995). Their metabolism is trying its hardest to fight back. There is no change in energy expenditure, but fat oxidation increases markedly. However, this change fails to bring the system back into regulation. Therefore, our experiments suggest that the intake side predominates.

Roberts: It may be possible to answer this question in a different way. It's difficult to see the effect of fat intake on energy balance when one controls for everything, and it's easy to see the effect of fat intake on energy intake and energy balance when one does not control for factors such as palatability, fibre content and energy density. This suggests that many of the effects of fatty diets are not metabolic. We should also be talking about fatty foods rather than fat because the so-called 'low fat' cakes that we see in supermarkets have a high carbohydrate content and they are easy to overconsume.

Blundell: We've tended to criminalize fat. It is a major contributor of overconsumption and weight gain. However, it should be kept in mind that a high fat diet is not a sufficient condition for weight gain. In other words, we're not dealing with a biological inevitability. Not everyone who eats a high fat diet is destined to become obese. Some people are protected, by whatever mechanism, from a high BMI. In the Leeds High Fat Study high fat consumers (> 45% energy from fat) are distributed across the range of BMIs: some underweight, some overweight and obese, and many of normal BMI. The difference between high BMI people and low BMI people is not the amount of food they are consuming. High fat consumers who are in the top 25% of the BMI range are more than 10 years older than those in the bottom 25% of the range. With low fat consumers (< 35% energy from fat) those with high BMIs are consuming a greater daily energy intake than those with low BMIs. We are working on the hypothesis that some high fat consumers are resistant to the weight-inducing effect of the diet for behavioural or metabolic reasons.

Bray: The rodents that David York and I have worked with are susceptible or resistant to becoming obese on a high fat diet. They have the ability to recognize a high level of fat that is contained within an otherwise invariant diet. When the fat is given in a more palatable form, they become fat; whereas when they are given a high energy-dense, high fat diet they adapt within a day or two by decreasing their food intake, and they do not gain weight. Therefore, palatability is a key component.

References

Eaton WW, Holzer III CE, Von Korff MV et al 1984 The design of the epidemiologic catchment area surveys: the control and measurement of error. Arch Gen Psychiatry 41:942–948

French SA, Jeffery RW 1994 Consequences of dieting to lose weight: effects of physical and mental health. Health Psychol 13:195–212

French SA, Perry CL, Leon GR, Fulkerson JA 1994 Weight concerns, dieting behavior, and smoking initiation among adolescents: a prospective study. Am J Publ Health 84:1818–1820

Heitmann BL, Lissner L, Sørensen TIA, Bengtsson C 1995 Dietary fat intake and weight gain in women genetically predisposed for obesity. Am J Clin Nutr 61:1213–1217

Horton TJ, Drougas H, Brachey A, Reed GW, Peters JC, Hill JO 1995 Fat and carbohydrate overfeeding in humans: different effects on energy storage. Am J Clin Nutr 62:19–29

Keys A, Brozek J, Henschel A, Mickelson O, Taylor HL 1950 The biology of human starvation. University of Minnesota Press, Minneapolis, MN

National Institutes of Health 1993 Methods for voluntary weight loss and control. National Institutes of Health Technology Assessment Conference. Ann Intern Med 119, no 7

Sawaya AL, Tucker K, Tsay R et al 1996 Evaluation of four methods for determining energy intake in young and older women: comparison with doubly labelled water measurements of total energy expenditure. Am J Clin Nutr 63:491–499

Simoneau JA, Bouchard C 1995 Skeletal muscle metabolism and body fat content in men and women. Obesity Res 3:23–29

Stubbs RJ, Harbron CG, Murgatroyd PR, Prentice AM 1995 Covert manipulation of dietary fat and energy density: effect on substrate flux and food intake in men eating *ad libitum*. Am J Clin Nutr 62:316–329

van Stratum P, Lussenburg RN, van Wezel LA, Vergroesen AJ, Cremer D 1978 The effect of dietary carbohydrate: fat ratio on energy intake by adult women. Am J Clin Nutr 31:206–212

The economic and psychosocial consequences of obesity

A. M. Rissanen

Department of Psychiatry, University of Helsinki, Tukholmankatu 8C, FIN 00290 Helsinki, Finland

Abstract. Obesity is a multifaceted problem with wide-reaching medical, social and economic consequences. These are partly determined by the wealth and disease pattern of the population. In less-developed societies overweight may be advantageous and socially acceptable. In affluent societies obesity is a well-recognized health hazard and a socially stigmatized condition. For the obese person, excess weight denotes an increased risk of disabling chronic diseases, lowered quality of life and loss of earnings. For the society, obesity is a major economic burden. Treatment costs of diseases directly attributable to obesity are estimated to correspond to about 4–5% of the total health care expenditure. The indirect costs arising from loss of productivity due to obesity may be even higher.

1996 The origins and consequences of obesity. Wiley, Chichester (Ciba Foundation Symposium 201) p 194–206

Obesity is a major risk factor for the development of common chronic and disabling conditions. The adverse consequences of obesity derive largely from these conditions, increasing the mortality, morbidity and disability of obese individuals.

The quality of life of obese people may be further impaired by the stigma of obesity. The obese may face prejudice and discrimination in most areas of social functioning, and obesity is associated with low levels of socioeconomic attainment and downward social mobility.

The societal costs of obesity

The most commonly used approach to estimate the costs of obesity in society is to measure the value of resources used or lost because of this condition. These calculations, based on the prevalence of obesity, estimate the direct and indirect costs. Direct costs are the medical costs of diagnosis, treatment and management of diseases attributable to obesity. These costs could have been prevented if obesity did not exist. Indirect costs reflect the value of loss of productivity due to obesity.

Direct costs

At present, relatively little information exists about the direct economic consequences of obesity-related diseases. The limited data available suggest that about 4–5% of total

194

health care expenditure can be attributable to obesity. Some of the data available from affluent countries are reviewed below.

The Netherlands. The excess use of medical care and associated costs due to obesity in the Netherlands have been estimated using data on 58 000 participants in the Health Interview Surveys from 1981 to 1989 (Seidell 1994). The health care costs included reported consultations of general practitioners and medical specialists, hospital admissions and use of prescribed drugs. Obese (body mass index [BMI] $> 30\,kg/m^2$) and overweight (BMI $25–30\,kg/m^2$) persons had an increased likelihood of having consulted a general practitioner. The cost of such consultations was 3–4% of the total costs attributable to obesity and overweight combined. The costs of hospitalizations were 3% and 2% for obesity and overweight, respectively. The excess use of medications by obese and overweight people was most conspicuous. Compared to non-obese people, obese persons were five times more likely to use diuretics and 2.5 times more likely to take drugs for cardiovascular diseases. It was estimated from these data that the direct costs of overweight and obesity are about 4% of the total health care costs in the Netherlands. This is of the same order of magnitude as the health care costs attributable to cancers.

France. To estimate the direct costs of obesity in France in 1992, Levy et al (1995) identified the costs of personal health care, hospital care physician services and drugs for diseases with well-established relationships with obesity (including non-insulin-dependent diabetes, hypertension, hyperlipidaemia, coronary heart disease, stroke, venous thromboembolism, osteoarthritis of the knee, gall bladder disease and certain cancers). The proportion of these diseases attributable to obesity (defined as BMI $\geqslant 27\,kg/m^2$) ranged from about 25% for hypertension and stroke to about 3% for breast cancer. The direct costs of obesity were almost Fr 12 billion, which corresponds to about 2% of the expenses of the French health care system. Costs of hypertension represented 33% of the total direct costs of obesity.

Finland. The impact of obesity on several indicators of health care utilization was assessed among about 10 000 adult Finns in the National Survey on Health and Social Security in 1987. The costs of medicines, physician consultations and hospital in-patient stay increased with increasing BMI (Table 1). The excess health care utilization was mainly due to an increased need for medication, the cost of which increased by about 120% when BMI increased from 25 to $40\,kg/m^2$. It was estimated on the basis of these data that if all Finns were of normal weight, the annual savings would be of the same order of magnitude as if all smokers in Finland were to permanently stop smoking.

Australia. The Australian Institute of Health and Welfare estimated that in 1989 the health care costs resulting from obesity (BMI $> 30\,kg/m^2$) accounted for about 4% of pharmaceutical expenditure, 2% of the cost of medical consultations and 1.6% of the

TABLE 1 The estimated effects of increase in body mass index (BMI) on selected measures of health care expenditure—the Finnish Survey on Health and Social Security 1987

	Per cent increase in			
Increase in BMI (kg/m²)	Cost of medicines	Hospitalization days	Physician consultations	Total cost
25–30	16.1	2.3	5.9	5.0
30–35	29.3	3.8	10.5	9.2
35–40	45.8	5.7	15.6	15.3
25–40	18.8	12.4	35.0	32.4

The estimates were obtained using the MIMIC (Multiple Indicators and Multiple Causes) model.

recurrent hospital expenditure (Segal et al 1994). Overall, at least 2% of the total recurrent health expenditure of some major obesity-related diseases (non-insulin-dependent diabetes, coronary artery disease, hypertension, gallstones, and cancers of the breast and colon) could be attributed to obesity. This is equal to 86% of the health care costs used for the management of alcohol-related diseases and 71% of the costs for the management of tobacco-related disease in Australia.

The USA.   Costs attributable to obesity were estimated on the basis of nation-wide prevalence data from 1986 (Colditz 1992). About 57% of the costs of non-insulin-dependent diabetes, 19% of the costs of cardiovascular diseases, 26% of those for hypertension and about 2.5% of the costs of cancers were estimated to be attributable to obesity. The total costs attributable to obesity for these disease conditions were calculated to represent 5.5% of the total cost of illness in 1986.

Sweden.   Preliminary observations from an ongoing nation-wide intervention study (SOS, the Swedish Obese Subjects) show dramatic reductions in the incidence of obesity-related diseases in severely obese persons after surgical weight loss (Sjöström et al 1995). For instance, the reduction for the incidence of diabetes in the first few years of follow-up has been about 17-fold (L. Sjöström, personal communication 1995). These findings suggest that impressive savings of the treatment costs of common diseases are achievable by effective treatment of severely obese persons.

The available estimates of health care costs are based mainly on cross-sectional data of selected obesity-related diseases. They do not include the costs of many of the diseases and conditions caused or worsened by obesity, such as the extra costs resulting from obesity-related complications of surgery and pregnancy. For instance, it was recently calculated that the hospitalization costs during pregnancy are more than twofold higher among overweight and obese French mothers, compared to the costs of pregnancies of normal weight French women (Galtier-Dereure et al 1995). The presented estimates on the direct costs of obesity are therefore likely to underestimate the magnitude of the true costs and of the savings achievable by the reduction of the prevalence of obesity in society.

Indirect costs

Losses of productivity due to premature death and disability from illness associated with obesity are considerable, but limited data on these costs are available. In the Swedish Obesity Study (Sjöström et al 1995) the frequencies of long-term sick-leave (over six months) were reported to be 1.4 and 2.4 times higher in obese men and women, respectively, than in the general Swedish population. Similarly, the rate of premature disability pensions were reported to be increased 1.5–2.8-fold among the SOS subjects. The total loss of productivity due to obesity was estimated to be about of 7% of the total costs of losses of productivity due to sick-leave and disability pensions in Sweden.

Using data from the National Health Interview Survey from 1988, Wolf & Colditz (1994) estimated that the cost of lost productivity as a result of obesity and associated diseases in the USA was about US$4 billion, or 52 391 480 annual lost work days. The same authors presented a conservative estimate of US$10 billion for the indirect costs arising from premature mortality due to diseases associated with obesity (including cardiovascular disease, non-insulin-dependent diabetes, gallbladder disease, cancers and musculoskeletal diseases).

In a large prospective Finnish study (Rissanen et al 1990), obesity was associated with a twofold increased risk of premature work disability in men, and a 1.5-fold greater risk in women. Most of the premature pensions attributable to obesity were due to cardiovascular and musculoskeletal diseases. One-quarter of all disability pensions from these diseases in women were solely attributable to overweight and obesity.

The future of the societal costs of obesity

Any change in the prevalence of obesity will have a major impact on the consumption and cost of medical care in society, and even a minor decline in the prevalence can be expected to result in substantial savings of the limited health care resources. Obesity represents a major avoidable contribution to the costs of illness in affluent countries. However, no such cost-containing prospects are evident. The prevalence of obesity is increasing. As advancing medical care reduces premature mortality of obese persons, the number of survivors with chronic diseases and premature disabilities will increase. The ageing populations of the western world are thus facing a mounting burden of costs arising from the sequelae of excess weight. These costs include the economic costs of the society and the personal costs of the obese individuals.

Economic and psychosocial consequences of obesity to the individual

Overweight has important social and economic consequences to the obese person (Enzi 1994, Sarlio-Lähteenkorva et al 1995). Negative attitudes toward obese subjects adversely affect their educational, employment, socioeconomic and marital status. Obesity and its treatment efforts may also induce psychological sequelae.

Social stigma, prejudice and discrimination

Numerous studies have documented prejudice and discrimination of obese persons in most areas of human functioning (Wadden & Stunkard 1985). The stigma of overweight is twofold, including the stigmatization of both the bodily appearance and the character of the obese person (Crocker et al 1993). The widespread view of obesity as a mark of personal inferiority is learned early. Children as young as six years of age describe obese children as 'ugly, lazy, dirty and stupid'. The negative attitudes towards obesity continue into adulthood and are apparent even in the teaching and medical professions.

Because of its visibility, obesity may affect most human interactions. Obese children and adolescents are less likely to be admitted to prestigious schools than their otherwise comparable non-obese peers. There is a bias against hiring an overweight job applicant, who is also likely to receive a lower pay for his work. Obese women are less likely to marry and be upwardly mobile in marriage.

The social and economic consequences of obesity are well illustrated by two recent studies of young adults. In the USA National Longitudinal Survey of Labor Market Experience (Gortmaker et al 1993), the relationships between overweight and subsequent educational attainment, marital status and household income were examined in subjects aged 16–24 in 1981. Seven years later, the initially obese women had completed fewer years at school, were less likely to be married and had lower household incomes than the women who had not been overweight, independent of their baseline socioeconomic status and aptitude test scores. Somewhat similar, but weaker, trends were observed among men.

In the National Child Development Study in Britain (Sargent & Blanchflower 1994), a national cohort of 16-year-olds was followed up for seven years. The men and women who had been obese at age 16 years had fewer years of schooling than their non-obese peers at age 23. There was a strong negative association between obesity and earnings in women, independent of parental social class and ability test. The inverse relationship between obesity at 16 years of age and earnings persisted whether the woman remained obese or moved to the non-obese category by age 23.

The studies cited above underscore the deleterious effects of overweight during adolescence. The adverse effects of obesity on socioeconomic status are most distinct in women, whereas in men and children they are apparent only at the heaviest weights (Stunkard 1996, this volume).

The observed strong association between low social class and obesity may have several explanations (Sörensen 1995). Obesity may lower socioeconomic status, low socioeconomic status may promote the development of obesity, and obesity and low socioeconomic status may share some of the causes that both promote the development of obesity and tend to reduce the socioeconomic status.

Adaptive responses and psychological consequences of obesity

Common coping mechanisms. Despite the social bias against obesity, many obese persons seem to cope well with their stigmatized condition. Population studies have generally failed to find differences between the psychological well-being of obese and normal weight persons (Wadden & Stunkard 1985). However, persons with abdominal fat accumulation may have more psychological problems than others. This form of obesity may, in fact, occur as a response to a chronically stressful environment (Björntorp 1993). Obese persons try to minimize obesity-related problems by adaptive behaviours, such as avoiding situations where being fat is a problem, earning social acceptance by overachieving in some areas of life, rejecting or reversing the societal definitions of obesity, or simply accepting the social stereotype of a 'fat person' (Hughes & Degher 1993).

Special problems of the obese. Some obese persons are likely to suffer from psychosocial ills and problems specific to their obesity and frequent dieting, including body image disparagement and binge eating (Stunkard & Wadden 1992). Body image disparagement is encountered in some obese persons and in non-obese women with eating disorders. Both obese and non-obese persons with disparagement of the body image view their bodies as grotesque and are often preoccupied with obesity and self-loathing. The disturbance most often occurs in adolescents and young women who have been obese since childhood. It is also common in persons from higher social groups in which sanctions against obesity are the strongest. Binge eating is a common problem among obese individuals (Spitzer at al 1992). Clinically problematic binge eating — frequent intake of large amounts of food, associated with a feeling of loss of control over eating and with quilt and depression — afflicts a substantial number of obese persons entering weight control programmes. Obese binge eaters show greater psychological distress than do obese people who do not binge. The aetiology of binge eating in obese subjects is not firmly established. It is possible that it develops in predisposed persons as a result of frequent unsuccessful efforts to lose weight (Wilson 1993).

Health-related quality of life in obese persons

The quality of life can be expected to be compromised in obese persons because of impaired physical and psychosocial functioning, but only a few studies have addressed this question (Sarlio-Lähteenkorva et al 1995). The most systematic approach of this kind (Sullivan et al 1993) found that severely obese Swedish people scored significantly lower than others in most measures of well-being, reporting more physical and obesity-related problems, impairment in social interactions, anxiety, depression and decreased mental well-being. In fact, the mental well-being of these people was worse than that of chronically ill or injured patients, e.g. survivors of cancers and spinal cord injuries.

The lowered quality of life of severely obese persons can be reversed. Dramatic changes in the quality of life after major weight loss by obesity surgery have been documented in several studies, reporting improvement in mood, self-esteem, interpersonal and vocational effectiveness, body-image, activity levels, and marital and sexual relations (Stunkard et al 1986). In contrast, the consequences of conventional dieting remain unknown. It is possible that failure to lose weight or to maintain weight loss may harm psychological functioning and the quality of life (Wilson 1993).

Little is known about the quality of life of moderately obese persons. Clinical experience suggests that they often seem to manage to adapt surprisingly well. Useful information could come from explorations of the means by which they remain psychologically intact and maintain a reasonably good quality of life despite an adverse social environment.

References

Björntorp P 1993 Visceral obesity: a 'civilization syndrome'. Obesity Res 1:206–222

Colditz GA 1992 Economic costs of obesity. Am J Clin Nutr 55:503S–507S

Crocker J, Cornwell B, Major B 1993 The stigma of overweight: affective consequences and attributional ambiguity. J Pers Soc Psychol 64:60–70

Enzi G 1994 Socioeconomic consequences of obesity. The effect of obesity on the individual. PharmacoEconomics (suppl 1) 5:54–57

Galtier-Dereure F, Montpeyroux F, Boulot P, Bringer J, Jaffiol C 1995 Weight excess before pregnancy: complications and cost. Int J Obes 19:443–448

Gortmaker SL, Must A, Perrin JM, Sobol AM, Dietz WH 1993 Social and economic consequences of overweight in adolescence and young adulthood. New Engl J Med 329:1008–1012

Hughes G, Degher D 1993 Coping with deviant identity. Deviant Behav 14:297–315

Levy E, Levy P, Le Pen C, Basdevant A 1995 The economic costs of obesity: the French situation. Int J Obes 19:790–792

Rissanen A, Heliövaara M, Knekt P, Reunanen A, Aromaa A, Maatela J 1990 Risk of disability and mortality due to overweight in a Finnish population. Br Med J 301:835 837

Sargent JD, Blanchflower DG 1994 Obesity and stature in adolescence and earnings in young adulthood: analysis of a British birth cohort. Arch Pediatr Adolesc Med 148:681–687

Sarlio-Lähteenkorva S, Stunkard AJ, Rissanen A 1995 Psychosocial factors and quality of life in obesity. Int J Obes 19:1S–5S

Segal CL, Cartre R, Zimmet P 1994 The cost of obesity. The Australian perspective. PharmacoEconomics (suppl 1) 5:45–52

Seidell JC 1994 Obesity in Europe. Prevalence and consequences for the use of medical care. PharmacoEconomics (suppl 1) 5:38–44

Sjöström L, Narbro K, Sjöström D 1995 Costs and benefits when treating obesity. Int J Obes 19:9S–12S

Sörensen TIA 1995 Socioeconomic aspects of obesity: causes or effects? Int J Obes 19:6S–8S

Spitzer RL, Devlin M, Walsh BT et al 1992 Binge eating disorder: a multisite field trial of the diagnostic criteria. Int J Eating Disord 11:191–203

Stunkard AJ 1996 Socioeconomic status and obesity. In: The origins and consequences of obesity. Wiley, Chichester (Ciba Found Symp 201) p 174–187

Stunkard AJ, Wadden T 1992 Psychological aspects of severe obesity. Am J Clin Nutr 55:524S–532S

Stunkard AJ, Stinnett JL, Smoller JW 1986 Psychological and social aspects of the surgical treatment of obesity. Am J Psychiatry 143:417–429

Sullivan M, Karlsson J, Sjöström L et al 1993 Swedish obese subjects (SOS): an intervention study of obesity. Baseline evaluation of health and psychosocial functioning in the first 1743 subjects examined. Int J Obes 17:503–512

Wadden TA, Stunkard AJ 1985 Social and psychological consequences of obesity. Ann Intern Med 103:1042–1067

Wilson GT 1993 Relation of dieting and voluntary weight loss to psychological functioning and binge eating. Ann Intern Med 119:727–730

Wolf AM, Colditz GA 1994 The cost of obesity. The US perspective. PharmacoEconomics (suppl 1) 5:34–37

DISCUSSION

Shaper: Aila Rissanen has shown us that there are strong measures of the costs of obesity. It has been suggested at this symposium that we should be thinking of a much lower ideal body mass index (BMI) in the range of 20–23 kg/m². Concerns have been expressed about the costs of aiming for this ideal BMI because of the pressure on people, and particularly on young women, to diet, which may result in anorexia, bulimia and other eating disorders. Aila Rissanen has shown us that the costs of overweight and obesity are high and that there is no good argument for not aiming towards a lower optimum BMI.

Allison: I disagree. There are at least two points that need to be considered. (1) Cost estimates are merely estimates, and they are based on numerous assumptions, such as that obesity has a causative role in the development of those diseases and that reducing obesity would reduce those costs. These assumptions may or may not be correct. (2) There are costs of trying to achieve a lower weight, such as medical, psychological, economical and social costs.

Bray: The cost analysis data were based on calculations using a BMI of at least 27 kg/m². For example, the Nurses' Health Study data were based on using a BMI of 29 kg/m² and the National Center for Health Statistics data were based on using a BMI of 27.3 kg/m² for women and 27.8 kg/m² for men. A grey zone occurs around a BMI of 25 to 27 kg/m². The risk associated with a BMI of 25 versus 27 kg/m² is small and the costs of moving it from 27 to 25 kg/m² may be far greater than any health care system can afford.

Rissanen: From the little we know, there seems to be an exponential increase in costs with increasing fatness. This starts at a BMI of 25–27 kg/m^2 and escalates sharply at around 30 kg/m^2.

Shaper: The majority of us here are not talking about a venture to decrease the BMI of everyone who is currently overweight or obese to 20–23 kg/m^2. We are considering future generations who should aim to have a BMI lower than 25–27 kg/m^2. Everyone who has a BMI of 25–29 kg/m^2 has passed through 21–23 kg/m^2 *en route*!

Ferro-Luzzi: The national cost of slimming in the USA is US$32 billion. Obviously, the best control strategy is prevention rather than treatment, and you made the point that the cost of prevention was much smaller than that of treating obesity. What proportion of the US$32 billion is absorbed by actions directed to assist non-obese or pre-obese people to keep their BMI within acceptable ranges?

Campfield: That figure includes everything from fitness gyms to exercise clothing and food.

Stunkard: US$1.5 billion is spent in health clubs, and most of the rest is spent on food. But there's no way of telling whether people would be more overweight without these foods.

Jackson: This appears to be an undesirable situation, and we need to look at whether the money spent on special foods is part of the solution rather than, as implied, part of the problem.

Shetty: We need to look at prevalence in terms of the median (or mean) BMI of a population. Rather than estimating costs based on definite numbers, such as by estimating costs of reducing the BMI of all overweight and obese people to 27 kg/m^2, we should attempt to estimate the costs on the basis of what would be achieved by reducing the median (or mean) BMI of a population. Rose & Day (1990) have shown that the close relationship between mean or median and prevalence implies that to help the 'deviant' minority within a population, the 'normal' majority must change.

Heitmann: We might learn something about decreasing the median BMI of a population from the Scandinavian experience. The data show that Scandinavian women are becoming leaner. It is difficult to determine why there are different trends in Scandinavian women, compared to women from other western societies, but if we could find out what mechanisms are operating in the Scandinavian female population we may be a step closer to defining intervention programmes aiming at shifting population distributions.

Rissanen: Danish women are smoking more heavily and the mortality rate is increasing. It is possible that some undesirable effect is occurring.

James: Norwegian women have been putting on weight very slightly on a secular basis over the last 10 years.

Heitmann: That depends on from where you have obtained your data, because data from the National Health Screening Service of Norway would suggest that the BMI of Norwegian women has been decreasing since 1967 whereas for men, in the same period, it has been increasing.

James: My information comes from Kaare Norum (personal communication), who is the current chairman of the Nutrition Council. We challenged these data because the evidence is that the levels of physical activity in Norway are high. I made the assumption from this that the weights had either stabilized or decreased. He denied this and informed us that they had been creeping up.

Rissanen: There are two main approaches for reducing the burden of obesity. One is the preventive population approach, calling for effective strategies to decrease the median BMI of a population. The other is the curative approach. Overweight people with obesity-related diseases and those at high risk for such diseases certainly deserve better treatments than they are getting at the moment. Population strategy is largely a political issue, whereas the other approach is more a medical issue.

Allison: The development of prevention strategies is an interesting notion for further research, but it's important to point out that, at least to my knowledge, there has not been a single study done showing the efficacy of a primary prevention trial for obesity. We can say that prevention is the obvious strategy to undertake, and hopefully we will develop appropriate methods in the future, but currently there's no way of telling whether prevention will be cost effective. It would be wonderful if in the future the median BMI was 20–23 kg/m^2 but to talk about doing that is fanciful at the moment.

Shaper: Societies currently exist that have BMIs in that range.

Swinburn: In the 1960s and 1970s the rates of coronary heart disease (CHD) were increasing, and there were no data on primary prevention trials. Even today, the data are slim, and the few trials that have been carried out have been done on a population basis. The Minnesota Heart Health Study, for example, had negative results, because heart disease declined similarly in the intervention and control populations. The secular changes were just overwhelming (Edlavitch et al 1991). Even if we don't have the trials for prevention of obesity, we have to follow the prevention of heart disease as an example.

Garrow: It seems to me that the reason why Boyd Swinburn is saying that the evidence we've got so far is poor, is that the various intervention trials were relatively ineffective and were carried out on old people. It would be nice to know the effect on health of preventing obesity in a random sample of young adults. The only way in which this can be done at a reasonable cost is to study populations, such as the Pima Indians, in whom the disease profile with increasing obesity is known. The opportunity for doing this sort of trial is slipping away. I hope that someone will fund a trial study of the primary prevention of obesity in young people, which would have to be followed for some time before the effects on health are observed.

Shaper: The follow-up period would not be that long for high risk groups such as the Pima Indians because one could look merely at the issue of weight gain. It is not necessary to look at the consequences because these have already been defined.

Garrow: But one would need to know the consequences of not gaining the expected amount of weight on the incidence of diabetes in Pima Indians, for example.

Stunkard: There have been five controlled trials in the USA and one in Finland. Not only did none of them prevent obesity, but in only two of them was there even a barely statistically significant decrease in the secular trend of weight gain. However, all of the cardiovascular trials were effective in controlling cigarette smoking and hypertension. This suggests that obesity is much more difficult to prevent or control than smoking and cardiovascular disease (Stunkard 1995).

Forrester: Modulating peoples' food choices given the variety available is extremely difficult. However, how malleable are people's food choices if agricultural and food policies are changed?

James: The development of food policy in most western societies post-war has, in terms of economics and food, been based on pre-war nutritional health concepts, i.e. that the most important point is to provide plenty of energy, particularly from meat and milk, at such a cheap cost that even the poorer sections of society can buy the commodities. The consequence of this is that billions of dollars have been put into agricultural systems supported by the national concern for food security, which has a defence security component. Therefore, at least in the whole of western Europe and the USA, there's always been a sense that we have to have enough home-grown food to keep us going. The costs of implementing that policy are gigantic. The policy has been associated with a massive health campaign, which has permeated the whole of society, encouraging people to eat high fat, high protein diets. Industries have been supported and sustained with huge subsidies for 50 years to try to achieve this. Therefore, in answer to the question: does agriculture drive the way in which we eat? It's probably true to say that we have all been driven by the same concepts. The investment in agriculture produces huge industrial combines, such as the dairy industry and the meat industry, that are promoted by their own advertising drives. To say that by changing agricultural policies we will miraculously solve the problem of obesity is a totally different proposition. In practice most agricultural policies are at present geared to producing food that we would consider less appropriate, given our current knowledge of health needs.

Forrester: Would it be worthwhile to do a cost–benefit analysis in this situation?

James: Economists will always come up with analyses that neglect the huge effect of the previous capital inputs to the dairy and meat industry. They actually talk about the flexibility of demand for foods. Short-term manipulations of flexibility of demand show that, for example, if the price of butter is increased in an attempt to reduce its consumption, this is achieved but the consumption of margarine increases instead, so economists then claim the responses are an intrinsic reflection of a demand for fat, which is untrue. Another possibility would be to tax these items, but governments would probably not manipulate the tax system in this way.

Jackson: You've painted a brilliant doomsday scenario. One has to add to your analysis that the productive end of the system has responded successfully in the past. There may well be considerable unwillingness to change because there are important costs associated with change, but that doesn't mean that there will not be change. Change will occur if the arguments for change are sufficiently sound and strong that it is worth the investment. Therefore, our responsibility is to demonstrate that the risk of the investment is sufficiently low and the benefits are sufficiently large that it is worthwhile driving that inertia forward. I am personally unimpressed with economists' approaches to this issue because they tend to be retrospective in terms of what has happened in the past, rather than being imaginative in terms of what might happen in the future.

Rissanen: A large population-based prevention programme was launched in the 1970s in North Karelia, Finland, where there was a record level of high mortality from CHD. The rate of cardiovascular disease declined in the region, but not appreciably more than in other parts of the country. The striking decline of cardiovascular disease in Finland has been accompanied by favourable changes in the national diet. These occurred despite the lack of health-oriented agricultural policies, which lagged well behind the increased public awareness of health values.

James: I've done an unpublished study for the Scottish office on precisely what's been happening in Finland. We've analysed data from a variety of sources. It's clear that agricultural change did occur, but the primary reason was the development of the industrial base in Finland. Seventy per cent of the population were dairy farmers and fisherman post-war, but there was then a shift of the population into the cities and a national policy whereby foods were imported to cope with the new demand for healthier foods. The largest increase in fruit consumption came with the increasing ownership of deep freezers, so that people were able to store soft fruit. A more deliberate agricultural policy was developed in Norway, where there was an organized scheme to ensure that every corner of Norway was able to purchase fruit and vegetables at the same cost as in Oslo. This is an example of what can be done. I'm not saying that the agricultural community will not respond, but it is rare to find policies being implemented at the primary agricultural level and geared to a primary health concern. The production policies post-war have helped the farmers to respond to concerns about food security and the need for cheap food. In both the meat and dairy industries there have been, since then, huge developments in response to consumer demand. It is possible for agriculture to respond, but this response tends to be in a sequential chain of consumer-to-government, consumer-to-industry, supermarket-to-food industry or food industry-to-primary producer. This sort of response involves huge investment costs.

Blundell: In many technologically advanced societies at the moment there is a premium on freedom of choice, including food choice, which is stimulated by the food industry. People working in the food industry know that the two factors which stimulate purchase and consumption of foods are: (1) taste; and (2) cost. People have to make difficult cognitive decisions in order to resist the temptation of these two factors. I believe we should not underestimate the power of palatability (good taste of food) to stimulate consumption, nor the difficulty people have in denying themselves the pleasure of eating.

Swinburn: We can look at car crashes and heart disease as models for how to bring about change. Car crashes used to be thought of as accidents, i.e. you couldn't do much to avoid them, apart from public education. Engineers then used the epidemiological triad of environment–host–vehicle, which was originally developed for the control of infectious diseases and then applied to car crashes. As a result they made substantial changes to the environment as a part of multidimensional approach to the problem. We need to adopt the same approach with obesity and ask people to make more rational decisions based on increased knowledge.

Bouchard: I am surprised by the universal trend that the discussion of body weight control or obesity reduction moves inevitably to nutrition. We know that despite a reduction in fat intake in the USA and the UK over the last decades, the prevalence of obesity continues to increase. I believe that the main culprit is the reduction in energy expenditure caused by automation and technological advances. We are barking up the wrong tree when we emphasize food choice, food labels, food production and related issues without first promoting a more active lifestyle.

References

Edlavitch SA, Crow R, Burke GL, Baxter J 1991 Secular trends in Q wave and non-Q wave acute myocardial infarction. The Minnesota Heart Survey. Circulation 83:492–503

Rose G, Day S 1990 The population mean predicts the number of deviant individuals. Br Med J 301:1031–1934

Stunkard A J 1995 Prevention of obesity. In: Brownell, KB, Fairburn CG (eds) Eating disorders and obesity: a comprehensive handbook. Guilford Press, New York, p 572–576

Obesity and physical activity

Anna Ferro-Luzzi and Laura Martino

National Institute of Nutrition, Via Ardeatina, 546–00178 Rome, Italy

Abstract. This paper discusses the epidemiological evidence linking obesity to physical activity. The underlying plausible hypothesis is that the feedback from energy expenditure to appetite may be weak at low levels of physical activity and that sedentary lifestyles therefore favour positive energy balance and weight gain. Obesity is widespread in developed countries and appears to have a marked secular trend. An analysis of time–budget surveys reveals that the time required for earning a living and domestic work has declined appreciably over recent decades. This negative secular trend is associated with a substantial decline in the energy spent on these activities. The contraction of work time has resulted in a converse expansion of free time, but the bulk of this is spent on passive leisure. Thus, at least for western societies, the overall energy expenditure has fallen for some decades and lifestyles have become increasingly more sedentary. The review of a large data set on energy expenditure under free-living conditions indicates that, despite their phenomenally diverse rates of obesity, there is no systematic difference between developed and developing societies. Multivariate regression analysis of body mass index on physical activity level (PAL) reveals a weak but statistically significant inverse relationship in men but not in women, and establishes that the risk of obesity increases sharply at a PAL of less than 1.80. In conclusion, a critical level of PAL has been identified, below which the chances of being overweight become substantial. The use of time is modelled contextually with its energy cost to show the extent to which energy expenditure may be modified. This has relevance from a policy standpoint, allowing a more focused approach for obesity prevention.

1996 The origins and consequences of obesity. Wiley, Chichester (Ciba Foundation Symposium 201) p 207–227

This paper addresses the issue of how physical activity relates to obesity. The underlying hypothesis is that at very low levels of physical activity, the feedback from expenditure to appetite may be weak (Ravussin et al 1988, Roberts et al 1988). A sedentary lifestyle therefore favours a positive energy balance and weight gain. Physical activity is not only one of the two major routes by which energy leaves the body but it is also the most flexible route, varying from near 0 (at rest in bed) to more than 10-fold the basal metabolic rate (BMR) for people engaging in vigorous exercise. The relationship between physical inactivity and obesity, however, is unlikely to be simple, and several confounders may complicate the picture, such as physical fitness, opportunities for exercise, diet and the temporal relationships between exercise and meals. In particular, cogent questions remain as to whether there is a threshold level of physical activity at which obesity is best prevented, whether the nature of the physical activity has a role to play and whether a sustained low cost activity is better, in terms of long-term maintenance of energy balance and the avoidance of obesity, than a short-lived, high cost activity.

When exploring the link between physical activity and body mass index (BMI), it is important to bear in mind that the supporting evidence comes from two different types of data sets (physical activity *per se* and energy expenditure) which are not synonymous. Physical activity denotes the amount of time dedicated to the various activities, whereas energy expenditure precisely denotes the calories that are spent either in any specific activity or over the whole day. Energy expenditure under free-living conditions is measured by indirect calorimetry or stable isotopic dilution, or is predicted on the basis of heart rates. Information on physical activity is generated by questionnaires or interviews, which define the length of time allocated to specified activities. Physical activity data are often translated into metabolic equivalents (METs) by applying generic coefficients such as multiples of BMR. In this case, the margin of approximation is relatively large and the reliability is low.

Despite these limitations, and the fact that we do not know whether various indices of physical activity represent a proxy for energy expenditure, rather than for other potentially important lifestyle variables, it is important to note that fairly good correlations have been obtained when the association between the length of time spent on specific activities and the degree of fatness has been tested. Thus, sedentary Americans have been found to weigh more than those who reported some physical activity (DiPietro et al 1993), and watching television for more than three hours per day was associated with twice the risk of obesity compared with watching television for less than one hour per day (Tucker & Friedman 1989). In North American adolescents the prevalence of obesity increased by 2% for each additional hour of television viewing per day (Dietz & Gortmaker 1985) and slimming successes were inversely proportional to the amount of television watched (Gortmaker et al 1990). In the UK the prevalence of obesity was inversely related to the level of physical activity in all age groups above 14 years (James 1996, this volume).

Four issues will be considered in the following sections of the paper: (1) given the positive secular trend for obesity throughout the world in recent decades, the evidence will be reviewed of a simultaneous negative time trend in the energy spent at work and during leisure; (2) the question will be addressed of whether the level of energy expenditure is appreciably higher in Third World countries, given that the rates of obesity there are phenomenally lower than in most western societies; (3) an analysis will be performed to establish whether energy expenditure rates measured directly are correlated with the body weights of individuals or groups; (4) an attempt will be made to establish whether there is a critical level of energy expenditure below which the probability of being obese rises appreciably.

Secular trends in physical activity

It is generally believed that physical activity in the western world has undergone a decline commensurate to the increasing mechanization of life. However, direct

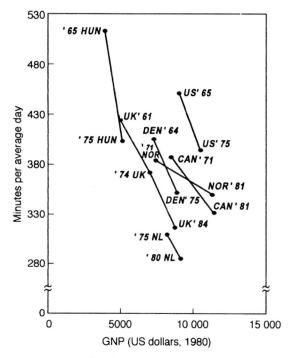

FIG. 1.   Changes over recent decades of the time spent in paid work by men in the various specified countries by level of Gross National Product (GNP) (modified from Gershuny 1995).

evidence of decreasing rates of energy expenditure over time is lacking. The only source of information is represented by the detailed data banks generated by time–budget surveys on how people allocate their daily time (Szalai 1972). These surveys are important tools of empirical sociological research, conducted for socioeconomic purposes rather than for establishing the level of energy expenditure. However, they lend themselves to a crude analysis of secular trends in physical activity. Time–budget surveys classify the activities of daily life under four major headings:

(1) personal needs, which includes sleep, time for meals and for personal hygiene;
(2) paid work;
(3) household work; and
(4) free time.

Although no change has taken place in the time dedicated to personal needs, all the evidence supports the view that throughout the industrial world the time needed to earn a living has dropped appreciably over recent decades (Gortmaker et al 1990). Figure 1 shows the reduction of the time dedicated to gainful work in several European and other countries between the early 1960s and the 1980s (Gershuny 1995). This decrease represents the outcome of changes in the labour market, such as

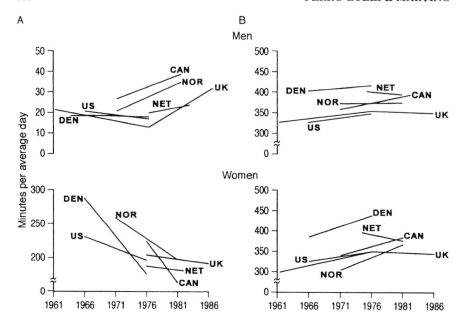

FIG. 2. Changes over recent decades of the time spent by men and women in domestic activities (A) and in leisure (B) (modified from Niemi 1995).

a shorter work shift, a shorter week and longer vacations. Concurrent with the decrease in the time dedicated to gainful work, there has been enormous technical progress resulting in the mechanization of most manual jobs, increased urbanization and the universal use of motor cars. These are just a few of the factors that decrease the energy cost of work. Thus, it appears highly plausible that the negative secular trend in the time dedicated to productive activities that has taken place in most industrial and post-industrial societies has been accompanied by a steady decline in the energy spent at work. Unfortunately, there is little if any information on what has happened in the developing countries.

The same sociological analyses also suggest that a similar substantial decline has taken place in the time spent in domestic activities (Fig. 2A, Niemi 1995). This has particularly affected women, on whom society still relies in the industrial world for carrying out most of the household work. There has been a negligible increase in the amount of time men spend doing household work.

The contraction of work time has resulted in a converse expansion of free time (Fig. 2B, Niemi 1995) and in a multiplication of the ways in which it can be used. In this paper, free time is classified into two broad categories: active leisure (such as outdoor activities and organized sports), which involves a certain degree of physical exertion; and passive leisure (such as watching television, reading and social visiting), where the energy cost may be close to the BMR (Klesges et al 1993).

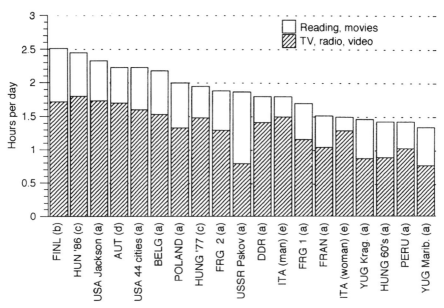

FIG. 3. Time spent in passive leisure, distinguishing watching television and videos and listening to the radio from reading and going to the movies. Sources of information: (a) Szalai (1972); (b) Anachkova & Pääkkonen (1992); (c) Central Statistical Office (1995); (d) ACSO (1995); and (e) ISTAT (1993).

What modern people choose to do with their free time, although studied by many sociologists, is not so well documented in energy terms. Nevertheless, it is fairly clear that the increase in television ownership has had the most striking and consistent impact on the amount of time dedicated to this medium, and it has altered the structure of leisure time, encroaching on the time allocated to other activities and even to weekday sleep (Niemi 1995). In the USA watching television has led to a steady decline of regular physical activity over recent decades and undesirable levels of sedentariness (Schlicker et al 1994). This has led to a public health policy of promoting physical activity to help curb the risk of cardiovascular disease (Brooks 1987, Folsom et al 1985). Also, in other countries mass media (televisions, radios, videos and movies) have come to occupy an increasingly large amount of time, at the expense of more active leisure (Fig. 3). Thus, in Finland, 2.5 hours are spent every day in front of the television or in similarly sedentary activities, and only 7–11% of free time is allocated to physically demanding leisure. At the other end of the spectrum the shortest duration of television watching, in countries such as France, Italy and Yugoslavia, is still about 1.5 hours per day. A similar scenario is found outside Europe. The Peruvians watch television for 1.5 hours per day, and in Japan Suzuki (1993) concludes that 'the Japanese have few leisure activities other than watching television'. He also reports that South Koreans watch television for more than three hours at weekends. The situation is particularly worrying for children because this medium substitutes for active playing. In Italy television is watched for almost two hours per day by the age of six, and this increases with age (Buratta & Sabbadini 1993). In the USA watching television by children has escalated by almost 100% over a period of about 15 years, i.e. between 1968 and 1982 (Gortmaker et al 1990).

In conclusion, a variety of evidence is concordant in suggesting a negative secular trend in work activity over recent decades in the western world, with a resultant expansion in leisure time. However, the bulk of the extra free time has been devoted to activities such as watching television and gainful work is to a large extent less physically demanding. Thus, the overall energy demand of modern life may have dropped appreciably.

Energy expenditure across the world

An earlier review of energy expenditure in free-living conditions in developed and developing countries concluded that there were no real differences between the two, once differences in body weight had been taken into account (Ferro-Luzzi 1988). Since then, other data on daily energy expenditure have been obtained, almost a quarter of which come from measures carried out by the $^2H_2$ ^{18}O technique. The tables in the appendix give the updated picture, which consists of 55 separate studies, selected for methodological reliability, including about 1550 individuals measured in more than 20 different countries. The appendix displays the number, age, weight, BMI, total energy expenditure and physical activity level (PAL, energy expenditure /BMR) values of the groups studied. PAL values, not to be confused with the information on physical activity derived from questionnaires on time use, express energy expenditure as a multiple of BMR. The use of PAL values allows a comparison of individuals of different sizes, although it is recognized that when grossly obese or simply larger individuals are compared with smaller ones, a small error will be introduced that attenuates the real differences in energy turnover (FAO–WHO Ad Hoc Expert Committee 1985). PAL values, however, are a universally accepted way of expressing energy expenditure and they also help to convey an easily understandable concept.

The average BMI and PAL values are given in Table 1. Data are also provided on the mean age, weight and energy expenditure. The entire sample, weighted for the numbers in each study group, has been combined into three broad classes: Third World subjects; western subjects; and elite athletes engaged in exceptionally vigorous exercises, such as marathon training, climbing the Himalayas or sledging across the Pole. The athletes are almost all males. The PAL value, when not given as such by the authors, is calculated from the measured BMR, if available, or from the predicted BMR (FAO–WHO Ad Hoc Expert Committee 1985). The differences in the number of subjects from one column to another reflect the omission of the relevant information in the respective papers; thus, although the PAL was measured in 973 men and 746 women, BMI data are available for only 807 men and 711 women.

Table 1 shows that the BMI is lowest in Third World subjects (as expected) with a mean of 20.9 kg/m^2 (17.2–23.3 kg/m^2) for men and 21.0 kg/m^2 (16.7–26.9 kg/m^2) for women. BMI is highest in the western subjects, with a mean of 25.2 kg/m^2 (21.2–28.6 kg/m^2) for men and 25.3 kg/m^2 (19.0–33.0 kg/m^2) for women. The athletes have values that are close to those of the Third World subjects. The PAL values of women are, in all classes, lower than those of men. The PAL values of the athletes are, as expected, the highest, reaching 1.96 (1.76–2.00) in women and 2.27 (1.73–5.1) in men. As for the comparison between Third World and western societies, after adjusting for BMI there is only a non-significant difference in the PAL value for men and no difference for women. We may conclude, therefore, that there are no systematic differences in the level of habitual activity between developed and developing countries.

This conclusion is difficult to reconcile with the profound difference in terms of mechanization of labour and home activities between Third World and industrial societies, and with the widespread belief that daily life in the less-developed countries demands a vastly superior physical effort. It seems counterintuitive that a Third World woman, who spends 30–150 min every day of her life simply fetching water (Fig. 4, UN 1991), or walks while attending to her daily chores for up to 1.5 hours (as in Ethiopia, India and New Guinea), should have a PAL value that is not dissimilar from that of a western housewife who just turns a tap to get water and drives to the shops. Several interpretations can be offered. A first possibility is that Third World women might compensate for the exertion associated with vital domestic chores by spending the rest of the day in low intensity activities, while western women employ more energy in their free time. Compensatory inactivity can occur for example in Ethiopia where seasonally higher PAL values are followed in the post-harvest season by lower values (Ferro-Luzzi et al 1990). An intra-week cycle in energy expenditure has also been recorded in ship-yard workers: white collar employees had lower energy expenditure during the week than those engaged in heavy manual labour, whereas during the weekend the level of energy output was reversed, with white collar workers engaging in vigorous exercises and the manual workers favouring quieter lifestyles. As a result, differences in overall energy expenditure between the two groups are small (Norgan & Ferro-Luzzi 1978).

Besides these physiological forms of compensation, Third World men and women may be less active simply because they are exposed to chronic energy deficiency (CED). Indeed, the curtailment of physical activity in order to spare energy represents the first line of defence when exposed to energy stress caused by insufficient dietary energy (Ferro-Luzzi & Branca 1996). Such a behavioural response is well exemplified by Viteri's findings that unsupplemented Guatemalan agricultural labourers, when coming home from work, were unable to do little else besides sitting and lying down, whereas a supplemented cohort displayed a much livelier lifestyle (Viteri 1982). Similarly, poorly nourished Rwandan women spend more time in low cost activities than their more nourished counterparts (Shetty & James 1994) and rural Indians with low BMIs engage less frequently in activities involving higher levels of physical exertion (A. Ferro-Luzzi, unpublished data from an ongoing research on the link between chronic energy deficiency and physical activity).

TABLE 1 Age, weight, body mass index (BMI), energy expenditure (EE) and physical activity level (PAL) by sex and population group (mean followed by S.D. between groups)

Population group	n	Age (years)	Weight (kg)	BMI (kg/m^2)	EE (kcal/day)	PAL (EE/BMR)
Men						
Third World	522[a]	31.4, 6.7	56.2, 3.8	20.9, 1.6	2794, 472	1.84, 0.31
Western countries	218[b]	37.7, 12.2	77.1, 4.0	25.2, 1.9	3107, 296	1.74, 0.15
Elite athletes	233[c]	28.6, 8.0	72.5, 7.1	21.6, 1.1	3899, 1175	2.27, 0.70
Total	973[d]	32.1, 9.1	64.7, 10.6	22.2, 2.4	3129, 824	1.92, 0.46
Women						
Third World	460[e]	31.9, 6.8	49.8, 6.0	21.0, 2.5	2076, 244	1.65, 0.17
Western countries	268	31.5, 6.4	68.0, 10.7	25.3, 4.0	2374, 321	1.64, 0.18
Elite athletes	18	31.5, 5.7	59.0, 6.9	20.8, 1.2	2769, 108	1.96, 0.08
Total	746[f]	31.8, 6.6	56.6, 11.8	22.6, 3.8	2199, 320	1.65, 0.18

[a]Number of subjects whose BMI was available is 393.
[b]Number of subjects whose EE was available is 203.
[c]Number of subjects whose BMI was available is 196.
[d]Total number of subjects whose BMI and EE were available is 807 and 958, respectively.
[e]Number of subjects whose BMI was available is 425.
[f]Total number of subjects whose BMI was available is 711.
BMR, basal metabolic rate.

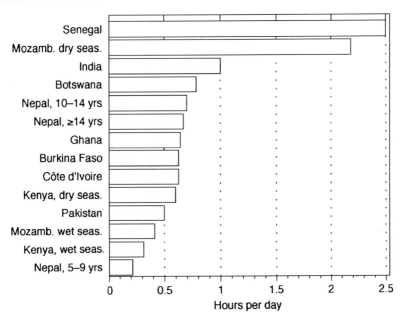

FIG. 4.   Time spent by Third World women fetching water (modified from UN 1991).

Energy expenditure and body mass index

A selected subset of the same worldwide data allows an analysis of the relationship between obesity and physical activity, namely whether fatter individuals tend to spend less energy. Only those data sets have been retained where weight, BMI, energy expenditure in kilocalories per day and PAL values were available. The elite athletes have been excluded because they are exceptional and would have biased the analysis. Table 2 illustrates the different PAL values of the groups in relation to BMI and sex. The PAL values of women remain much the same at all BMIs whereas those of men drop from a PAL of 1.91 for individuals with a BMI below 18.5 kg/m^2 to 1.70 for BMIs above 25.0 kg/m^2. Multivariate regression analyses of BMI on PAL by sex, with athletes omitted and with dummy variables for less developed (0) and developed (1) countries, shows that the model explains a significant proportion of the total variance of BMI, with an adjusted R^2 of 0.6 in men ($P = 0.00$) and 0.3 in women ($P = 0.00$) (Table 3). However, only a modest proportion of the total variance of BMI is explained by the PAL alone, the largest part being accounted for by ecological variables. In men the standardized β coefficients are -0.08 ($P = 0.00$) for the PAL and 0.76 ($P = 0.00$) for the country variable. In women, after controlling for the country, the PAL was no longer a statistically significant factor. An analysis of the residuals confirms these results showing the absence of systematic bias. Thus, for an increase of energy expenditure, e.g. from a PAL of 1.55, denoting a very sedentary lifestyle, to a PAL of

TABLE 2   Mean physical activity level (PAL) by sex and body mass index (BMI) class (athletes excluded)

BMI class	n	Mean, S.D.
Men		
< 17.0	0	ND
17.0–18.5	26	1.91, 0.00
18.5–25.0	491	1.84, 0.31
25.0–30.0	94	1.70, 0.12
30.0–40.0	0	ND
Total	611	1.82, 0.29
Women		
< 17	9	1.87, 0.08
17.0–18.5	76	1.65, 0.14
18.5–25.0	449	1.64, 0.20
25.0–30.0	103	1.66, 0.12
30.0–40.0	56	1.66, 0.10
Total	693	1.65, 0.18

ND, not determined.

2.05, which is a rather intense lifestyle, the BMI would drop by only 0.36 kg/m^2 (95% confidence interval 0.12–0.59). Substituting energy expenditure in kilocalories per day for the PAL and co-varying for body weight does not change the results.

Men's results are consistent with the significant inverse associations found by other authors exploring the links between physical activity as assessed by questionnaires and BMI (Bullen et al 1964, Fontvieille et al 1993, Ravussin et al 1988, Bandini et al 1990, Roberts 1993, DiPietro et al 1993), although contrary results have also been published (Blair & Buskirk 1987, Romanella et al 1991, Prentice et al 1996).

Levels of energy expenditure and obesity prevention

The last point is whether a critical threshold level of energy expenditure exists below which energy intake is less tightly down-regulated. In other words, the question is asked of how active should one be in order to avoid becoming obese? Being active is fatiguing, and most people would prefer to limit the exertion to the minimum level required.

The odds ratio of being overweight or obese, denoted as BMI > 25 kg/m^2, have been calculated for progressively higher PAL values as thresholds between sedentary and active lifestyles (Table 4). Odds ratios have not been calculated for women, given their insignificant association between PAL and BMI after controlling for the country effect.

TABLE 3   Multiple regression of body mass index on physical activity level (PAL), controlling for country

Source of variance	B	S.E. of B	β	S.E. of β	P
Men[a]					
Intercept	22.27	0.45	0.00	0.00	0.00
PAL	−0.71	0.24	−0.08	0.03	0.00
Country[b]	4.13	0.14	0.76	0.03	0.00
Women[c]					
Intercept	19.34	1.12	0.00	0.00	0.00
PAL	0.98	0.67	0.05	0.03	0.14
Country[b]	4.30	0.25	0.55	0.03	0.00

[a]Adjusted $R^2 = 0.60$ ($P = 0.00$).
[b]Dummy variable: 0 for developing country; 1 for developed country.
[c]Adjusted $R^2 = 0.30$ ($P = 0.00$).
B, non-standardized regression coefficient; β, standardized regression coefficient.

The results suggest that there is a critical level of physical activity below which the risk of being overweight increases sharply. Table 4 shows that the risk of being overweight or obese is about sevenfold lower at a PAL of more than 1.8. The observation that lower PALs are dissociated to a large extent from higher risks of obesity may be explained by an overriding effect of other more powerful factors which, at such low levels of PAL, would easily obscure the effect of inactivity *per se*. These have been discussed elsewhere in this volume (Bouchard 1996, Blundell & King 1996, Astrup 1996). Similarly, one could argue that the lack of a relationship between PAL and obesity in women might result from their mean level of energy expenditure being low enough (PAL = 1.60) to allow other factors (such as diet and genetics) to exert a more powerful influence.

TABLE 4   Odds ratios and 95% confidence intervals of being overweight /obese (body mass index >25 kg/m^2) if sedentary. Progressively higher physical activity level (PAL) values have been used to discriminate sedentary from active lifestyles

Sedentary level	Odds ratio	95% confidence interval
PAL ≤ 1.60	2.8	1.8–4.4
PAL ≤ 1.70	1.3	0.8–2.0
PAL ≤ 1.80	7.6	4.4–13.3

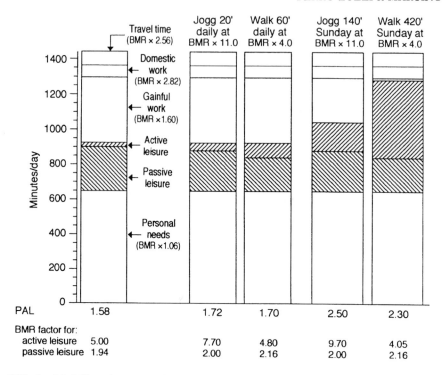

FIG. 5. Modelling the nature, duration and timing of active leisure required to achieve an overall mean physical activity level (PAL) of about 1.70. The activity profile of the average Italian adult male, aged 30–60 years, is taken as the basis for the exercise (first column, ISTAT 1993). He is assumed to weigh 70 kg and to have a predicted basal metabolic rate (BMR) of 1690 kcal/day. He is sedentary, being employed in a light-activity job (BMR factor = 1.60, FAO–WHO Ad Hoc Expert Committee 1985), and he spends only 24 min per day in active leisure at a BMR factor of 5.00. The other 252 min are spent in passive leisure (BMR × 1.94). Daily jogging (BMR × 11.0) for 20 min (second column) or brisk walking (speed 4 km/hr; BMR × 4.0) for 60 min (third column) will raise his daily PAL to about 1.70. If this man chooses instead to concentrate his exercise into one day per week, he will have to jog for 140 min (fourth column) or walk for about 7 hours (fifth column) on that day to achieve the same average weekly PAL of 1.70.

Modelling activity profiles

The previous analysis has provided us with at least a vague idea of the level of energy expenditure at and above which the chances of becoming obese are reduced. Therefore, it is now possible to look into how this desirable level of physical activity can be achieved. Figure 5 displays a profile of the activity pattern of an individual. The time-frame is that of the average Italian adult male (ISTAT 1993); the energy costs of the activities carried out in the various segments of the day are expressed as multiples of BMR and represent intelligent guesses based on literature data (Ainsworth et al 1993) and on actual measures (James & Schofield 1990). These figures do not claim to be a true value of PAL, but they provide a useful comparative basis for the subsequent modelling exercise. The man is aged 30 to 60 years, weighs 70 kg and has a BMR of 1690 kcal/day. This man is assumed to be fairly sedentary and employed in a low energy cost occupation, e.g. as an office worker. As a result, his PAL is only 1.58, much lower than the critical level of 1.8. His chances of becoming obese are therefore appreciable. He can increase his PAL to at least 1.7 by using his plentiful free time. It is easily calculated that to go from a PAL of 1.55 to 1.70, this person needs to spend 300 extra calories per day. To achieve this amount of energy, the man has to walk or run for about 4 km. If he does this every day, it will take him 20 minutes to jog quite rapidly (12 km/h) or one hour if he walks (4 km/h). Both these options are feasible but undoubtedly they require motivation, perseverance, a minimum of physical fitness and the right environment. Therefore, it is appropriate to consider the implication of skipping the daily routine and instead transfer the exercise to the weekend. To maintain the target average of PAL 1.7 with only weekend exercise means that a person must jog for almost 2.5 h or walk for up to 7 h, a prospect that goes well beyond what would motivate normal people. The same reasoning can be applied to other sports, such as tennis, golf and swimming. One option is to modify the transport system, which would allow a level of activity as part of the normal daily routine and not as a specially intended exercise. This is a logical proposition, as it is easy to skip one or more sessions if the exercise is dissociated from one's normal lifestyle.

General conclusions

Although activity and obesity are part of the same equation describing the flow of energy in humans, the link is fairly complicated and the existing epidemiological evidence is inconclusive, with a margin of error in the data that is, at present, too large to allow firm conclusions.

Despite these limitations, it is reasonable to conclude that: (a) the overall level of energy expenditure in the western world appears to have been falling for some decades; (b) the seemingly obvious conclusion that energy expenditure is systematically higher in Third World countries is not supported by the evidence; (c) there is a modest but significant inverse association between a group's energy expenditure and the prevalence of obesity, although this is more clearly established for men than for women; and (d) there appears to be a critical level of energy expenditure below which it may be difficult to down regulate energy intake.

Finally, from a policy standpoint, advice to the population aimed at promoting physical activity should:

(1) be based on actual evidence on how people spend their time;
(2) specify the level of physical activity recommended for obesity prevention; and
(3) diversify the means to achieve it in the targeted population.

Acknowledgements

We thank G. Catasta and E. Toti for invaluable assistance in the elaboration and tabulation of time–budget surveys. This analysis and part of the background information was obtained with the financial support of DGXII of the EU within the STD1, STD2 and STD3 Framework Programmes.

References

ACSO 1995 Zeitverwendung 1992/1981. Austrian Central Statistical Office, Wien

Ainsworth BE, Haskell WL, Leon AS et al 1993 Compendium of physical activities: classification of energy costs of human physical activities. Med Sci Sports 25:71–80

Anachkova B, Pääkkonen H 1992 Housework time in Bulgaria and Finland. Studies no. 193, Statistics, Helsinki

Astrup A 1996 Obesity and metabolic efficiency. In: The origins and consequences of obesity. Wiley, Chichester (Ciba Found Symp 201) p 159–173

Bandini LG, Schoeller DA, Dietz WH 1990 Energy expenditure in obese and nonobese adolescents. Pediatr Res 27:198–203

Blair D, Buskirk ER 1987 Habitual daily energy expenditure and activity levels of lean and adult-onset and child-onset obese women. Am J Clin Nutr 45:540–550

Blundell JE, King NA 1996 Overconsumption as a cause of weight gain: behavioural–physiological interactions in the control of food intake (appetite). In: The origins and consequences of obesity. Wiley, Chichester (Ciba Found Symp 201) p 138–158

Bouchard C 1996 Genetics of obesity in humans: current issues. In: The origins and consequences of obesity. Wiley, Chichester (Ciba Found Symp 201) p 108–117

Brooks CM 1987 Leisure time physical activity assessment of American adults through an analysis of time diaries collected in 1981. Am J Physiol 77:455–460

Bullen BA, Reed RB, Majer J 1964 Physical activity of obese and nonobese adolescent girls appraised by motion picture sampling. Am J Clin Nutr 14:211–223

Buratta V, Sabbadini LL 1993 Can time use statistics describe the life of children? Time use methodology: towards consensus. Note e relazioni no. 3 Istituto di Statistica, Rome, p 51–66

Central Statistical Office 1995 Changes in the way of life of the Hungarian Society. 1. Social time use. Department of Social Statistics, Budapest

Dietz WH, Gortmaker SL 1985 Do we fatten our children at the television set? Obesity and television viewing in children and adolescents. Paediatrics 75:807–812

DiPietro L, Williamson DF, Caspersen CJ, Eaker E 1993 The descriptive epidemiology of selected physical activities and body weight among adults trying to lose weight: the behavioural risk factor surveillance system survey, 1989. Int J Obes 17:69–76

FAO–WHO Ad Hoc Expert Committee 1985 Energy and protein requirements. WHO, Geneva (Technical Report Series 724)

Ferro-Luzzi A 1986 Range of variation in energy expenditure and scope for regulation. In: Taylor TG, Jenkins NK (eds) Proc of the XIII International Congress of Nutrition. J Libbey Press, London, p 393–399

Ferro-Luzzi A 1988 Marginal energy malnutrition: some speculations on energy sparing mechanisms. In: Collins KJ, Roberts DF (eds) The capacity for work in the tropics. Cambridge University Press, New York (Soc Study Human Biol Symp Series 26) p 141–164

Ferro-Luzzi A, Branca F 1996 Coping with poverty: the biological impact of nutrition insecurity. In: Livi-Bacci M, De Santis G, Cornia A (eds) Demography and poverty. Oxford University Press, in press

Ferro-Luzzi A, Scaccini C, Taffese S, Aberra B, Demeke T 1990 Seasonal energy deficiency in Ethiopian rural women. Eur J Clin Nutr (suppl 1) 44:7–18

Folsom AR, Carpersen CJ, Taylor HL et al 1985 Leisure time physical activity and its relationship to coronary risk factors in a population-based sample. Am J Epidemiol 121:570–579

Fontvieille AM, Kriska A, Ravussin E 1993 Decreased physical activity in Pima Indian compared with Caucasian children. Int J Obes 17:445–452

Gershuny J 1995 Economic activity and women's time use. In: Niemi I (ed) Time use of women in Europe and North America. United Nations, Geneva, p 23–54

Gortmaker SL, Dietz WH Jr, Cheung LW 1990 Inactivity, diet and the fattening of America. J Am Diet Assoc 90:1247–1252

ISTAT 1993 Indagine Multiscopo sulle famiglie, Anni 1987–1991. No. 4 L'uso del tempo in Italia. Istituto di Statistica, Roma

James WPT 1996 The epidemiology of obesity. In: The origins and consequences of obesity. Wiley, Chichester (Ciba Found Symp 201) p 1–16

James WP, Schofield EC 1990 Human energy requirements: a manual for planners and nutritionists. Oxford University Press, New York

Klesges RC, Shelton ML, Klesges LM 1993 Effect of television on metabolic rate: potential implications for childhood obesity. Pediatrics 91:281–286

Niemi I 1995 A general view of time use by gender. In: Niemi I (ed) Time use of women in Europe and North America. United Nations, Geneva, p 1–22

Norgan NG, Ferro-Luzzi A 1978 Nutrition, physical activity, and physical fitness in contrasting environments. In: Parizkova J, Rogozkin VA (eds) International series on sport sciences, vol 7: Nutrition, physical fitness, and health. University Park Press, New York, p 167–193

Prentice AM, Black AE, Coward WA, Cole TJ 1996 Energy expenditure in overweight and obese adults in affluent societies: an analysis of 319 doubly-labelled water measurements. Eur J Clin Nutr 50:93–97

Ravussin E, Lillioja S, Knowler WC et al 1988 Reduced rate of energy expenditure as a risk factor for body-weight gain. N Engl J Med 318:467–472

Roberts SB 1993 Energy expenditure and the development of early obesity. Ann N Y Acad Sci 699:18–23

Roberts SB, Savage J, Coward WA, Chew B, Lucas A 1988 Energy expenditure and intake in infants born to lean and overweight mothers. N Engl J Med 318:461–466

Romanella NE, Wakat DK, Loyd BH, Kelly LE 1991 Physical activity and attitudes in lean and obese children and their mothers. Int J Obes 15:407–414

Schlicker SA, Borra ST, Regan C 1994 The weight and fitness status of United States children. Nutr Rev 52:11–17

Shetty PS, James WPT 1994 Body mass index. A measure of chronic energy deficiency in adults. Unipub, Lanham, MD (FAO Food and Nutrition Paper Series 56)

Suzuki Y 1993 Time use surveys and research in Asia. Time use methodology: towards consensus. Note e relazioni, no. 3. Istituto di Statistica, Rome, p 351–358

Szalai A (ed) 1972 The use of time: daily activities of urban and suburban populations in twelve countries. Mouton de Gruyter, Hawthorne, NY

Tucker LA, Friedman GM 1989 Television viewing and obesity in adult males. Am J Public Health 79:516–518

UN 1991 The world's women 1970–1990: trends and statistics. United Nations, New York

Viteri F 1982 Nutrition and work performance. In: Scrimshaw NS, Wallerstein MB (eds) Nutrition policy implementation: issues and experience. Plenum, New York, p 3–13

DISCUSSION

Ravussin: There are different approaches for looking at the impact of physical activity on body weight. First, cross-sectional data often reveal an inverse relationship between body mass index (BMI) and physical activity (Rising et al 1994), indicating that obese and overweight subjects are less active than their lean counterparts. However, such correlations do not provide cause and effect relationships, and it is impossible to know whether obese individuals are less active because of their obesity or whether a low level of physical activity caused obesity. Secondly, the secular trend in the increased prevalence of obesity seems to parallel a decrease in physical activity. One of the best examples of this is by Prentice & Jebb (1995), who used crude proxies for inactivity, such as amount of time viewing television or number of cars per household. Both types of studies indicate that physical inactivity may play an important role in the development of obesity. However, only prospective studies will indicate the role of physical inactivity in the aetiology of obesity. For example, Dietz & Gortmaker (1985) have clearly documented that in young children the amount of television watching is predictive of BMI some years later. There have also been three important studies showing the protective effect of physical activity on the development of non-insulin-dependent diabetes mellitus (NIDDM) (Helmrich et al 1991, Manson et al 1991, 1992). However, in those studies, if physical activity had a significant impact on reducing the incidence of diabetes, it had little impact on BMI, especially when the data were corrected for initial BMI. One can say, therefore, that more prospective data are urgently needed.

Roberts: Intervention studies don't change body composition appreciably when those interventions are exclusively focused on physical activity without changing the diet. Body composition in those intervention studies changes as you would expect based on the cross-sectional relationships between fitness and fatness, suggesting that body composition is in equilibrium with the levels of physical activity (Roberts 1995). However, there are genetic differences influencing the capacity for physical activity between different people that can account for much of the individual variability seen in cross-sectional studies.

Prentice: I would like to endorse Eric Ravussin. We have to be careful when using a power ratio, particularly when looking specifically for differences between different BMIs, because we know that the analyses may easily be invalid. Eric has described a statistical point of view, but another way to look at it is just to ask what is the best exponent that corrects for body weight in different activities? It's a complex issue. We have a paper coming out shortly showing that it's invalid to use a power ratio to look at differences in activity over different BMIs (Prentice et al 1996). Anna Ferro-Luzzi also showed some time and motion studies, which is the approach that we recommend should be used. Statistically, there is no way that one can make the body weight correction because the correction itself is dependent on the proportion of weight-dependent and weight-independent exercise that a person does, which cannot be measured unless time-and-motion studies are done. There's abundant evidence using this approach supporting a relationship between physical activity and BMI. In my opinion, there is a cut-off point, so that those people who do absolutely nothing are particularly at risk.

Ferro-Luzzi: Let me reply in order to the various points raised. Eric Ravussin has mentioned that cross-sectional data have revealed the existence of an inverse relationship between BMI and physical activity. Although this is true, it is important to mention that almost all the epidemiological studies that have investigated such a relationship have based their assessment of physical activity on a questionnaire, mostly self-administered, which established the number of working hours people engage in specific leisure activities that were classified into three or more categories of intensity. This approach is far from accurate and cannot provide a true estimate of the level of energy expenditure. Thus, in my view, physical activity is likely to be a proxy for something else that relates to BMI, such as lifestyle or perhaps a concern for keeping lean. It does not prove that BMI is low because people spend more energy. Eric Ravussin also mentioned secular trends of obesity and crude proxies for physical activity. I have reviewed these studies, and I have found them of general value, but in my presentation I have made a deliberate effort to move away from these proxies and to explore the impact of total energy expenditure. He also expressed concern about the use of the physical activity level (PAL) measurement in my analyses. This manner of expressing activity levels has been used in all studies that have found correlations between BMI and physical activity. There are some limitations of relating energy expenditure to BMI. Controlling for body weight by covariance analysis does not provide us with more meaningful results, either when using PAL or energy expenditure.

Andrew Prentice commented on the best exponent for correcting body weight when expressing energy expenditure data. This was a proposition advanced by Heusner (1985), who developed the Kleiber idea of a mass exponent (Kleiber 1947). We have also investigated the possibility of using a specific power for body weight, developing it from measures of dynamic and non-dynamic standard activities in individuals who differed markedly in stature. We found that the power function for body weight of short and tall people in stationary activity was 0.80 and 0.73, respectively. However, there are little available data addressing how energy is allocated to different activities, and it is impossible to assign diverse powers to body weight according to the type of activity carried out. In other words, one is limited in what one can do by the amount of information that is provided. I was interested in identifying the existence of a threshold of activity that was protective, and my analysis of the data in the literature, despite the incomplete information, demonstrated that it did exist, at least for males. I believe this is a good starting point, although it warrants more data.

Swinburn: Physical activity may have an impact on body weight through mechanisms other than those related to energy expenditure; for example, through oxidative changes in muscle or effects on appetite. Many problems are generated if energy expenditure is included in the calculations, so I suggest that we should discard it from those calculations.

Garrow: Carolyn Summerbell and I have attempted to do a systematic survey of all the exercise studies of overweight people in which the control groups were people on the same diet who did not exercise (Garrow & Summerbell 1995). There are 28 such studies (but no studies of the obese), and the mean weight loss by exercising (in combination with dieting) was of the order of 3 kg in 30 weeks. Pinning our faith on exercise as a method of reducing obesity is unrealistic.

Bouchard: We have repeatedly heard the figure of a 3 kg weight loss over 30 weeks. Let us keep in mind that it may take years, perhaps as much as 20 years, to become overweight or obese. A 30-week period of a one-year intervention study is probably not a good time-frame to consider the role of any behavioural change in weight control. There are data showing a stronger relationship between the level of physical activity and BMI than those considered here. For example, Eric Ravussin and his colleagues, and Peter Davies and his colleagues have shown that energy expenditure was significantly and negatively correlated with per cent body fat in children (Zurlo et al 1992, Ferraro et al 1991, Davies et al 1995). Others have also shown the same phenomenon in adults (Schulz & Schoeller 1994). These correlations are in the range of -0.5 to -0.8.

Ravussin: We have two lines of evidence to suggest that a low level of physical activity may play a role in the development of obesity. First, in adults, there is an inverse relationship between physical activity measured by double-labelled water and body composition (Rising et al 1994). Secondly, 10-year-old Pima Indians (a population prone to obesity) have lower levels of physical activity when compared to age-matched Caucasians. Unfortunately, these are only cross-sectional studies.

Bouchard: There are also prospective data based on questionnaire assessments of PAL which indicate that the inactive people gain more weight over time. However, at this time, we have no prospective studies based on double-labelled water assessment of energy expenditure of activity.

Ferro-Luzzi: You mentioned that in children PAL correlates fairly strongly with per cent body fat. I find it astonishing that correlation coefficients as high as -0.8 could be obtained. We are considering an indicator that may be a crude proxy for something else which is important in determining whether BMI is high or low and whether it is possible to gain weight over time or not. Thus, Williamson et al (1993) were unable to find any correlation between physical activity at baseline and subsequent weight gain, but the correlation was present if the analysis was cross-sectional rather than longitudinal. Also, the Finnish study (Rissanen et al 1991) was only based on an estimation using questions relating to the frequencies of certain leisure activities.

James: Aila Rissanen, were those studies (Rissanen et al 1991) performed in men or women?

Rissanen: Both.

James: Was there a strong relationship in both cases?

Rissanen: Yes.

James: What are the levels of activity in which there was a decrease in weight gain?

Rissanen: I can't answer that question from the data.

Prentice: I endorse what Claude Bouchard, Boyd Swinburn and Aila Rissanen have said. The evidence is overwhelming from questionnaire time-and-motion studies that inactivity predisposes people to excess weight gain. The double-labelled water experiments are riddled with methodological flaws, so it doesn't surprise me that you're not finding those relationships. All the existing analyses are severely flawed (see Prentice et al 1996). They all make the assumption that when the cost of physical activity is calculated as total energy expenditure minus the basal metabolic rate (BMR) then the appropriate denominator is body weight. We can demonstrate that this is simply not the case by using measurements of people across different body weights to show that the appropriate denominator depends entirely on the activity. That is, if a person is climbing upstairs all day the appropriate exponent for the denominator is one, and if a person is cycling the appropriate denominator is weight to the power zero because the cost of doing that work is virtually independent of the person's weight. If the person is performing light household chores the exponent is 0.8, and if they are sitting down the exponent is 0.3. Therefore, the correct exponent is somewhere between zero and one, it is certainly not one and for most people the average is about 0.5, i.e. the square root of body weight. This means that whenever you look at the cost of physical activity in a heavy person and divide by weight to the power of one you are over-correcting and you automatically create the negative correlation with body fatness. We and others have demonstrated this by random number generations.

Allison: I would like to ask for some clarification of some of the points that Andrew Prentice has raised. Am I correct in saying that in order to obtain a measure of activity one has to control for body size, so one must divide the measure of physical activity by body size, but that the difficulty arises in working out the exponent of body size?

Prentice: Yes. The exponent will be different for each of us depending on the mixture of activities we do. We know that fatter people will expend more energy because they carry more weight around, but we want to know whether they are expending more or less energy proportionate to their body weight. To do this people have tended to divide activity energy expenditure by body weight, but I'm saying that that is a serious over-correction, so that overweight people look as if they're less active.

Allison: So you want to ask 'Is something related to body weight after controlling for body weight?', but isn't that a contradiction?

Prentice: That's the problem I'm raising.

James: The fundamental problems of just using body weight were recognized in the original analyses during the development of PAL use (WHO 1985). The challenge was to choose the simplest way of standardizing data, hence the development of PAL in relation to BMR, which has a direct weight relationship and recognizes the need for different values if one is looking at specific physical activities. In common with David Allison I can't get my mind round the precise issue you are addressing.

Prentice: The PAL measurement is not a bad index unless there is a lot of body fat. BMR is closely related to fat-free mass, so one is assuming that there is a constant relationship between fat-free mass and fat mass. This relationship breaks down in overweight people.

Roberts: I'm personally less overwhelmed by the prospective data for two reasons. (1) It's easier to obtain unbiased measures of physical activity than it is dietary intake or dietary composition. (2) Although I accept Claude Bouchard's point that intervention studies have been carried out over a relatively short time period, if one compares the magnitude of the effect of these intervention studies with dietary intervention studies, then it is clear that dietary intervention studies are more effective in changing body composition than the physical activity interventions over a similar time period.

Ravussin: I would like to add one piece of information that I believe is important. We have measured spontaneous physical activity (fidgeting) in a whole-body calorimeter (Zurlo et al 1992). We first found that the level of spontaneous physical activity is a strong familial trait which may be genetically determined. But more importantly we found that male subjects with a low level of spontaneous physical activity were more likely to gain weight than those with a high level of spontaneous physical activity. Also, the variability in physical activity accounts for 100–800 kcal/day, depending upon the body weight of the subjects. This aspect of physical activity has often been ignored in the past.

Ferro-Luzzi: I would like to return to the issue of the way to account for body mass when comparing people that have different body weights, different compositions of fat-free mass or different proportions of body fat. This is an old, as yet unresolved question, where statistical and numerical corrections can only resolve what is a biological issue. Field studies are epidemiological in nature and also cannot answer this question. The approximation that is achieved by standardizing for body weight or controlling body weight by co-varying for it and, finally, when using the BMI expression, is the best that can be achieved with those data. In my opinion, the entire literature so far cited in this discussion and the results of my analyses all point to a link between energy expenditure expressed as PAL (or metabolic equivalents) and BMI.

References

Davies PS, Gregory J, White A 1995 Physical activity and body fatness in pre-school children. Int J Obes Relat Metab Disord 19:6–10

Dietz WH, Gortmaker SL 1985 Do we fatten our children at the television set? Obesity and television viewing in children and adolescents. Pediatrics 75:807–812

Ferraro R, Boyce VL, Swinburn B, De Gregorio M, Ravussin E 1991 Energy cost of physical activity on a metabolic ward in relationship to obesity. Am J Clin Nutr 53:1368–1371

Garrow JS, Summerbell CD 1995 Meta-analysis: effect of exercise, with or without dieting, on the body composition of overweight subjects. Eur J Clin Nutr 49:1–10

Helmrich SP, Ragland DR, Leung RW, Paffenbarger RS 1991 Physical activity and reduced occurrence of non-insulin dependent diabetes mellitus. N Engl J Med 325:147–152

Heusner AA 1985 Body size and energy metabolism. Ann Rev Nutr 5:267–293

Kleiber M 1947 Body size and metabolic rate. Physiol Rev 27:511–541

Manson JE, Rimm EB, Stampfer 1991 Physical activity and incidence of non-insulin-dependent mellitus in women. Lancet 338:774–778

Manson JE, Nathan DM, Krolewski AS, Stampfer MJ, Willett WC, Hennekens CH 1992 A prospective study of exercise and incidence of diabetes among US male physicians. JAMA 268:63–67

Prentice AM, Jebb SA 1995 Obesity in Britain: gluttony or sloth? Br Med J 311:437–439

Prentice AM, Goldberg GR, Murgatroyd PR, Cole TJ 1996 Physical activity and obesity: problems in correcting expenditure for body size. Int J Obes 20:688–691

Rising R, Harper IT, Fontvielle AM, Ferraro RT, Spraul M, Ravussin E 1994 Determinants of total daily energy expenditure: variability in physical activity. Am J Clin Nutr 59:800–804

Rissanen A, Heliövaara M, Knekt P, Reunanen A, Aromaa A 1991 Determinants of weight gain and overweight in adult Finns. Eur J Clin Nutr 45:419–430

Roberts SB 1995 Abnormalities of energy expenditure and the development of obesity. Obesity Res (suppl 2) 3:155S–163S

Schultz LO, Schoeller DA 1994 A compilation of total daily energy expenditures and body weight in healthy adults. Am J Clin Nutr 60:676–681

WHO 1985 Energy and protein requirements. Report of a Joint FAO/WHO/UNU Expert Consultation. World Health Organization, Geneva (Technical Report Series 724)

Williamson DF, Madans J, Anda RF, Kleinman JC, Kahn HS, Byers T 1993 Recreational activity and ten-year weight change in a US national cohort. Int J Obes 17:279–286

Zurlo F, Ferraro RT, Fontvieille AM, Rising R, Bogardus C, Ravussin E 1992 Spontaneous physical activity and obesity: cross-sectional and longitudinal studies in Pima Indians. Am J Physiol 263:296E–300E

Coherent, preventive and management strategies for obesity

George A. Bray

Pennington Biomedical Research Center, Louisiana State University, 6400 Perkins Road, Baton Rouge, LA 70808-4124, USA

Abstract. The increased risk of morbidity and mortality from obesity, central body fat and weight gain, and the benefits of weight reduction argue that the cost associated with obesity could be beneficially affected by prevention of weight gain or induction of weight loss. Genetic, metabolic and demographic predictors of weight gain have been identified that allow the selection of high risk individuals. Among the metabolic predictors are a low metabolic rate, insulin sensitivity and a high respiratory quotient. Demographic predictors include current smokers, certain dieting behaviours, lower socioeconomic class, a low level of education, use of contraceptives, status post-partum and rapid weight gain in childhood. Several studies suggest that weight gain can be prevented. Targets for such strategies might be high risk families, current smokers, those who are planning to stop smoking and those with a low metabolic rate. For those who fail primary prevention, treatment may be appropriate. The greater the degree of excess weight, the greater the risk and the more appropriate treatment becomes to reduce body weight.

1996 The origins and consequences of obesity. Wiley, Chichester (Ciba Foundation Symposium 201) p 228–254

The adage 'an ounce of prevention is worth a pound of cure' applies to obesity more than to any other disease. This chapter will examine coherent strategies for the prevention and management of obesity. They will be coherent in the sense that the approaches for identifying at-risk populations and preventing the development of obesity in those at high risk for developing this problem will be evaluated in terms of the risk/benefit ratio, which will also be the strategy used for evaluating management strategies for individuals who are failures of primary prevention. Such a series of strategies has both a chronological and socioeconomic strategy. Preventive efforts must be aimed at children and adolescents identified as at high risk. At later stages in life, high risk groups would include pregnant women, status post-partum, individuals developing sedentary lifestyles, and weight gain associated with the menopause and in the elderly. Socioeconomic status and gender also play important roles, with women having higher prevalence rates for obesity, yet having lower mortality rates from diseases associated with obesity. Lower socioeconomic and educational status increase the prevalence of obesity.

Are the resources to be used for preventive and management strategies justified by the potential outcomes?

Obesity, weight gain and central fat distribution all contribute to increased mortality and morbidity. The general shape of the relationship between increasing weight and risk from obesity is curvilinear. It is frequently described as J-shaped, although in other studies it may appear to be only the monotonic ascending part of a parabolic curve. This general shape is similar for both men and women. The data adapted from the American Cancer Society Study are shown in Fig. 1 (Lew & Garfinkel 1979, Bray & Gray 1988a,b), together with data for the relationship between diastolic blood pressure and mortality (Stamler et al 1989) and the relationship between cholesterol and mortality (Stamler et al 1986). The three data sets have been aligned to show the levels at which there is 'low risk', 'moderate risk' and 'high risk'. Data for all-cause mortality in smokers and non-smokers from the Nurses' Health Trial (Manson et al 1995) are similar, as are other long-term studies (Manson et al 1987, Waaler 1984, Lindsted et al 1991). Using these risk curves from Manson et al (1995), G. M. Faich (personal communication 1995) calculated that a body mass index (BMI) difference of $5\,kg/m^2$ more (BMI $27\,kg/m^2$ to $32\,kg/m^2$) would be associated with 122 more deaths/ million women per year in the obese group. In a review of the health costs associated with this risk, Colditz (1992) estimated that in the USA they accounted for 7.8% of total health care costs in 1992 (Table 1). Data from several other countries where estimates of the impact of obesity have been made are similar.

Weight gain in adult life also increases health risks for both men and women. A weight gain of 10 kg or more even within the normal weight range is associated with a significant degree of excess risk (Willett et al 1995). Likewise, fat located in the visceral and abdominal regions also significantly increases risk of overall mortality, coronary heart disease, stroke, diabetes and certain cancers (Bray 1994). This is most evident for diabetes, where even small degrees of excess weight or central body fat increase the risk of developing diabetes substantially (Ohlson et al 1987). It would thus appear that prevention of weight gain, prevention of obesity and prevention of central fat accumulation would significantly reduce the overall rates of mortality and morbidity associated with obesity.

These data on morbidity and mortality suggest that weight loss should produce significant health benefits. The most impressive data supporting this proposition have been published by Williamson et al (1995) using data from the American Cancer Society Study (Lew & Garfinkel 1979).

Intentional weight loss of more than 9.1 kg within the past year in 28 388 obese women aged 40–64 with no pre-existing illness was associated with a 25% reduction in all-cause mortality and in deaths from heart disease. In the same study 15 069 women, with a BMI above $27\,kg/m^2$ and co-morbid conditions such as a coronary heart disease,

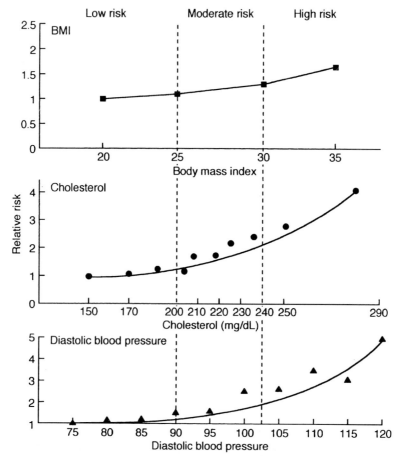

FIG. 1.   Relationship of body mass index (BMI, kg/m²), cholesterol and diastolic blood pressure to relative risk of mortality. Data from the American Cancer Society Study (Lew & Garfinkel 1979) have been replotted for the BMI data, and tables in papers by Stamler et al (1986, 1989) are used to construct the relationship between cholesterol and blood pressure. (Copyright 1995, George A. Bray.)

hypertension, stroke, diabetes, cancer and cirrhosis, who intentionally lost any amount of weight experienced a 20% decrease in all-cause mortality, a 30–40% reduction in mortality associated with diabetes and a 40–50% reduction in mortality from cancers linked to obesity (Williamson et al 1995).

Other sources of data also support this proposition. In the Swedish Obesity Study, Sjöström and his colleagues (L. Sjöström, personal communication 1995) have evaluated the prevalence of hypertension and diabetes before intervention by gastric bypass surgery with the cure rate and prevalence of new cases over two years after treatment. The prevalences of hypertension were 44% and 51%, respectively, in the

TABLE 1   Obesity increases health costs

Disease	Cost attributable to obesity (US$ billion)
Cardiovascular disease	22.2
Musculoskeletal disease	17.0
Diabetes	11.3
Gallbladder disease	2.3
Cancer	1.9
Hypertension	1.5
Total	56.2

From Colditz (1992).

two groups at baseline (Table 2). Two years later 43% of the surgical cases had been cured but only 21% of the control cases. In contrast, only 5% of those without hypertension developed high blood pressure over two years after gastric bypass surgery, compared to 15% in the control group. The impact of treatment on diabetes is even more striking (Table 2). Here the prevalences at baseline were 13% and 16%. In those treated surgically, 69% of the cases were cured. Of those who did not have diabetes at baseline, only 0.5% developed diabetes over the next two years. In the control group, where essentially no weight was lost, only 16% showed a cure of diabetes, while 7.8% of those without diabetes at baseline developed it in two years. Blackburn & Kanders (1994) have also shown the improvement in diabetes and hypertension in patients treated with a low energy diet for 18 months. These data are similar to those of Sjøström and colleagues.

Against the benefits of weight loss are the potential risks associated with weight loss and weight regain. Several studies have argued that weight loss is associated with increased risk of mortality (Pamuk et al 1992). In most of these studies, the question of whether weight loss was intentional or unintentional could not be answered. It has been known since the time of Hippocrates that weight loss is a bad prognostic sign and

TABLE 2   Swedish Obesity Study

Disease	Treatment	Prevalence at baseline (%)	Two-year follow-up	
			Cured (%)	New cases (%)
Hypertension	surgery	51	43	5.0
	control	44	16	15.0
Diabetes	surgery	16	69	0.5
	control	13	16	7.8

these data confirm that proposition. When intentional weight loss was examined by Williamson et al (1995), it appeared that weight loss was beneficial, suggesting that the weight losses in these other studies were, in both normal and overweight subjects, in most instances unintentional.

Weight regain after weight loss is another imputed risk to weight loss programmes. In a careful evaluation of the data, the US Task Force on Obesity concluded that the detrimental effects of weight cycling had not been effectively demonstrated and should not serve as a barrier to preventive or management strategies (Atkinson et al 1994).

Can we identify predictors of weight gain?

If the propositions that obesity, weight gain and central fat deposition are hazardous to health and that intentional weight loss is beneficial, can we identify and predict those at risk of weight gain to effectively target strategies towards those at high risk? A growing number of approaches will allow prediction of some individuals who are at high risk for obesity. Among these are genetic, metabolic and demographic predictors.

Genetic predictors

It has long been recognized that obesity runs in families (Bouchard 1994). Children from overweight families have a substantially increased risk of developing obesity from both genetic and environmental components. In twin studies heritability estimates are high, ranging from 50–80%. In nuclear families the heritability estimates range from 30–50% and in adoption studies from 10–30%. Regardless of the paradigm used, genetic factors play a significant role with an overall heritability estimated as 0.34 (Vogler et al 1995).

A number of genetic markers are beginning to appear that are associated with obesity or with weight gain. In experimental mice and rats it is well recognized that several single-gene defects can produce obesity. In humans these loci have not been shown to be associated with any but the most severe forms of obesity, and then with some uncertainty (Reed et al 1995). Also from studies of animal models susceptible to dietary obesity, it has been possible to identify upwards of 12 chromosomal locations that are strongly associated with this susceptibility to increased total and regional body fat (Warden et al 1995, West et al 1994). As yet, the precise genes involved in these animal models are unknown. In humans a number of genetic loci have been identified with various levels of significance (Bouchard & Pérusse 1996). Clearly, the future is open to identifying individuals at higher risks because of their genetic make up, which may provide the basis for a preventive strategy by targeting overweight families and screening their children.

Metabolic factors

A number of metabolic predictors for obesity have been suggested. In intensive studies of the Pima Indians, Ravussin & Swinburn (1992) have identified several predictors. A low metabolic rate, or low level of total energy expenditure, predicts weight gain in obese individuals. A high respiratory quotient indicating carbohydrate oxidation is also predictive of future weight gain. Finally, increased insulin sensitivity, measured by a euglycaemic hyperinsulinaemic clamp, also predicts subsequent weight gain. Griffiths et al (1990) have proposed that a more rapid fall in the basal metabolic rate per kilogram of body weight in infants puts them at higher risk for developing obesity than in infants where the metabolic rate falls more slowly. In women, contraceptive users and women at the end of pregnancy are at particularly high risk for developing obesity (Korkeila et al 1995). Similarly, children who show rapid weight gain in childhood are more likely to enter adolescence and adulthood with increased body fat stores.

Demographic factors

A number of demographic factors can be identified from clinical studies. One of the strongest is the association, particularly in women, with social class and particularly with the level of education. There is also a reduced level of obesity in subgroups with increased levels of physical activity, suggesting that this is a second important factor (Rissanen et al 1990). The decline in physical activity during this century may be an important contributor to the development of the rising incidence of obesity, particularly the increasing frequency of watching television. Diet has also been proposed as an important factor in the development of obesity. The consumption of a high fat diet in a number of epidemiological studies has been related to increased obesity (Lissner & Heitman 1995). In a six-year follow-up of risk factors for weight gain in twins, Korkeila et al (1995) found that current smoking in both men and women was associated with an increased six-year risk for weight gain. Dieting at baseline in both men and women was also associated with increased risk for subsequent weight gain. Among men, a high level of stress and a low level of education were additional demographic risk factors. For women, additional factors included getting less than six hours of sleep per night, and neurotic behaviour.

Can we prevent obesity?

Two sets of data suggest that long-term positive changes in weight status can occur. The first is a non-intervention study in Framingham, Massachusetts. Cohorts of women and men have been followed since 1948. In an early publication by Ashley & Kannel (1974), the weight curves for men and women can be seen to go in opposite directions, with women's weight on average decreasing and men's weight increasing. This suggests that the two genders are responding differently to the environmental factors acting on their genetic substrate, and it raises the potential for social marketing of weight control messages to gender-specific audiences.

A second study is by Epstein et al (1990), which examines the effect of behavioural change techniques for overweight children. Their trial involved comparing a nontreated group with a group in which parent and child were treated together and a third group in which parent and child were treated separately. At five and 10 years following the initial study the children treated together with their parents showed significantly less weight gain and were below the relative weight at which they started the study 10 years earlier. This maintenance of a lower relative weight occurred throughout the adolescent period when weight gain can be a major problem. Of considerable interest is that the parents of these children returned to their initial weight whereas the children did not, suggesting that age-specific strategies may also be important tools in a coherent strategy for the prevention of obesity. This study has been replicated three times. It appears to apply to pre-pubertal children, where an increased height leads to a lesser degree of obesity when they reach their adult height. Similar studies in adolescents who have already achieved their adult height do not produce these results.

Targets for preventive strategies

From the predictors of weight gain, it is obvious that children from families where one or both parents are overweight are at higher risk. This may be for genetic or environmental reasons, or for both. Identifying these children in their pre-school years allows the potential for applying techniques similar to those of Epstein et al (1990) focused on the child/parent relationship. Children from lower socioeconomic groups, particularly those from families with rapid weight gain in childhood, should be targeted for intervention (Lissau & Sørenson 1994).

Probably the most significant association is with socioeconomic status (Sobal & Stunkard 1989). Higher levels of education and income reduce the risk significantly. Thus, we can target the high risk, lower socioeconomic groups. The phenomenon of 'restrained' eating is common among the higher socioeconomic groups (Lawson et al 1995). Therefore, the behavioural and social techniques that might introduce 'restraint' into the lower social and educational levels may be another way to target high risk groups.

Another high risk group are those currently smoking, and in particular those who are attempting to stop smoking. Weight gain is a common event during cessation of smoking and, in heavy smokers, this weight gain can be more than 10% of initial body weight (Klesges et al 1991). Strategies aimed at this group might be particularly effective in preventing weight gain and reducing the desire to start smoking again to induce weight loss. Based on the information available, efforts to reduce the level of fat in the diet below 30%, to reduce the level of saturated fat and to replace the sedentary lifestyle with a more active one would all be valuable strategies because they would attack not only obesity, but also the high prevalence of heart disease. The selection and evaluation of targets can be broadened, but the costs of evaluation of the metabolic and genetic factors at present would make it prohibitive to use these as part of a cost-effective programme.

Failures from primary prevention

The rising prevalence of obesity in the USA (Kuczmarski et al 1994), the UK (Prentice & Jebb 1995) and much of the western world implies that current preventive strategies are ineffective for many people. Thus, secondary prevention and treatment are essential and will remain so until our ability to identify and target primary preventive strategies becomes more effective.

Risk–benefit assessment of obesity

Risks of obesity

In evaluating the currently available agents for treatment of obesity and whether new ones are to be developed, a paradigm is needed to assess the risks and benefits of treatment versus no treatment. As overweight increases, the risk from excess weight increases (Bray & Gray 1988a,b). These risks are distributed over a number of causes, including heart disease, diabetes mellitus, gallbladder disease and some forms of cancer.

Benefits of treatment for obesity

Benefits of treating obesity fall into two categories, a reduction in risks of ill-health and an improvement in the quality of life. Caloric restriction of mice and rats also supports the hypothesis that avoiding fattening will prolong life (Masoro 1985).

Effects of weight reduction on morbidity are congruent with the data on mortality. Toeller et al (1982) reported that over 10 years, the risk of diabetes was reduced when individuals maintained or preferably lost small amounts of weight as opposed to when they gained weight. L. Sjøström (personal communication 1995) has reported that over two years, 7.8% of individuals with an average BMI of $38 \, \text{kg/m}^2$ developed diabetes, compared with 0.5% of those whose BMI was lowered following gastric bypass surgery. Long et al (1994) have provided similar data. In monkeys, diabetes does not develop over more than nine years when their weight is restricted, compared with the development of diabetes in nearly half the monkeys that are allowed to become obese (Hansen & Bodkin 1993). Weight reduction also has significant positive benefits on blood pressure in more than half of the treated patients, and it also lowers lipid levels. In the Framingham Study, Kannel & Gordon (1979) reported that a 10% change in body weight produced parallel changes in cholesterol of 11 mg/dL, in glucose of 2 mg/dL, in uric acid of 0.4 mg/dL and in systolic blood pressure of 5 mmHg.

Risks of treatment

Treatments for obesity, whether by drugs or other modalities, can have detrimental effects of their own. Of the currently available drugs, most have minor side-effects, many of which diminish with treatment. For short-term use in individuals who wish to lose small amounts of weight (probably the majority of the overweight population) these side-effects should not be a deterrent because the drugs will only be used for a short period. When the magnitude of the obesity carries more significant risks, such as when an individual has a BMI of above 30 mg/kg², chronic treatment will be needed and potential risks of any drug need to be evaluated carefully.

Algorithm

An algorithm for starting with BMI and arriving at an overall assessment of risk is shown in Fig. 2 (Bray & Gray 1988b). The initial relative risk is established from the BMI. As shown in Fig. 1, the lowest risk is with a BMI of 25 kg/m². A higher BMI

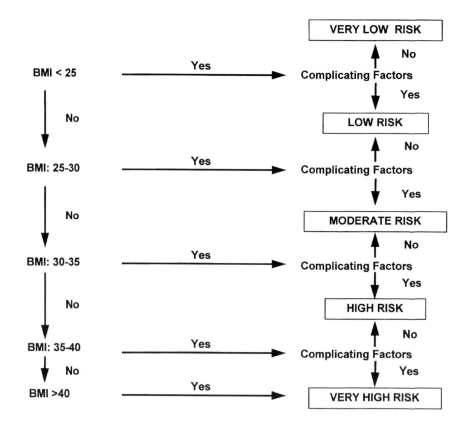

FIG. 2. Algorithm for evaluating the risk from obesity and complicating factors. The complicating factors include young age, male, family history of early heart disease or diabetes mellitus, and hyperlipidaemia or hypertension. BMI, body mass index (kg/m²). (Copyright 1988, George A. Bray.)

carries an increased risk. This risk can be further adjusted, particularly at the lower levels of BMI by using the waist circumference. In men a waist circumference of 90–100 cm and in premenopausal women of 80–90 cm would increase the risk by an equivalent amount to a gain in BMI of 1–2 kg/m², and a waist circumference of above 100 cm in men and above 90 cm in women would increase the risk by an equivalent amount to a gain in BMI of 2–4 kg/m². Similarly, the presence of hypertriglyceridaemia, low levels of high density lipoprotein–cholesterol, fasting hyperglycaemia, diabetes mellitus, or strong family histories of early heart disease or diabetes would increase the risk. Young individuals and individuals who have gained more than 10 kg since the age of 18 are also at higher risk than older individuals at stable weight with the same BMI.

Analogy with hypertension

I return to the comparison with hypertension. The year 1958 was a watershed in the treatment of hypertension; it was the year that thiazides became available. The treatments available for managing the hypertensive patient prior to introduction of chlorothiazide were the use of a low sodium diet, lumbar sympathectomy or ganglionic-blocking drugs. These were analogous in many ways to treatments for obesity that utilize low calorie diets, gastric bypass operations or the mitochondrial uncoupling agent, dinitrophenol. In 1958 the diuretic chlorothiazide was introduced into clinical practice. Its effect in reducing blood pressure was immediately recognized, and this drug became a cornerstone for the treatment of hypertension. Its effect on sodium excretion might be analogous to agents for the treatment of obesity that are designed to reduce digestion of food or reduce its absorption and thus increase fat loss in the faeces. Orlistat fits this category. It is a potent inhibitor of pancreatic lipase and an anti-obesity drug that has a dose–response effect on weight loss (Drent et al 1995).

The sympathetic nervous system and its central connections have been utilized for the treatment of hypertension as well as obesity. α-Methyldopa and clonidine are two centrally acting adrenergic drugs used in the treatment of hypertension. The centrally active adrenergic drugs — such as amphetamine, diethylpropion, phentermine and mazindol, as well as the α-1 adrenergic agonist phenylpropanolamine — might be considered as analogous agents for treatment of obesity (Bray 1995a).

Unique to the treatment of obesity, and not present in the armamentarium for treatment of hypertension, are serotonergic (5-HT) drugs of which fenfluramine, dexfenfluramine and fluoxetine are the current examples. These drugs work by augmenting the extracellular concentration of serotonin, which depresses food intake by acting at serotonin receptors ($5-HT_{1B}$ or $5-HT_{2C}$) (Bray 1995a).

The importance of the sympathetic nervous system for the control of blood pressure is further emphasized by the development of α-1 adrenergic antagonists such as prazosin and terazosin, as well as the use of propranolol, a blocker of β-1 and β-2 adrenergic receptors. The adrenergic analogue for treatment of obesity might be β-3 adrenergic agonists that act on β-3 adrenergic receptors located in brown adipose tissue and white fat cells (Arch & Kaumann 1993).

Angiotensin I-converting enzyme (ACE) inhibitors have proven to be the most effective anti-hypertensive medications yet developed. In evaluating the current search for agents to treat obesity, the key question is by which mechanism will an agent with the effectiveness of the ACE inhibitors be developed to treat obesity? I believe that the β-3 adrenergic agonists, drugs that can modulate glucocorticoid effects on the feeding system, or selective antagonists to neuropeptide Y may have these features.

Treatments currently available for obesity

Obesity has many causes and, as might be expected, different kinds of treatments have been used to reduce the risks that are believed to result from excess fatness. These treatments include behaviour modification, diet, exercise, pharmacotherapy and surgery.

Behaviour modification

Beginning with its introduction by Stuart (1967), behaviour modification has grown to become a cornerstone of treatment for obesity (Brownell & Kramer 1989). As with all treatments for obesity except surgery, weight regain is the expected result when treatment is stopped. Among the longest treatments using behavioural approaches are studies in which these techniques have been applied to 'non-pharmacological' treatments of hypertension. The results of three such published studies are shown in Fig. 3. Note that over the 18–36 months of follow-up there was a slow gain of weight in the control groups, compared to the initial loss and subsequent regain in the experimental groups. This suggests that even with continued treatment there is a reduction in effectiveness.

Diet

Dietary approaches to the treatment of obesity have been used since the time of Hippocrates (Bray 1990). Popular dietary books and pamphlets to aid obesity also have a long history dating from the mid-nineteenth century (Banting 1863). Diets can be divided into three broad groups: (1) low calorie; (2) very low calorie; and (3) low fat.

Low calorie diets, or diets based on calorie counting have been in vogue for a long time. One of the most popular is the 'prudent diet' (Jolliffe 1963). If any of these diets alone had been successful in producing long-term changes in body weight, new diets would no longer have the appeal that greets them with each new year.

Very low calorie diets recommend levels below 800 kcal per day. Most very low calorie diets come as 'formula' diets. Comparison studies have shown no increased

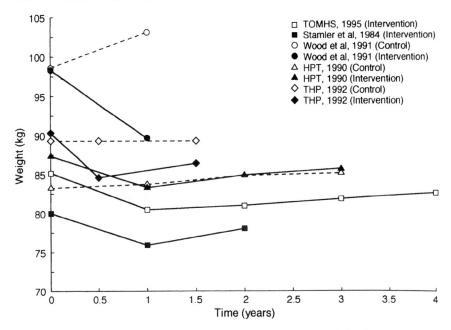

FIG. 3. Weight loss in control and experimental groups receiving behaviour modification. HPT, Hypertension Prevention Trial Research Group; THP, Trials of Hypertension Prevention Collaborative Research Group.

weight loss when the diet contains 400 versus 800 kcal per day. Comparison of a low calorie diet, referred to as a balanced deficit diet, and a very low calorie diet showed more weight loss during treatment for the latter, but at 12 months of follow-up the two groups were identical due to the more rapid regain in the very low calorie diet group (Wadden et al 1990).

Low fat diets in short-term clinical trials have been shown to reduce weight (Lissner & Heitman 1995). There are also suggestive data that low fat diets, if adopted by the population at large, might reduce the risk of obesity, together with heart disease and some forms of cancer.

Exercise

If obesity is the result of a positive energy balance, then exercise, as a mechanism for increasing energy expenditure, should reduce weight. In spite of this logic, the use of exercise regimes as primary approaches to the treatment of obesity have been met with little success (Ballor & Keesey 1991). In contrast, exercise as a method of keeping weight down can be much more effective. The 18-month follow-up by Pavlou et al (1989) showed that policemen who maintained their physical activity after a weight loss programme were more successful in the long run. This would fit with the data showing the lower rates of obesity in subgroups of the population who are less sedentary (Rissanen et al 1990). Higher exercise levels have also been associated with lower rates of heart disease and overall death (Paffenbarger et al 1993, Blair et al 1995). Thus, together with a low fat diet, recommendations for exercise to prevent and maintain a lower weight make good sense.

Pharmacotherapy

All of the currently approved drugs for the treatment of obesity are derivatives of β-phenethylamine (except mazindol, which is a tricyclic compound). Recent data suggest that the current aversion to these drugs and the restrictions placed on their use by many health authorities may be leading to inadequate use of drugs that are potentially more successful than recognized. The current group of drugs can be divided into those that act on the adrenergic neurotransmission system and those that act on the serotonergic system of neurotransmission. The lengths of drug trials last up to 3.5 years, but most are 60 weeks or less. When the medications are stopped, weight regain is the rule. This observation proves that the drugs work when taken, but that drugs don't work when not taken. The analogy with hypertension is again pertinent. When an anti-hypertensive drug is used, blood pressure can be reduced. When the drug is stopped, the blood pressure is expected to rise because the anti-hypertensive drugs treat, but do not cure, hypertension. The same is true of obesity. Drugs work when used, but when the treatment is terminated patients regain weight.

Noradrenergic appetite suppressants. The drugs currently available in this group include benzphetamine, diethylpropion, mazindol, phendimetrazine and phentermine. All, except mazindol, are β-phenethylamine derivatives. Mazindol is a tricyclic compound. Data from a multicentre trial using mazindol and placebo are shown in Fig. 4 (Walker et al 1977). Figure 4A shows three centres in which the effect of the placebo was minimal, and Fig. 4B shows one centre that had a vigorous effect of the placebo. The weight loss in the drug-treated groups was comparable in both panels. However, the effect of the placebo was much greater in Fig. 4B than in Fig. 4A. The interpretation of the effect of the drug depends on how one makes the comparison.

The maximal effect of an appetite suppressant would be to lower food intake to zero, i.e. starvation. No known drug does this, but very low calorie diets and vigorous behaviour modification programmes can produce major reductions in food intake on an acute basis. The closer the effect of the placebo is to zero the less the maximal effect of any appetite suppressant will be. In Fig. 4 the effect of the drug is identical, and the same conclusion of drug effectiveness would be reached if the baseline weights were used for comparison. The difference between Figs 4A and 4B would then be that the effect of the placebo was much greater in Fig. 4B. If the drugs are compared with placebo, the drug is effective in Fig. 4A but not in Fig. 4B. For these reasons, I believe that drug treatment should be compared to the baseline weights (Bray 1995b).

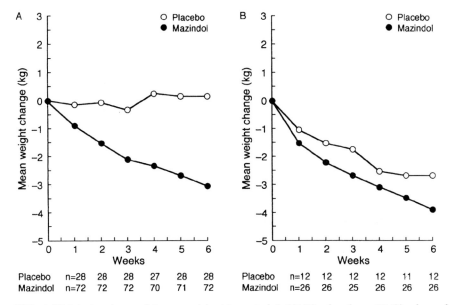

FIG. 4. Weight loss in a multi-centre trial with mazindol. (A) Placebo alone. (B) Placebo and behaviour modification. (From Walker et al 1977, with permission.)

Serotonergic drugs. The only approved serotonergic drug for the treatment of obesity is fenfluramine, which like the noradrenergic drugs is a β-phenethylamine derivative. Fenfluramine differs from the other β-phenethylamines in having no noradrenergic effects. Therefore, it is not an amphetamine-like drug because it has no addictive potential. Indeed, none of the noradrenergic agents are amphetamine-like drugs because, unlike amphetamine, they do not affect the dopaminergic system. The potential for their abuse is also very weak (if at all), in contrast to the clear-cut addictive potential of amphetamine.

The largest study with fenfluramine is the International Dexfenfluramine (INDEX) Study, a multi-centre trial conducted in Europe (Guy-Grand et al 1989) (Fig. 5). Note that the placebo-treated group had significant weight loss, making the decision about whether to compare the weight loss in the drug-treated group from the baseline or from the placebo an important one. The placebo effect can be highly variable. Figure 6 shows the weight loss of placebo-treated groups in several trials of appetite suppressant drugs lasting 31–60 weeks. It is obvious that the placebo groups lost different amounts of weight from one study to another. In the more effective placebo-treated groups there was no detectable effect from the addition of a drug. However, this is to be expected because an appetite suppressant cannot produce more weight loss than starvation itself. The closer the placebo effect is to zero calories, the less likelihood it is to see a drug effect.

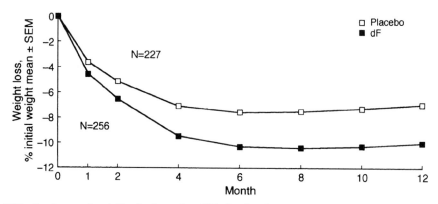

FIG. 5. International Dexfenfluramine (dF) Study. Groups are treated with placebo or dexafenfluramine for 12 months (for those who completed the trial; N dF = 227, N placebo = 256). Baseline (i.e. those who began the trial) N dF = 404, baseline N placebo=418 (Guy-Grand et al 1989).

In evaluating new drugs, the placebo effect needs to be kept in mind (Bray 1995b). I recommend a study design to minimize weight loss with a placebo, unless the comparison is from baseline, when it makes no difference. The hypertension analogy is again informative. Weight loss and a low sodium diet can reduce blood pressure. If new anti-hypertensive drugs had to be shown to be effective in patients placed on a severe weight loss diet, and with a sodium intake of less than 10 mmoles/day, it would be difficult to show any drug effect.

Combined treatment. Both noradrenergic and serotonergic mechanisms are involved in regulating food intake. Recognizing this, Weintraub et al (1992) reasoned that it might be more productive to combine agents acting on each system. In their study, patients received fenfluramine and phentermine for periods of up to 3.5 years. In the initial double-blind period, the patients treated with the drug lost nearly 15% of their initial weight compared to less than 5% for the group treated with the placebo. With continued treatment in either intermittent or continuous dosage, Weintraub et al (1992) concluded that many patients achieved a significant long-term benefit. For nearly 20% there was little benefit, and for the others there was a modest effect. The analogy with hypertension is again relevant. Different patients respond to different drugs. Combinations have proven more effective than single agents for many patients, and the same appears likely to be true for the treatment of obesity.

Sibutramine. Sibutramine is a new appetite suppressant which is currently under trial. Like most of the other appetite-suppressing drugs, it is a β-phenethylamine, but it has the novel property of reducing the uptake of both norepinephrine and serotonin. In

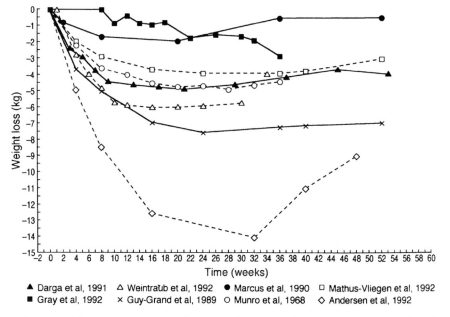

FIG. 6.   Weight loss in groups treated with placebos in anti-obesity drug trials of 31–60 weeks are plotted against time.

clinical trials, there is a dose–response effect with weight loss for up to two years (Bray et al 1996).

Surgery

Surgical treatment for obesity has been used for more than 40 years (Sugerman et al 1992). It is currently reserved for individuals with BMI values above 35–40 kg/m² i.e. high risk obesity. Three operations are currently in use, the most widely used of which is gastric restriction. The involves producing a small upper pouch drained into the jejunum. A second common procedure is vertical-banded gastroplasty. In comparative studies, the gastric bypass operation has been shown to produce more weight loss with less likelihood of regain. The final type of operation is a double-channel operation in which the stomach and the intestine are transected, and the two channels reconnected at various distances. This operation is technically more difficult and has had numerous problems. The principal value of the surgical approaches is that the patient cannot reverse them. Thus, recidivism is rare.

Acknowledgements

I thank M. Cutrer and T. Hodges for preparation of the manuscript.

References

Andersen T, Astrup A, Quaade F 1992 Dexfenfluramine as adjuvant to low-calorie formula diet in the treatment of obesity: a randomized clinical trial. Int J Obes 16:35–40

Arch JRS, Kaumann AJ 1993 Beta (3)-adrenoceptor and atypical beta-adrenoceptor. Med Res Rev 13:663–729

Ashley FW, Kannel WB 1974 Relation of weight change to changes in atherogenic traits: the Framingham Study. J Chronic Dis 27:103–114

Atkinson RL, Dietz WH, Foreyt JP et al 1994 Weight cycling. JAMA 272:1196–1202

Ballor DL, Keesey RE 1991 A meta-analysis of the factors affecting exercise-induced changes in body mass, fat mass and fat-free mass in males and females. Int J Obes 15:717–726

Banting W 1864 Letter on corpulence, addressed to the public, 3rd edn. Harrison, London

Blackburn GL, Kanders BS 1994 Obesity. Pathophysiology, psychology and treatment. Chapman & Hall, New York

Blair SN, Kohl HW, Barlow CE et al 1995 Changes in physical fitness and all-cause mortality: a prospective study of healthy and unhealthy men. JAMA 273:1093–1098

Bouchard C (ed) 1994 The genetics of obesity. CRC Press, Boca Raton, FL

Bouchard C, Pérusse L 1996 Current status of the human obesity gene map. Obesity Res 4:80–89

Bray GA 1990 Obesity: historical development of scientific and cultural ideas. Int J Obes 14:909–926

Bray GA 1994 Topography of body fat. Adv Endocrinol Metab 5:297–322

Bray GA 1995a Pharmacologic treatment of obesity: symposium overview. Obesity Res 3:415S–417S

Bray GA 1995b Evaluation of drugs for treating obesity. Obesity Res 3:425S–434S

Bray GA, Gray DS 1988a Obesity, part I: Pathogenesis. West J Med 149:429–441

Bray GA, Gray DS 1988b Obesity, part II: Treatment. West J Med 149:555–571

Bray GA, Ryan DH, Gordon D, Heidingsfelder H, Cerise F, Wilson K 1996 A double-blind randomized placebo-controlled trial of sibutramine. Obesity Res 4:263–270

Brownell KD, Kramer FM 1989 Behavioral management of obesity. Med Clin North Am 73:185–201

Colditz GA 1992 Economic costs of obesity. Am J Clin Nutr 55:503S–507S

Darga LL, Carroll-Michals L, Botsford SJ, Lucas CP 1991 Fluoxetine's effect on weight loss in obese subjects 1–3. Am J Clin Nutr 54:321–325

Drent ML, Larsson I, William-Olsson T et al 1995 Orlistat (RO-18-0647), a lipase inhibitor, in the treatment of human obesity: a multiple dose study. Int J Obes 19:221–226

Elmer PJ, Grimm R, Laing B et al 1995 Life-style intervention: results of the treatment of mild hypertension study (TOMHS). Prev Med 24:378–388

Epstein LH, Valoski A, Wing RR, McCurley J 1990 Ten-year follow-up of behavioral, family-based treatment for obese children. JAMA 264:2519–2523

Gray DS, Fujioka K, Devine W, Bray GA 1992 Fluoxetine treatment of the obese diabetic. Int J Obes 16:193–198

Griffiths M, Payne PR, Stunkard AJ, Rivers JPW, Cox M 1990 Metabolic-rate and physical development in children at risk of obesity. Lancet 336:76–78

Guy-Grand B, Apfelbaum M, Crepaldi G, Gries A, Lefebvre P, Turner P 1989 International trial of long-term dexfenfluramine in obesity. Lancet II:1142–1144

Hansen BC, Bodkin NL 1993 Primary prevention of diabetes mellitus by prevention of obesity in monkeys. Diabetes 42:1809–1814

Hypertension Prevention Trial Research Group 1990 The hypertension prevention trial: three-year effects of dietary changes on blood pressure. Arch Intern Med 150:153–162

Jolliffe NJ 1963 Reduce and stay reduced on the prudent diet, 3rd edn. Simon & Schuster, New York

Kannel WB, Gordon T 1979 Physiological and medical concomittants of obesity: the Framingham study. In: Bray GA (ed) Obesity in America. Department of Health, Education and Welfare, Washington, DC, p 125–153

Klesges RC, Benowitz NL, Meyers AW 1991 Behavioral and biobehavioral aspects of smoking and smoking cessation: the problem of postcessation weight gain. Behav Ther 22:179–199

Korkeila M, Kaprio J, Pissanen A, Koskenvuo M 1995 Consistency and change of body mass index and weight: a study on 5967 adult Finnish twin pairs. Int J Obes 19:310–317

Kuczmarski RJ, Flegal KM, Campbell SM, Johnson CL 1994 Increasing prevalence of overweight among US adults: the National Health and Nutrition Examination Surveys, 1960 to 1991. JAMA 272:205–211

Lawson OJ, Williamson DA, Champagne CM et al 1995 The association of body weight, dietary intake, and energy expenditure with dietary restraint and disinhibition. Obesity Res 3:153–161

Lew EA, Garfinkel L 1979 Variations in mortality by weight among 750,000 men and women. J Chronic Dis 32:563–576

Lindsted K, Tonstad S, Kuzma JW 1991 Body mass index and patterns of mortality among Seventh-day Adventist men. Int J Obes 15:397–406

Lissau I, Sørensen TIA 1994 Parental neglect during childhood and increased risk of obesity in young adulthood. Lancet 343:324–327

Lissner L, Heitmann BL 1995 Dietary fat and obesity: evidence from epidemiology. Eur J Clin Nutr 49:79–90

Long SD, O'Brien K, Macdonald KG Jr et al 1994 Weight loss in severely obese subjects prevents the progression of impaired glucose tolerance to type II diabetes. Diabetes Care 17:372–375

Manson JE, Stampfer MJ, Hennekens CH, Willett WC 1987 Body weight and longevity. A reassessment. JAMA 257:353–358

Manson JE, Willett WC, Stampfer MJ et al 1995 Body weight and mortality among women. N Engl J Med 333:677–685

Marcus MD, Wing RR, Ewing L, Kern E, McDermott M, Gooding W 1990 A double-blind, placebo-controlled trial of fluoxetine plus behavior modification in the treatment of obese binge-eaters and non-binge-eaters. Am J Psychiatry 147:876–881

Masoro EJ 1985 Aging and nutrition: can diet affect life span? Trans Assoc Life Insur Med Dir Am 67:30–44

Munro JF, MacCuish AC, Wilson EM, Duncan LJP 1968 Comparison of continuous and intermittent anorectic therapy in obesity. Br Med J 1:352–354

Ohlson LO, Larsson B, Eriksson H, Svärdsudd K, Welin L, Tibblin G 1987 Diabetes mellitus in Swedish middle-aged men: the study of men born in 1913 and 1923. Diabetologia 30:386–393

Paffenbarger RS Jr, Hyde RT, Wing AL, Lee I-M, Jung DL, Kampert JB 1993 The association of changes in physical-activity level and other lifestyle characteristics with mortality among men. N Engl J Med 328:538–545

Pamuk ER, Williamson DF, Madans J, Serdula MK, Kleinman JC, Byers T 1992 Weight-loss and mortality in a national cohort of adults, 1971–1987. Am J Epidemiol 136:686–697

Pavlou KN, Krey S, Steffee WP 1989 Exercise as an adjunct to weight loss and maintenance in moderately obese subjects. Am J Clin Nutr 49:1115–1123

Prentice AM, Jebb SA 1995 Obesity in Britain: gluttony or sloth? Br Med J 311:437–439

Ravussin E, Swinburn BA 1992 Pathophysiology of obesity. Lancet 340:404–408

Reed DR, Ding Y, Xu W, Cather C, Price RA 1995 Human obesity does not segregate with the chromosomal regions of Prader–Willi, Bardet–Biedl, Cohen, Borjeson or Wilson–Turner syndromes. Int J Obes 19:599–603

Rissanen A, Heliövaara M, Knekt P, Reunanen A, Aromaa A, Maatela J 1990 Risk of disability and mortality due to overweight in a Finnish population. Br Med J 301:835–837

Sobal J, Stunkard A J 1989 Socioeconomic status and obesity: a review of the literature. Psychol Bull 105:260–275

Stamler R, Stamler J, Gosch FC, McDonald AM 1984 Primary prevention of hypertension: a randomized controlled trial. Ann Clin Res 43:136–142

Stamler J, Wentworth D, Neaton JD 1986 Is relationship between serum cholesterol and risk of premature death from coronary heart disease continuous and graded? JAMA 256:2823–2828

Stamler J, Neaton JD, Wentworth DN 1989 Blood pressure (systolic and diastolic) and risk of fatal coronary heart disease. Hypertension 13:2I–12I

Stuart RB 1967 Behavioral control of overeating. Behav Res Ther 5:357–365

Sugerman H J, Kellum JM, Engle KM et al 1992 Gastric bypass for treating severe obesity. Am J Clin Nutr 55:560S–566S

Toeller M, Gries FA, Dannehl K 1982 Natural history of glucose tolerance in obesity. A ten year observation. Int J Obes 6:145–149

Trials of Hypertension Prevention Collaborative Research Group 1992 The effects of non-pharmacologic interventions on blood pressure of persons with high normal levels: results of the trials of hypertension prevention. JAMA 267:1213–1220

Vogler GP, Sørensen TIA, Stunkard A J, Srinivasan MR, Rao DC 1995 Influences of genes and shared family environment on adult body mass index assessed in an adoption study by a comprehensive path model. Int J Obes 19:40–45

Waaler HT 1984 Height, weight and mortality: the Norwegian experience. Acta Med Scand 679:1–56

Wadden TA, Foster GD, Letizia KA, Mullen JL 1990 Long-term effects of dieting on resting metabolic rate in obese outpatients. JAMA 264:707–711

Walker BR, Ballard IM, Gold J A 1977 A multicentre study comparing mazindol and placebo in obese patients. J Int Med Res 5:85–90

Warden CH, Fisler JS, Shoemaker SM et al 1995 Identification of 4 chromosomal loci determining obesity in a multifactorial mouse model. J Clin Invest 95:1545–1552

Weintraub M, Sundaresan PR, Schuster B et al 1992 Long-term weight control: the National Heart, Lung and Blood Institute-funded multimodal intervention study. I–VII. Clin Pharmacol Ther 51:581–646

West DB, Goudey-Lefevre J, York B, Truett GE 1994 Dietary obesity linked to genetic-loci on chromosome-9 and chromosome-15 in a polygenic mouse model. J Clin Invest 94:1410–1416

Willett WC, Manson JE, Stampfer M J et al 1995 Weight, weight change, and coronary heart disease in women: risk within the 'normal' weight range. JAMA 273:461–465

Williamson DF, Pamuk E, Thun M, Flanders D, Byers T, Heath C 1995 Prospective study of intentional weight-loss and mortality in never-smoking overweight US white women aged 40–64 years. Am J Epidemiol 141:1128–1141

Wood PD, Stefanick ML, Williams PT, Haskell WL 1991 Effects on plasma lipoproteins of a prudent weight-reducing diet, with or without exercise, in overweight men and women. N Engl J Med 325:461–466

DISCUSSION

Hitman: What do you mean by a cure for diabetes?

Bray: A glucose concentration falling below 7.8 mM.

Hitman: This represents an optimal control of diabetes, which might be defined as not requiring the use of pharmacological methods to maintain normoglycaemia, but it doesn't necessarily mean a cure for diabetes. It's a semantic argument because what you want to know is whether the person is cured of the long-term complications. My guess is that they aren't. The microvascular complications may be cured but some of the macrovascular complications may not be.

Bray: Only time will tell. I take your point.

Campfield: A more appropriate term may be remission.

Roberts: I have two questions. Firstly, are there any data on the people who don't respond to drugs? When they are taken off drugs are they worse or has the drug had no long-term effect?

Secondly, could you comment on the possible side-effects of drug treatment, such as memory loss?

Bray: I can't give you any data on the long-term follow-up of people who fail to respond to drugs. In Weintraub's data they maximized the dosage of medication in the group that failed to respond, and they found that their weights remained high (Weintraub et al 1992).

There have been press reports of memory loss in individuals taking appetite-suppressing drugs. In the controlled trials there's no difference in memory loss between the placebo group and the group treated with drugs. The reports of memory loss were based on uncontrolled trials and it's difficult to assess these uncontrolled self-reported data.

Blundell: We should be aware that the reduction of food intake by voluntary dieting produces disadvantageous changes that can be called risks or side-effects. A number of studies have demonstrated that dieting and high levels of dietary restraint are associated with impairments of cognitive performance (Green et al 1994). This means that sustained dieting carries a risk of impaired attention, short-term recall (memory) and reaction time.

Jackson: Are these side-effects transient or permanent?

Blundell: I can't answer that question because the studies were carried out at particular time points. However, it does seem that the impairments are not due to the short-term energy deficit itself. The effects are probably caused by the worry or stress of dieting which interferes with the efficiency of information processing.

Shaper: Do people stay on the anti-obesity drugs for life?

Bray: The four-year trial that Weintraub has done is the longest trial that exists. The International Dexfenfluramine Study is the second longest (Guy-Grand et al 1989), and there are two other one-year-long trials but that's about all.

Shaper: Is it the intention that patients would stay on the treatment for life?

Bray: That is the intention for high risk people. The data on recidivism are clear. If the medication is stopped the patients gain weight, because drugs don't work when they're not taken.

James: The concept of long-term therapy is not accepted by all medical authorities and drug agencies, although I do agree with you.

Bray: We're currently persuading the Food and Drug Administration (FDA) to accept the concept that chronic therapy is appropriate for some overweight people.

Campfield: The FDA's current guidelines are that a large number of people should be exposed to a drug for one year and a smaller number of people exposed for two years. Therefore, newly approved drugs in the USA will come with two-year treatment data, with the implication that they can be used for long-term treatment or at least intermittent treatment throughout life when weight gain becomes a risk.

Allison: But we don't really know the side-effects of life-long treatment on these drugs. On the other hand, if we ran a trial for 40 years it would be 40 years before anyone received a drug. How is it possible to deal with these considerations?

Bray: That's a fair question. I can make an analogy with hypertension and with drugs that lower cholesterol. In these cases the efficacy and safety of drugs are tested for one-year and two-year periods. The drug is then marketed and monitored for possible low risk events that could not be detected even in large clinical trials. All we're asking for from anti-obesity drugs is that their criteria for evaluation be comparable to those of other chronic high risk conditions like hypertension and hypercholesterolaemia.

Stunkard: It's not yet possible to decide that we will enforce lifetime treatment. It's an iterative process that will be continued if there is continued success. Let me propose that if the treatment is limited to people who are also receiving treatment for hypertension or diabetes, for example, then it may not be necessary to demonstrate the absolute safety of the drug. It may simply be sufficient to demonstrate that it is safer than the treatments for the other disorders.

In the Weintraub data there were people who didn't respond at all, but were there also people who responded and then regained weight on treatment?

Bray: Yes, there were.

Stunkard: What happened when the treatment was stopped in these people?

Bray: In the Weintraub study treatment stopped at three and a half years, so for the last six months all of the people were off treatment. Most of the patients tended to regain weight during this period.

Stunkard: Were there people who regained weight while still on treatment?

Bray: Some people didn't lose much weight, and some were non-responders. About a third of the people who lost weight maintained this loss. Another third put the weight back on, and the remaining third had a response that was in-between.

Stunkard: Was the rebound in body weight when they stopped treatment similar in those who had begun to regain weight on drugs and those who hadn't begun to regain weight on drugs?

Bray: That's a difficult question to answer because of the way they performed the trial. It was really a series of trials. One group were on intermittent treatment, i.e. three months on and three months off. When this group were on the treatment their weight decreased and when they came off the treatment their weight increased. Another group were on continuous treatment, and their weight was relatively stable. When the treatment was terminated at three and a half years, and when a readjustment was done for their second double-blind trial, they regained weight because many peoples' dose levels were decreased back to the initial dose levels. Therefore, people tended to regain weight after the initial weight loss. When the treatment was stopped the weight regain was larger.

McKeigue: Is there a subgroup of patients with hypertension, diabetes or both who could be treated simply with anti-obesity agents and not with blood pressure-lowering agents or sulfonylureas?

Bray: If you could prevent weight gain you would prevent most cases of non-insulin-dependent diabetes mellitus (NIDDM) and many cases of hypertension.

Campfield: The studies where weight loss has been achieved were recently reviewed by the Food and Nutrition Board of the Institute of Medicine (Thomas 1995). The idea that people can be taken off hypertensive medication if they achieve 10% weight loss has implications for the use of these medications. If the treatment was started with caloric restriction and continued with anti-obesity agents, only non-responders to the anti-obesity agents would need to take specific anti-hypertensive medications, for example. We have not yet tested this hypothesis. The prospective NIDDM trial being planned in the USA that George Bray mentioned may address this issue. In terms of NIDDM, we know that if we could achieve and maintain weight loss in a significant number of patients, the amount of hypoglycaemic medication they would have to take in addition to anti-obesity medication would be reduced.

McKeigue: The pay-off of treating something that is further back in the causal pathway of obesity, rather than treating one of the complications of it, is likely to be much greater simply because by treating obesity you don't just lower blood pressure but you lower the risk of several other conditions as well.

York: Is it possible to estimate the relative costs of long-term treatment with drugs as opposed to the cost of non-treatment? Because in persuading health care people to take up this strategy, one would have to be able to convince them that treatment is cheaper.

Prentice: This is currently being studied in the UK.

Campfield: The market projections for each of these anti-obesity drugs are about US$500 million in year five, so if three drugs need to be taken then the pharmaceutical companies would hope to gain US$1.5 billion in sales. One would have to add patient visits to that to come up with a reasonable cost estimation.

Forrester: Bearing in mind the concerns about the side-effects of long-term treatment with active agents, have any trials been done with placebos to monitor long-term behaviour modifications?

James: A placebo group is being incorporated into a number of the drug trials, and behavioural modifications are being used.

Forrester: And do they work?

James: Yes, and it varies according to the centre as to whether that weight loss is maintained. It seems to be a feature of the way the centre handles their general support for patients.

Jackson: Is it possible to get a sense of the nature of the input for the behavioural modification?

Bray: The long-term trials using behaviour and lifestyle modifications come mainly from trials to prevent hypertension. The treatment group loses about 5 kg, but then gradually regains this in spite of continued maximal efforts of behaviour modification. After three years, when they're still in the treatment programme, they're back to their original weight. The untreated placebo control group at this time are heavier than their original weight, so there's a small advantage but the personnel cost of treatment is quite high.

Campfield: In the trials with Xenical™ (Orlistat) where there was a large placebo effect, the goal was about a 500 kilocalorie reduction, depending on initial body weight (Drent et al 1995). Weight maintenance is the goal for pharmacotherapy, rather than the initiation of weight loss. In the fluoxetine trial for weight loss, everyone regained weight in the second half of the trial (Goldstein et al 1994). They didn't overshoot, they went back to their initial weight. George Bray's position that anti-obesity drug trials be designed so that the placebo group loses only a small amount of weight may be correct for appetite suppressants, e.g. sibutramine. In my opinion, drugs should only be used to assist the lifestyle changes (diet, exercise) that should be permanently incorporated into daily routines.

Shaper: There has been a battle in the UK for the last 20–25 years as to whether the lower levels of blood cholesterol are biologically normal i.e. associated with low mortality. Those against this argument presented U-shaped and J-shaped curves to indicate the increased mortality in those with lower blood cholesterol, although over the last decade it has been shown convincingly that the relationship between blood cholesterol and mortality is linear when you correct for the appropriate confounders, such as pre-existing disease and early cancer. At last we have accepted that the only approach to the blood cholesterol problem is a reduction of population blood cholesterol levels, and we are now beginning to identify the high risk groups that should be on lifetime treatment. These groups are becoming smaller and smaller as they are becoming more clearly defined. One can write a similar scenario for blood pressure and hypertension. Therefore, we're back to the issue that when the appropriate confounders are controlled for, the relationship between BMI and mortality is linear. Having 20% of the population in the USA on lifetime appetite suppressants and on drugs for the prevention of diabetes and hypertension is not ideal. We have to think in terms of a lower optimal BMI being preventative.

James: Do you think that all drug therapy is nonsense?

Shaper: No, there will be clearly defined, at-risk individuals who will need this kind of treatment.

Campfield: The general direction of obesity prevention is being steered towards pharmacotherapy. The pharmaceutical industry first has to show the efficacy and safety of anti-obesity drugs, and then show that they cause a significant reduction in morbidity and a prolongation of life. The next logical step would then be to use anti-obesity drugs to prevent obesity in high risk young people.

Shaper: I'm not talking about trying to decrease an obese individual's BMI to a lower and optimal BMI. We are stuck with the problems that you're talking about in therapeutic terms. I am talking about the prevention of weight gain in the next generation.

Campfield: But young people have an increasing prevalence of obesity, even though diet and exercise are freely available to them. We need new approaches, such as using medication to reset the optimal BMI.

Swinburn: What are we trying to prevent? If we're trying to prevent obesity, then talking about the individual high risk approach is essentially treating existing obesity. Cholesterol is a good analogy. It is wrong to think that we will be able to reduce the mean cholesterol level of a population just by treating all those with a high level. If we want to deal with a population, we have to have a population-based approach. The individual high risk approach involves asking individuals to make large changes in lifestyle, whereas small changes spread across a whole population is what has worked for cholesterol.

Another problem with the individual high risk approach is that we need to identify who these high risk people are. This is not the case for the population approach, although it does require the involvement of policy legislation, industry and environmental issues.

Ravussin: I agree with Boyd Swinburn that actions should be taken at the population level. However, one has to remember that it took centuries for humans to achieve what they were aspiring to, i.e. plenty of food and less gruelling physical activity. It is, therefore, going to take more than five years to reverse that and to have people willing to give up part of the conveniences of our modern lifestyles. In my opinion, we still need to identify the high risk groups within a population because it is clear that genetic differences cause the variability in BMI within a given environment. George Bray talked about identifying high risk people using biochemical and physiological markers that cannot be used on a large scale because of the cost and labour involved in such characterization. However, we can now use genetic methods to screen large numbers of people for variants in genes playing a role in the development of obesity. Obviously, such an approach will be difficult or impossible if hundreds of genes are involved but realistic if only a few genes are involved.

Hitman: I would like to respond to this comment that genetics will solve everything. We should exercise caution whilst studying these multifactorial diseases. There will be individual cases where a single gene marker or variant will be beneficial and will be selected, but it is more likely that we're dealing with genes which determine susceptibility to disease rather than when present always lead to disease (so-called 'necessary' genes). Not only will the number of genes involved be important, but also the interactions between the individual genes and the gene—environment interaction. For example, we are beginning to identify many of the genes involved in insulin-dependent diabetes. The strategies that people are adopting are to screen blood with genetic markers as a first step and then test the genetically susceptible individuals for evidence of disease activation using humoral markers (i.e. islet cell antibodies). This would then identify a high risk group of individuals for which one could design strategies to prevent insulin-dependent diabetes. Furthermore, the identification of some of the susceptibility genes may also give us some clues about the development of rational pharmacological therapies.

Shaper: What age group would be screened?

Hitman: It depends on the intervention. If a very toxic drug was the only way to prevent the disease, then one could say that screening would not be done because the effects of the drug are worse than the disease itself. On the other hand, if a non-toxic drug was available, then it may be possible to screen children. However, we must have a marker that shows the disease has been initiated. It is not possible to use genetic markers alone as a means for intervention.

Bouchard: I agree, it would not be advisable to use such a drug, particularly if the disease was influenced by numerous susceptibility genes, each with only a small effect.

James: On the subject of future research, where are the studies of physical activity and dietary changes going to lead us?

Blundell: I believe we can agree that being sedentary constitutes a risk factor for developing a positive energy balance and for weight gain. It follows that more active individuals are more likely to resist weight gain. I feel very comfortable to advocate increasing physical activity as a way of combating obesity. People opposing this idea argue that increased physical activity will simply stimulate people to eat more. However, my understanding of the evidence is that there exists a rather weak coupling between physical activity and energy intake. The bad news from this is that when people reduce physical activity (lapse into a sedentary lifestyle) then food intake is not down-regulated; the good news is that increasing physical activity (and therefore energy expenditure) does not up-regulate food intake.

It is important to recognize that both physical activity and energy intake are usually forms of voluntary behaviour. Consequently, if optimal and detrimental patterns of behaviour can be identified then it should be possible to devise strategies to maximize useful behaviours and minimize behaviours that constitute a risk for positive energy balance. Considering this, it is important to convert statements about energy balance into statements about behaviour. As I have mentioned elsewhere, 'people do not eat megajoules, they eat foods'. Knowledge about weight gain over a certain number of years can be reduced to a statement about an average energy excess per day (say 30 kcal). However, it will be difficult to do anything about this until this average energy value has been transformed into a behaviour pattern. Indeed, an average positive energy balance of 30 kcal per day could be achieved through a variety of behavioural profiles involving different patterns of eating and food choices. For example, it has been suggested that one particularly unhelpful pattern would involve an occasional eating episode of high fat foods (Horton et al 1995). This would not give the body time to adapt by, for example, increasing fat oxidation, and the fat would be more likely to be stored. This type of high risk behaviour pattern could be a target for preventive strategies.

James: I would like to put in a snapshot the implications of our policy analyses on physical activity. We're not going to be able to convert everybody to become moderately active. We described this in detail in a report on obesity for the Department of Health (DOH 1995). We showed that active adults tended to have been active as children, and that sedentary adults that had been active as children were more likely to be persuaded to become active. This implies that children should adopt an active lifestyle. One of the major determinants of inactivity in children, apart from watching television, is the terror of parents about their children playing outside. It's been shown in Leicester, UK that if the appropriate environment is provided, such as removing traffic in the vicinity of their homes, children go outside and are active. Town planning over the last two or three decades has favoured the use of the car. The number of children who cycle or walk to school has decreased markedly over this period. Sixty per cent of normal journeys are within the distance of an easy cycle ride for most people in western societies, but it is easier to drive the car. Town planning measures in Holland that favour cycle paths show that people will take up cycling if it is easy and safe. It may not be that difficult to organize an increased level of activity in everyone's daily life if town planning and traffic policies are changed.

Björntorp: Are there any differences in the responses of men and women to exercise?

Shaper: There are no differences.

Allison: I am in favour of using environmental restructuring to elicit behavioural modifications. However, there is a prevalent notion that for any particular phenotype, such as the pattern of activity, tracking through age (i.e. a consistency in relative ranking from age to age) suggests that childhood interventions will be preventive and will persist throughout life. This assumes that an environmental influence at one point in time is able to change the phenotype and that this phenotype is maintained. We have to bear in mind that all of the tracking we observe on any of these phenotypes may be due to the influence of a constant genotype. Claude Bouchard's group have shown that there is a genetic influence on physical activity patterns. Therefore, this may solely account for any tracking over time.

Garrow: Prevention, long-term treatment and maintenance of weight loss, the efficacy of the placebo, and behavioural modification all have one thing in common, which is the prevention of unconscious eating or unconscious weight gain. The device that I suggest will prevent unconscious weight gain is the inexpensive waist cord (Garrow 1992). We have done some pilot trials of the waist cord, and we have obtained some moderately good results (Garrow & Webster 1986). I am surprised that its use has not been incorporated into some of the more expensive trials.

Heymsfield: The future of obesity lies in its prevention. However, I'm pessimistic about achieving this because living in New York City, I've been overexposed to Madison Avenue and Wall Street, and I've learned how business people think. Gradually over the last few years I've realized that obesity is a tremendous economic engine. Many people profit from obesity; for example, those who sell diet foods, run health centres and make television commercials. Even I profit from obesity because I take care of obese patients. Obesity is built into the very fabric of our economic system, and therefore I see it as an essentially irreversible state.

James: You have a wonderful North American approach to what I see as the need for socialized medicine.

Prentice: I understand what Steve Heymsfield is saying, but I'm rather distraught by this nihilism about preventive medicine. We may have said the same thing about the increase in coronary heart disease (CHD) 30 years ago, and a great deal has been achieved since then. There is also a lot we can do in the field of obesity. In this very room there are numerous people who may have a natural propensity to obesity, but because they're well informed they have managed to fight against the environmental issues. Low fat intake and physical activity are two of the key answers. We have to show the consumers these answers because there has to be a consumer-led change. There is room for a great deal of optimism.

Allison: Unfortunately, I share some of Steve Heymsfield's pessimism. You made an analogy with cardiovascular disease but, at least from statistics in the USA, it is not clear to me that there has been a reduction in the prevalence of cardiovascular disease, although there has been a reduction in death from cardiovascular disease.

Swinburn: There has been a clear reduction in mortality associated with cardiovascular disease, particularly amongst the middle-aged, and that has resulted from a decreased incidence of cardiovascular disease rather than an increase in saving the lives of those with CHD.

References

DOH 1995 Obesity. Reversing the increasing problem of obesity in England. A report from the Nutrition and Physical Activity Task Forces (The Health of the Nation). Department of Health, London

Drent ML, Larsson I, William-Olson T et al 1995 Orlistat (RO 18–0647), a lipase inhibitor, in the treatment of human obesity: a multiple dose study. Int J Obes 19:221–226

Garrow JS 1992 The management of obesity. Another view. Int J Obes (suppl 2) 16:59S–63S

Garrow JS, Webster JD 1986 Long-term results of treatment of severe obesity with jaw wiring and waist cord. Proc Nutr Soc 45:119A

Goldstein DJ, Rampey AH Jr, Enas GG, Potvin JH, Fludzinski LA, Levine LR 1994 Fluoxetine: a randomized clinical trial in the treatment of obesity. Int J Obes 18:129–135

Green MW, Rogers PJ, Elliman NA, Gatenby SJ 1994 Impairment of cognitive performance associated with dieting and high levels of dietary restraint. Physiol Behav 55:447–452

Guy-Grand B, Apfelbaum M, Crepaldi G, Gries A, Lefebvre P, Turner P 1989 International trial of long-term dexfenfluramine in obesity. Lancet II:1142–1144

Horton TJ, Drongas H, Brachey A, Reed GW, Peters JC, Hill JO 1995 Fat and carbohydrate overfeeding in humans: different effects on energy storage. Am J Clin Nutr 62:19–29

Thomas PR 1995 Weighing the options: criteria for the evaluating weight-management programs. Food and Nutrition Board, Institute of Medicine, National Academy Press, Washington DC

Weintraub M, Sundaresan PR, Schuster B 1992 Long term weight control: the National Heart, Lung and Blood Institute-funded multimodal intervention study. I–VII. Clin Pharmacol Ther 51:581–646

Summary

W. P. T. James

The Rowett Research Institute, Greenburn Road, Bucksburn, Aberdeen AB2 9SB, UK

Obesity is clearly emerging as a global epidemic and it has been generally accepted at this symposium that obesity is arising almost wherever we look in the world. The Caribbean data presented by Terrence Forrester and Rainford Wilks were particularly illuminating because of the amazing differences in the prevalence of obesity between the islands. The African diaspora study is also extremely important in that it demonstrated, in epidemiological terms, the relationships between an increasing body weight of a population and the prevalences of diabetes, hypertension, coronary heart disease and other adult chronic conditions seen so prevalently in western societies. Gerry Shaper highlighted the close link between weight gain and an increase in blood pressure and how by simply concentrating on hypertension or hypercholesterolaemia we downgrade the real importance of weight gain.

Despite the evident public health problem, one of the conclusions of this symposium is that surprisingly few groups in medicine or public health are studying the issue. The subject of weight gain has been a Cinderella in medical science and it is only in the last 10 years that we have really begun to start unravelling the factors conducive to the weight gain of children and adults.

In assessing the basis for the epidemic of obesity, this symposium has clearly recognized the multiplicity of factors that interact in an age-dependent manner to produce excess weight gain. Alan Jackson highlighted the importance of childhood and adolescence obesity and how fetal events may be an important determinant of susceptibility late in life. Everyone at this symposium also seems to agree on the importance of visceral adiposity, which Claude Bouchard emphasized is under strong genetic control. The issue is how best to identify the non-genetic determinants of visceral obesity and the amplifiers of this selective accumulation of fat. Are factors such as smoking or alcohol in adult life, genetics and fetal programming involved? The prospects for developing new genetic probes for both the susceptibility to general weight gain and to visceral adiposity have been stimulated by the discovery of leptin and its receptors. Per Björntorp also outlined his suggestion that programming of the hypothalamic-pituitary-adrenal (HPA) axis may be involved in abdominal adiposity and that we may need to recognize that tonic amplification of this axis results from stress. Paul McKeigue highlighted the fundamental importance of visceral fat in determining the insulin resistance and propensity to diabetes of Asian immigrants to many parts of the world, so we need to consider the sociobiology of a society as well as the genetic variation in the propensity to amplify the HPA axis and accumulate abdominal fat.

We had a substantial input on the metabolic features of obesity and on the control of food intake at this symposium. Arne Astrup and others who set out the metabolic issues were essentially, once they had converted it into energetic terms, discussing the question of whether the differences in the metabolic efficiency of an individual could account for the development of their obesity and how a high fat diet might promote fat storage in susceptible individuals with a seemingly reduced ability to oxidize fat. There are indeed metabolic markers of individual propensities to weight gain, but they do not seem to offer a complete explanation. John Blundell reminded us of the importance of the passive overconsumption of energy-dense diets and its interaction with a low level of physical activity, and Anna Ferro-Luzzi presented the first attempt to analyse objectively the worldwide data on physical activity and derived a cut-off point below which weight gain is likely. Albert Stunkard also presented a fascinating analysis of the socioeconomic aspects of obesity. The educational level of an individual does seem to be a useful marker of an adult's response to any tendency to weight gain and this response seems to be reflected in their constrained eating as well as their conscious increase in leisure-time activity.

Aila Rissanen's collation of recent analyses of the true economic costs of obesity suggests that they are far higher than we had originally envisaged. Obesity should not be viewed simply as the outcome of an individual disturbance in behavioural responses to environmental change but in public-health terms as a reflection of societal changes that affect the whole of the population, suggesting that societal issues have economic importance. To pick out individuals as in some way suffering from a distinctive disturbance in energy balance is to ignore the epidemiological analyses that show the smooth spectrum of individual body mass indices (BMIs) that shift as societal factors change. On this basis the analysis and discernment of the optimum average BMI of a population has to be seen in a different light from that of working out the implications for individual management of overweight individuals. George Bray emphasized the need to tackle this multi-dimensional problem of obesity in many different ways. Individual management and the selection of high risk groups for specific targeting is an essential component of any new strategy and we should face up to the fact that effective therapies may need to include the use of appropriate drugs. As obesity rates escalate, the problem of how best to manage obese patients will be accentuated; several drugs are on the horizon because there have been a number of exciting developments in our understanding of the metabolic basis of obesity, particularly in relation to leptin, the appetite suppressant hormone derived from adipocytes. Then we will need to see how best to integrate both prevention and management in the strategies for dealing with severe obesity. If we also develop a strategy for preventing further weight gain in overweight patients, then we might be able to start shifting the perception of how best to manage the condition. By accumulating the evidence on the pathophysiology of obesity we are all hoping that over the next few decades we can make sufficient progress to persuade the medical profession of the major medical significance of obesity, the importance of societal change for its prevention and the value of coherent programmes of individual therapy.

This symposium recognized early that we need to collaborate much more effectively and combine expertise from different areas, e.g. molecular biology with epidemiology, and to compile proper epidemiological questionnaires of physical activity with metabolic validation studies so that we obtain a true index of physical activity. We also need to assess the energy density of the diet and not simply its fat content because the two features are very different and have very different industrial implications — an energy-dense diet can reflect the use of syrups and maltodextrins as well as sugars such as sucrose. All the factors relating to weight gain therefore have to be brought together to develop effective preventive strategies because, in the absence of effective prevention policies, we are going to witness an explosion in obesity rates.

I would like to end on a note of optimism. We have made considerable progress over the last 10 years, with several hypotheses being developed and then revised. From this symposium it is clear that we have many research opportunities which we must grasp if we are to make enough progress to understand and then reverse the escalating incidence of obesity and improve its therapy.

Appendix

TABLE 1 Physical activity level (PAL) of adult males from selected studies on energy expenditure (EE) under free-living conditions. Age, number of subjects, weight, body mass index (BMI), total EE and PAL (EE/basal metabolic rate) are indicated, as well as a brief description of the population and the method of measuring EE

Age (y)	n	Weight (kg)	BMI (kg/m²)	EE (kcal/d)	PAL	Population[a]
22	17	68.4	22.1	2849[b]	1.73	USA volunteers, constant activity (27)
38	10	51.4	19.0	3840[c]	2.60	Burma farmers, monsoon (50)
38	10	52.8	19.5	2940[c]	1.97	Burma farmers, harvest (50)
38	10	54.0	19.9	2230[c]	1.48	Burma farmers, summer (50)
32	16	79.7	25.7	3401[b]	1.88	UK normal people (32)
68	7	77.1	25.2	2675[b]	1.58	USA retired rural people (26)
69	15	76.1	24.3	NA[b]	1.75	USA elderly (43)
30	60	53.4	20.8	3202[c]	2.14	Machiguenga horticulturalists (33)
42	30	83.6	28.6	2870[b]	1.56	USA Pima Indians (40)
31	6	78.3	24.4	4558[b]	3.23	USA soldiers high altitude exercise (30)
41	4	84.6	26.5	3215[b]	1.73	USA Beltsville normal people (47)
25	6	73.3	23.0	3040[c]	1.69	USA Ohio university students (5)
24	20	61.1	20.9	2360[c]	1.46	Nigeria students (10)
33	8	48.3	18.6	2285[c]	1.59	India farmers (22)
35	3[e]	ND	21.2	3513[b]	2.20	Mt. Everest climbers (54)
41	2	81.2	NA	7209[b]	4.00	North Pole sledging expedition (49)
30	4	69.2	NA	7027[b]	4.18	Tour de France cyclists (53)
30	4	69.2	NA	8604[b]	5.11	Tour de France cyclists (53)

Age (y)	n	Weight (kg)	BMI (kg/m²)	EE (kcal/d)	PAL	Population[a]
30	4	69.2	NA	8532[b]	5.07	Tour de France cyclists (53)
37	8	71.0	22.4	2772[b]	1.63	Netherlands normal people (55)
38	4	72.6	22.9	3250[b]	1.88	Netherlands marathon trainers 0–30 min/day (55)
38	4	72.6	22.9	3489[b]	2.03	Netherlands marathon trainers 20–60 min/day (55)
37	8	71.0	22.0	3322[b]	1.95	Netherlands marathon trainers 30–90 min/day (55)
28	10	53.9	NA	2199[c]	1.46	Philippines typists (16)
26	10	56.3	NA	2701[c]	1.76	Philippines shoemakers (14)
32	10	54.8	NA	2486[c]	1.64	Philippines drivers (15)
25	25	54.8	NA	2486[c]	1.64	Philippines textile mill workers (17)
25	33	56.0	NA	2390[c]	1.56	Philippines fishermen (12)
25	32	54.0	NA	3035[c]	2.02	Philippines sugarcane workers (12)
28	9	51.5	NA	3298[c]	2.25	Philippines rice farmers (13)
45	11	56.5	19.8	2127[c]	1.39	Upper Volta farmers (4)
36	23	58.5	19.8	2414[c]	1.55	Upper Volta farmers dry season (7)
36	16	58.5	19.8	3466[c]	2.23	Upper Volta farmers wet season (7)
18–29	19	57.4	21.9	2629[c]	1.69	New Guinea Kaul young farmers (37)
18–29	28	58.3	22.5	2557[c]	1.58	New Guinea Lufa young farmers (37)
30+	32	55.1	21.8	2151[c]	1.42	New Guinea Kaul older farmers (37)
30+	15	56.0	22.4	2581[c]	1.69	New Guinea Lufa older farmers (37)
39	10	56.0	20.6	3288[c]	2.15	Iran Varanin farmers, spring (6)
38	14	56.0	21.6	3469[c]	2.27	Iran Varanin farmers, summer (6)
35	10	59.0	21.0	3625[c]	2.32	Iran Varanin farmers, autumn (6)

Age (y)	n	Weight (kg)	BMI (kg/m²)	EE (kcal/d)	PAL	Population[a]
38	12	59.0	21.2	2619[c]	1.68	Iran Varanin farmers, winter (6)
30	18	60.1	23.2	3705[c]	2.32	Guatemala farmers (51)
30	5	53.8	20.8	2892[c]	1.93	Machiguenga horticulturalists dry season (34)
25	8	51.8	20.8	3322[c]	2.26	Machiguenga horticulturalists wet season (34)
36	38	75.6	24.9	2855[c]	1.62	Italy shipyard sedentary work (35)
39	37	77.9	26.2	3137[c]	1.76	Italy shipyard moderate work (35)
37	75	76.1	20.9	3309[c]	1.88	Italy shipyard heavy work (35)
22	6	64.0	21.2	2820[c]	1.70	UK students (36)
19	59	63.3	21.2	3776[c]	2.29	UK army recruits (21)
27	23	79.8	NA	4919[b]	2.59	USA marines winter exercise (29)
22	14	72.6	23.2	3493[b]	1.98	USA sedentary students (42)
24	7	76.3	24.0	3317[b]	1.84	USA student staff, normal intake (41)
24	7	76.3	24.0	3503[b]	1.89	USA student staff, normal intake + 1000 kcal (41)
24	7	76.3	24.0	3331[b]	1.79	USA student staff ad libitum intake (41)
23	4	73.8	21.8	4750[b]	2.63	Australia soldiers training for jungle warfare (24)
29	26	51.2	17.2	2461[d]	1.91	Gambia low BMI farmers (19)
29	28	67.7	23.3	3034[d]	1.95	Gambia normal BMI farmers (19)
33	8	76.6	22.6	3160[c]	1.79	Australia large eaters (9)
37	8	77.3	24.8	3937[c]	2.22	Australia small eaters (9)
27	16	75.9	24.2	3400[b]	1.85	USA soldiers training (18)

[a]Numbers in brackets refer to reference list.
[b]Double-labelled water.
[c]Factorial method (time allocation + EE).
[d]Heart rate.
[e]Males and females.
NA, not available.

TABLE 2 Physical activity level (PAL) of adult females from selected studies on energy expenditure (EE) under free-living conditions. Age, number of subjects, weight, body mass index (BMI), total EE and PAL (EE/basal metabolic rate) are indicated, as well as a brief description of the population and the method of measuring EE

Age (y)	n	Weight (kg)	BMI (kg/m²)	EE (kcal/d)	PAL	Population[a]
35	16	62.7	24.5	2359[b]	1.77	UK normal people (32)
29	13	57.5	22.1	1910[b]	1.41	UK normal people (39)
26	9	52.4	19.7	2826[b]	1.99	USA elite runners (46)
64	6	65.2	23.9	2092[b]	1.43	USA retired people rural (26)
20	20	51.3	19.6	1641[c]	1.31	Nigeria students (11)
36	22	45.1	18.9	1948[c]	1.51	Ethiopia farmers yearly maximum (23)
36	22	44.3	18.3	1820[c]	1.43	Ethiopia farmers yearly minimum (23)
25–29	NA	58.0	NA	118–226[c]	1.47–1.68	Ivory Coast farmers (1)
27	NA	43.3	16.9	1924[c]	1.67	Machiguenga horticulturalists (33)
26	7	50.2	20.0	2308[b]	1.87	Gambia rural people(28)
34	11	49.6	22.9	2203[c]	1.75	Colombia Amazonia horticulturalists (20)
23	6	56.0	21.7	2283[c]	1.73	USA Ohio students (5)
37	19	46.7	20.7	179–250[c]	1.77–2.01	Nepal 1870 m farmers (38)
28	8	36.9	16.7	1968[c]	1.90	India farmers (22)
33	12	59.6	21.2	2261[b]	1.67	USA Rochester normal people (52)
36	38	85.2	31.7	2677[b]	1.73	USA Rochester obese people (52)
37	5	64.3	21.5	2366[b]	1.70	Netherlands normal people (55)
37	2	67.4	22.5	2725[b]	1.93	Netherlands marathon trainers 10–30 min/day (55)
37	2	67.4	22.5	2486[b]	1.76	Netherlands marathon trainers 20–60 min/day (55)
37	5	64.3	21.5	2796[b]	2.01	Netherlands marathon trainers 30–90 min/day (55)
25	10	46.9	NA	1888[c]	1.60	Philippines typists (16)
33	14	48.7	NA	2032[c]	1.63	Philippines textile mill workers (17)

Age (y)	n	Weight (kg)	BMI (kg/m²)	EE (kcal/d)	PAL	Population[a]
34	10	54.0	NA	2032[c]	1.57	Philippines housewives (14)
31	12	50.6	20.6	2127[c]	1.68	Upper Volta farmers wet season (3)
31	12	50.6	20.6	2653[c]	2.10	Upper Volta farmers dry season (3)
31	14	49.9	19.6	1936[c]	1.54	Upper Volta farmers end of harvest (4)
23	6	49.0	21.2	1960[c]	1.62	Guatemala peasants (45)
28	18	49.2	22.2	2008[c]	1.65	Guatemala peasants lactating (45)
18–29	23	49.8	21.6	1932[c]	1.57	New Guinea Kaul young farmers np-nl (37)
30–49	17	45.9	20.4	1692[c]	1.38	New Guinea Kaul adult farmers np-nl (37)
27	7	51.0	21.8	1857[c]	1.49	New Guinea Kaul farmers pregnant (37)
18–29	31	51.1	22.1	2268[c]	1.82	New Guinea Lufa farmers young np-nl (37)
30–49	7	46.3	20.6	2141[c]	1.74	New Guinea Lufa farmers adult np-nl (37)
25	7	53.5	22.9	2277[c]	1.78	New Guinea Lufa farmers pregnant (37)
25	20	44.5	21.4	1984[c]	1.73	Machiguenga horticulturalists wet season (34)
27	8	44.3	21.4	1960[c]	1.71	Machiguenga horticulturalists dry season (34)
26	13	63.7	23.4	2103[c]	1.47	USA housewives pregnant first trimester (2)
26	12	70.4	25.9	2294[c]	1.50	USA housewives pregnant second trimester (2)
26	14	77.0	28.3	2366[c]	1.46	USA housewives pregnant third trimester (2)
26	12	62.4	22.9	1840[c]	1.31	USA housewives lactating first trimester (2)
26	6	54.8	22.0	1845[c]	1.54	Italy institute staff (A. Ferro-Luzzi, unpublished results 1995)

Age (y)	n	Weight (kg)	BMI (kg/m²)	EE (kcal/d)	PAL	Population[a]
35	8	49.1	21.8	1925[b]	1.58	Guatemala urban resettled lower SES (48)
37	7	59.8	26.9	2253[b]	1.67	Guatemala urban resettled upper SES (48)
35	9	87.9	32.9	2443[b]	1.52	UK obese people (39)
41	18	44.9	17.6	2143[c]	1.74	Benin farmers post-harvest BMI < 18 kg/m² Jan–Feb (44)
39	16	65.0	26.2	2422[c]	1.66	Benin farmers post-harvest BMI > 23 kg/m² Jan–Feb (44)
41	18	44.1	17.3	2041[c]	1.73	Benin farmers pre-harvest BMI < 18 kg/m² (44)
39	16	63.3	25.5	2453[c]	1.70	Benin farmers pre-harvest BMI > 23 kg/m² (44)
41	18	44.3	17.3	2165[c]	1.76	Benin farmers post-harvest BMI < 18 kg/m² Aug–Sept (44)
39	16	63.6	25.8	2521[c]	1.73	Benin farmers post-harvest BMI > 23 kg/m² Aug–Sept (44)
29	13	57.5	22.2	1909[b]	1.42	UK Cambridge lean people (39)
35	9	87.9	33.0	2441[b]	1.52	UK Cambridge obese people (39)
21	16	54.2	21.3	1735[b]	1.34	Swaziland agricultural school applicants (31)
29	22	61.0	22.3	2484[b]	1.86	Sweden before pregnancy (25)
29	22	63.7	23.3	2293[b]	1.60	Sweden gestational week 16–18 (25)
29	22	70.2	25.7	2986[b]	1.81	Sweden gestational week 30 (25)
37	9	53.6	19.0	2192[c]	1.69	Australia large eaters (8)
34	9	60.9	23.1	2912[c]	2.14	Australia small eaters (8)

[a]Numbers in brackets refer to reference list.
[b]Double-labelled water.
[c]Factorial method (time allocation + EE).
NA, not available; np-nl, non-pregnant/non-lactating; SES, socioeconomic status.

References

1. Berio A-J 1984 The analysis of time allocation and activity patterns in nutrition and rural development planning. Food Nutr Bull 6:53–68
2. Blackburn MW, Calloway DH 1976 Energy expenditure and consumption of mature, pregnant and lactating women. J Am Diet Assoc 69:29–37
3. Bleiberg FM, Brun TA, Goihman S 1980 Duration of activities and energy expenditure of female farmers in dry and rainy seasons in Upper-Volta. Br J Nutr 43:71–81
4. Bleiberg FM, Brun TA, Goihman S, Lippman D 1981 Food intake and energy expenditure of male and female farmers from Upper-Volta. Br J Nutr 45:505–515
5. Borel MJ, Riley RE, Snook JT 1984 Estimation of energy expenditure and maintenance energy requirements of college-age men and women. Am J Clin Nutr 40:1264–1272
6. Brun TA, Geissler CA, Mirbagheri I, Hormozdiary H, Bastani J, Hedayat H 1979 The energy expenditure of Iranian agricultural workers. Am J Clin Nutr 32:2154–2161
7. Brun TA, Bleiberg F, Goihman S 1981 Energy expenditure of male farmers in dry and rainy seasons in Upper-Volta. Br J Nutr 45:67–75
8. Clark D, Tomas F, Withers RT et al 1992 Differences in energy metabolism between normal weight 'large-eating' and 'small-eating' women. Br J Nutr 68:31–44
9. Clark D, Tomas F, Withers RT et al 1993 No major differences in energy metabolism between matched and unmatched groups of 'large-eating' and 'small-eating' men. Br J Nutr 70:393–406
10. Cole AH, Ogbe JO 1987 Energy intake, expenditure and pattern of daily activity of Nigerian male students. Br J Nutr 58:357–367
11. Cole AH, Ogungbe RF 1987 Food intake and energy expenditure of Nigerian female students. Br J Nutr 57:309–318
12. De Guzman PE 1981 Energy allowances for the Philippine population. Proc Workshop 'Energy expenditure under field consitions'. Prague, Czechoslovakia
13. De Guzman PE, Dominguez SR, Kalaw JM, Basconcillo RO, Santos VF 1974 A study of the energy expenditure, dietary intake, and pattern of daily activity among various occupational groups, I: Laguna rice farmers. Phil J Sci 103:53–65
14. De Guzman PE, Dominguez SR, Kalaw JM, Buning MN, Basconcillo RO, Santos VF 1974 A study of the energy expenditure, dietary intake and pattern of daily activity among various occupational groups, II: Marikina shoemakers and housewives. Phil J Nutr 27:21–30
15. De Guzman PE, Kalaw JM, Tan RH et al 1974 A study of the energy expenditure, dietary intake and pattern of daily activity among various occupational groups, III: Urban jeepney drivers. Phil J Nutr 27:182–188
16. De Guzman PE, Cabrera JP, Basconcillo RO et al 1978 A study of the energy expenditure, dietary intake and pattern of daily activity among various occupational groups, V: Clerk-typist. Phil J Nutr 31:147–156
17. De Guzman PE, Recto RC, Cabrera JP et al 1979 A study of the energy expenditure, dietary intake and pattern of daily activity among various occupational groups, VI: Textile-mill workers. Phil J Nutr 32:134–148
18. DeLany JP, Schoeller DA, Hoyt RW, Askew EW, Sharp MA 1989 Field use of $D_2^{18}O$ to measure energy expenditure of soldiers at different energy intakes. J Appl Physiol 67:1922–1929
19. Della Bianca P, Jequier E, Schutz Y 1994 High level of free-living energy expenditure in rural Gambian men: lack of behavioral adaptation between low and normal BMI groups. Eur J Clin Nutr 48:273–278
20. Dufour DL 1984 The time and energy expenditure of indigenous women horticulturalists in the northwest Amazon. Am J Phys Anthropol 65:37–46

21. Edholm OG, Adam JM, Heavy MJR, Wolff HS, Goldsmith R, Best TW 1970 Food intake and energy expenditure of army recruits. Br J Nutr 24:1091–1107
22. Edmundson WC, Edmundson SA 1989 Energy balance, nutrient intake and discretionary activity in a South Indian village. Ecol Food Nutr 22:253–265
23. Ferro-Luzzi A, Scaccini C, Taffese S, Aberra B, Demeke T 1990 Seasonal energy deficiency in Ethiopian rural women. Eur J Clin Nutr 44:7–18
24. Forbes-Ewan CH, Morrisey BLL, Gregg GC, Waters DR 1989 Use of a doubly labeled water technique in soldiers training for jungle welfare. J Appl Physiol 67:14–18
25. Forsum E, Kabir N, Sadurskis A, Westerterp K 1992 Total energy expenditure of healthy Swedish women during pregnancy and lactation. Am J Clin Nutr 56:334–342
26. Goran MI, Poehlman ET 1992 Total energy expenditure and energy requirements in healthy elderly persons. Metabolism 41:744–753
27. Goran MI, Beer WH, Wolfe RR, Poehlman ET, Young VR 1993 Variation in total energy expenditure in young healthy free-living men. Metab Clin Exp 42:487–496
28. Heini A, Schutz Y, Diaz E, Prentice AM, Whitehead RG, Jequier E 1991 Free-living energy expenditure measured by two independent techniques in pregnant and nonpregnant Gambian women. Am J Physiol 261:9E–17E
29. Hoyt RW, Jones TE, Stein TP et al 1991 Doubly labeled water measurement of human energy expenditure during strenous exercise. J Appl Physiol 71:16–22
30. Hoyt RW, Jones TE, Baker-Fulco CJ et al 1994 Doubly labeled water measurement of human energy expenditure during exercise at high altitude. Am J Physiol 266:966R–971R
31. Huss-Ashmore R, Goodman JL, Sibiya TE, Stein TP 1989 Energy expenditure of young Swazi women as measured by the doubly-labelled water method. Eur J Clin Nutr 43:737–748
32. Livingstone MBE, Strain JJ, Prentice AM et al 1991 Potential contribution of leisure activity to the energy expenditure patterns of sedentary populations. Br J Nutr 65:45–155
33. Montgomery E 1978 Towards representative energy data: the Machiguenga study. Proc Fed Am Soc Exp Biol 37:61–64
34. Montgomery E, Johnson A 1977 Machiguenga energy expenditure. Ecol Food Nutr 6:97–105
35. Norgan NG, Durnin JVGA 1980 The effect of six weeks of overfeeding on the body weight, body composition, and energy metabolism of young men. Am J Clin Nutr 33:978–988
36. Norgan NG, Ferro-Luzzi A 1978 Nutrition, physical activity, and physical fitness in contrasting environments. In: Parizkova J, Rogozkin VA (eds) International series on sport sciences, vol 7: Nutrition, physical fitness, and health. University Park Press, New York, p 167–193
37. Norgan NG, Ferro-Luzzi A, Durnin JVGA 1974 The energy and nutrient intake and the energy expenditure of 204 New Guinean adults. Phil Trans R Soc Lond B 268:309–348
38. Panter-Brick C 1993 Seasonality of energy expenditure during pregnancy and lactation for rural Nepali women. Am J Clin Nutr 57:620–628
39. Prentice AM, Black AE, Coward WA et al 1986 High levels of energy expenditure in obese women. Br Med J 292:983–987
40. Rising R, Harper IT, Fontvielle AM, Ferraro RT, Spraul M, Ravussin E 1994 Determinants of total daily energy expenditure: variability in physical activity. Am J Clin Nutr 59:800–804
41. Roberts SB, Young VR, Fuss P et al 1990 Energy expenditure and subsequent nutrient intakes in overfed young men. Am J Physiol 259:461R–469R
42. Roberts SB, Heyman MB, Evans WJ, Fuss P, Tsay R, Young VR 1991 Dietary energy requirements of young adult men, determined by using the doubly labeled water method. Am J Clin Nutr 54:499–505
43. Roberts SB, Fuss P, Evans WJ, Heyman MB, Young VR 1993 Energy expenditure, aging and body composition. J Nutr 123:474–480

44. Schultink JW, Van Raaij JMA, Hautvast JGAJ 1993 Seasonal weight loss and metabolic adaptation in rural Beninese women: the relationship with body mass index. Br J Nutr 70:689–700
45. Schulz LO, Alger S, Harper I, Wilmore JH, Ravussin E 1992 Energy expenditure of elite female runners measured by respiratory chamber and doubly labeled water. J Appl Physiol 72:23–28
46. Schutz Y, Lechtig A, Bradfield RB 1980 Energy expenditures and food intakes of lactating women in Guatemala. Am J Clin Nutr 33:892–902
47. Seale JL, Rumpler WV, Conway JM, Miles CW 1990 Comparison of doubly labeled water, intake-balance, and direct- and indirect-calorimetry methods for measuring energy expenditure in adult men. Am J Clin Nutr 52:66–71
48. Stein TP, Johnston FE, Greiner L 1988 Energy expenditure and socio-economic status in Guatemala as measured by the doubly labeled water method. Am J Clin Nutr 47:196–200
49. Stroud MA, Coward WA, Sawyer MB 1993 Measurements of energy expenditure using isotope-labeled water ($^2H_2{}^{18}O$) during an Arctic expedition. Eur J Appl Physiol Occup Physiol 67:375–379
50. Tin-May-Than, Ba-Aye 1985 Energy intake and energy output of Burmese farmers at different seasons. Hum Nutr Clin Nutr 39:7C–15C
51. Viteri FE, Torun B, Galicia JC, Herrera E 1971 Determining energy costs of agricultural activities by respirometer and energy balance techniques. Am J Clin Nutr 24:1418–1430
52. Welle S, Forbes GB, Statt M, Barnard RR, Amatruda JM 1992 Energy expenditure under free-living conditions in normal-weight and overweight women. Am J Clin Nutr 55:14–21
53. Westerterp KR, Saris WHM, van Es M, ten Hoor F 1986 Use of the doubly labeled water technique in humans during heavy sustained exercise. J Appl Physiol 61:2162–2167
54. Westerterp KR, Hayser B, Brouns F, Herry JP, Saris WHM 1992 Energy expenditure climbing Mount Everest. J Appl Physiol 73:1815–1819
55. Westerterp KR, Meijer GA, Janssen EME, Saris WH, ten Hoor F 1992 Long-term effect of physical activity on energy balance and body composition. Br J Nutr 68:21–30

Index of contributors

Non-participating co-authors are indicated by asterisks. Entries in bold type indicate papers; other entries refer to discussion contributions.

Indexes compiled by Liza Weinkove.

Subject index

Other Ciba Foundation Symposia:

No. 194 **Genetics of criminal and antisocial behaviour**
Chairman: Sir Michael Rutter
1996 ISBN 0 471 95719 4

No. 197 **Variation in the human genome**
Chairman: Kenneth M. Weiss
1996 ISBN 0 471 96152 3

No. 206 **The rising trends in asthma**
Chairman: Stephen Holgate
1997 ISBN 0 471 97012 3